£2

Urodynamics

Springer

*London
Berlin
Heidelberg
New York
Barcelona
Budapest
Hong Kong
Milan
Paris
Santa Clara
Singapore
Tokyo*

Paul Abrams

Urodynamics

Second edition

With 145 Figures
Including 3 Colour Plates

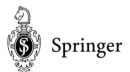 Springer

Paul Abrams, MD, FRCS
Bristol Urological Centre, Southmead Hospital,
Westbury-on-Trym, Bristol BS10 5NB, UK

ISBN 3-540-19678-1 2nd Edition Springer-Verlag Berlin Heidelberg New York
ISBN 0-387-19678-1 2nd Edition Springer-Verlag New York Berlin Heidelberg

ISBN 3-540-11903-5 1st Edition Springer-Verlag Berlin Heidelberg New York
ISBN 0-387-11903-5 1st Edition Springer-Verlag New York Berlin Heidelberg

British Library Cataloguing in Publication Data
Abrams, Paul, 1947 -
    Urodynamics. - 2nd ed.
    1. Urodynamics
    I. Title
    616.6'2'0754
ISBN 3540196781

Library of Congress Cataloging-in-Publication Data
Abrams, Paul, 1947 -
    Urodynamics/Paul Abrams. - 2nd ed.
        p.   cm.
    Includes bibliographical references and index
    ISBN 3-540-19678-1 (hardback: alk paper)
    1. Urodynamics. I. Title
    [DNLM: 1. Urodynamics. 2. Urologic Diseases - diagnosis. WJ 102
A161u 1997]
RC901.9.A25 1997
616.6'07-dc21
DNLM/DLC
for Library of Congress   96-51999

First published 1983
Second Edition 1997
Reprinted 1998

Typeset by EXPO Holdings, Malaysia
Printed and bound by Bell and Bain Ltd, Glasgow, Scotland
28/3830-54321 Printed on acid-free paper

Preface

Lower urinary tract dysfunction produces a huge burden on sufferers in particular and on society in general. Lower urinary tract symptoms have a high prevalence in the community: 5% of children aged 10 wet the bed, while 15% of women and 7% of men have troublesome incontinence; and in elderly men of 75, benign prostatic hyperplasia occurs in more than 80% of individuals, with benign prostatic enlargement coexisting in up to half this group and half of these having bladder outlet obstruction.

The confusion felt in many people's minds as to the role of urodynamics has receded for the most part. The need to support the clinical assessment with objective measurement has become accepted by most clinicians specialising in the care of patients with lower urinary tract symptoms (LUTS). Since the first edition of this book in 1983, urodynamics has become more widely accepted. In the last ten years the number of urodynamic units in Britain and Europe has increased rapidly and almost every hospital of any significance embraces urodynamic investigations as an essential part of the diagnostic armamentarium of the urology and gynaecology departments. Further, specialists in geriatrics, paediatrics and neurology recognise the importance of urodynamics in the investigation of a significant minority of their patients.

Despite the technological innovations that have seen the introduction of computerised urodynamics, the development of neurophysiological testing and the introduction of new techniques such as ambulatory monitoring, the objectives of this book remain unchanged. Urodynamics may appear complicated, and one of the objectives of this book is to put the subject over simply but in enough detail to allow urodynamic investigation to be accepted, on its own merit, as a fundamental contribution to the management of many patients. To do this means not only describing the tests but also showing in which clinical areas they help management and in which they are pointless. It means concentrating on the common clinical problems and on the presenting symptom complexes, not the diagnosis; and it means pointing out any limitations and possible artifacts of investigation.

We hope that a clinician with no previous experience in urodynamics will, after reading this book, appreciate the value and limitations of the subject, and will have obtained the necessary practical advice on the use of the appropriate equipment in the correct situations. Because this book is based on personal experience, references in the text are relatively few.

Bristol Urological Institute   Paul Abrams
April 1997

References

Brocklehurst JC (1993). Urinary incontinence in the community – analysis of a MORI poll. Br Med J 306:832–834.

Burgio KL, Matthews KA, Engel BT (1991). Prevalence, incidence and correlates of urinary incontinence in healthy, middle-aged women. J Urol 146:1255–1259.

O'Brien J, Austin M, Sethi P, O'Boyle P (1991). Urinary incontinence: prevalence, need for treatment, and effectiveness of intervention by nurse. Br Med J 303:1308–1312.

Sandvik H, Hunskaar S, Seim A, Hermstad R, Vanvik A, Bratt H (1993). Validation of a severity index in female urinary incontinence and its implementation in an epidemiological survey. J Epidemiol Community Health 47:497–499.

Torrens MJ (1974). The control of the hyperactive bladder by selective sacral denervation. ChM Thesis, Bristol University.

Turner Warwick R, Milroy E (1979). A reappraisal of the value of routine urological procedures in the assessment of urodynamic function. Urol Clin N Am 6:63–70.

Whiteside CG (1979). Symptoms of micturition disorders in relation to dynamic function. Urol Clin N Am 6:55–62.

Contents

List of Abbreviations

AUDS	ambulatory urodynamic studies
BOO	bladder outlet obstruction
BPE	benign prostatic enlargement
BPH	benign prostatic hyperplasia
BPO	benign prostatic obstruction
DFV	dysfunctional voiding
DHR	detrusor hyperreflexia
DI	detrusor instability
DSD	detrusor sphincter dyssynergia
DUA	detrusor underactivity
GP	general practitioner (family physician)
GSI	genuine stress incontinence
ICS	International Continence Society
IDSO	isolated distal sphincter obstruction
ISC	intermittent self-catheterisation
LUTD	lower urinary tract dysfunction
LUTS	lower urinary tract symptoms
MUCG	micturating cystourethrography
MUCP	maximum urethral closure pressure
p_{abd}	intra-abdominal pressure
p_{det}	detrusor pressure
pQS	pressure–flow studies
p_{ves}	intravesical pressure
PVR	post-void residual
Q_{ave}	average flow rate
Q_{max}	maximum flow rate
TURP	transurethral resection of the prostate
UDS	urodynamic studies
UFS	urine flow studies
UPP	urethral pressure profile
VUDS	videourodynamic studies
VUR	vesico-ureteric reflux

Measurement Units

Quantity	Unit		Symbol
volume	millilitre	(ml)	V
time	second	(s)	t
flow rate	millilitres/second	(ml/s)	Q
pressure	centimetres of water	(cmH$_2$O)	p

Urodynamic Qualifiers

Intra vesical (bladder)	ves
Intra urethral	ura
Detrusor	det
Intra abdominal (usually rectal)	abd

Chapter 1
Principles of Urodynamics

There are two basic aims of urodynamics:

- To reproduce the patient's symptomatic complaints.
- To provide a pathophysiological explanation for the patient's problems.

Implicit in these aims is the acceptance that whilst the patient's symptoms are important, because they bring the patient to the clinician, they are often misleading. Most patients with lower urinary tract dysfunction present to their doctor with symptoms, but in all branches of medicine symptoms have been shown to be misleading to a varying degree. Were symptoms reliable, then further investigation would not need to precede active management. At one time the elderly male patient with lower urinary tract symptoms (LUTS) would automatically have been offered a prostatectomy and, similarly, a woman with LUTS would have had an anterior repair with or without a hysterectomy. Most of the published literature indicates that the symptoms of lower urinary tract dysfunction (LUTD) are unreliable. Previously clinicians appreciated the need for some investigations and chose to assess the lower urinary tract using "static" investigations such as intravenous pyelography (IVP) and cystourethroscopy. However, the lower urinary tract, both during filling and emptying, is a dynamic system. Hence it is appropriate to use dynamic investigations for the investigation of lower urinary tract problems.

The statement "the bladder is an unreliable witness" was made by Bates in 1970 in one of the early papers on urodynamics (Bates et al., 1970). Two important papers appeared in 1980, one by a gynaecologist, Gerry Jarvis, who found (Jarvis et al., 1980) that, of 100 patients diagnosed by symptoms as having stress incontinence, on urodynamics only 68 were shown to have genuine stress incontinence. This was supported by the findings of Powell (working in the Bristol unit; Powell et al., 1980) that only 50% could be shown to have genuine stress incontinence. Both authors also looked at patients with apparent detrusor instability and Jarvis confirmed this diagnosis in only 51% of cases whilst Powell's showed detrusor instability in only 33% of such patients. Further work in women has shown that in women with apparently genuine stress incontinence, 12% had another cause for their apparent stress incontinence: in most patients the provocation factors leading to the apparent stress incontinence were provoking detrusor instability, leading to the reported incontinence. Clearly in this group of patients, with apparent stress incontinence, surgery would have been unsuccessful in at least the 12% who were suffering from an altogether different type of problem. These papers illustrate the difficulty of assessing women with lower tract dysfunction by symptoms alone. As in women, LUTS in the males are of poor diagnostic value, and furthermore the findings from IVP and cystoscopy have been shown to be poor indicators of bladder outlet obstruction. Both Abrams (1978) and Andersen (1979) have shown that the symptoms of apparent prostatic obstruction are misleading. Of the many symptoms that the textbooks attribute to prostatic outlet obstruction they could show that only slow stream and hesitancy bore any correlation with the urodynamic findings of obstruction, that is, high voiding pressure and low urine flow rate. Because symptoms have been shown to lack diagnostic specificity in all clinical groups, it is not surprising to find that when surgery was based on symptoms alone the results were less than satisfactory. The decision to recommend prostatic surgery was previously indicated by an assessment of symptoms backed by the findings from IVP and cystourethroscopy. Early audit of prostatectomy assessed by these means showed a cure rate of only 72%, poor for an elective procedure. Urodynamic studies provided alternative explanations for many symptoms and, when dynamic investigations of function (urodynamics) rather than static investigations of structure (IVP and cystoscopy) were used in preoperative evaluation, the results of surgery improved to 88%.

The preceding discussion relates to men and women who are neurologically normal and therefore able to appreciate sensation from their lower urinary tract. In patients who have neurological conditions affecting the lower urinary tract, it is common for sensation to be absent or abnormal, making their symptomatic complaints even more difficult to interpret.

Faced with the unpalatable fact that patients submitted for surgery without objective confirmation of their condition did rather poorly, surgeons reacted in different ways. Many became ostrich-like, and dismissed those who published these results as poor surgeons bereft of clinical acumen and operative skills, while making no effort to assess their own results. Others, who had always been uneasy about patient assessment by symptoms and non-functional studies, such as intravenous pyelography, seized the opportunity to study these large groups of patients by urodynamic means. Hence in the 1970s there was a rapid expansion of clinical and research urodynamics. The wider acceptance of urodynamics has allowed us to look at LUTS from a different perspective.

The Urodynamic History

Despite having discussed the shortcomings of symptoms it must be conceded that the patient's symptoms are important; they trouble the patient sufficiently for him or her to seek medical help, and LUTS should be assessed in a systematic way.

In some quarters there has been a nihilistic approach to urodynamic investigations, based on the alleged inadequacy of this method of assessment, and on the premise that if the patient's symptoms are improved by an intervention, for example an operation, then that is all that matters! However, because the patient's symptoms and the objective urodynamic findings bear little relationship to each other, this approach has several major drawbacks. Already mentioned are the less than adequate results from elective surgery, when only symptoms were considered in diagnosis. Second, it is now well established that there is a very large placebo effect in patients with LUTS. The symptoms of men with proven bladder outlet obstruction, secondary to benign prostatic hyperplasia, can be improved by placebo treatment to such an extent that 40 to 60% of men in the placebo arm of drug studies consider themselves considerably improved.

Nevertheless, it is apparent that those doctors and nurses familiar with urodynamic techniques, and with a functional appreciation of bladder and urethral physiology, are able to take a history from the patient that gives a much more accurate picture of the patient's real problems. The significance of individual symptoms and groups of symptoms is discussed in detail in Chapter 4.

The Urodynamic Physical Examination

Patients referred for urodynamics will have been examined in a general way, either in the hospital clinic from which the referral emanated, or by the patient's general practitioner (primary care physician). Hence the efforts of the urodynamic staff should be to concentrate on a physical examination that will shed light on the patient's symptomatic complaints and the underlying pathophysiological processes that could have caused these complains. We consider that one of the great advantages of the Bristol unit is that adequate time is given for close questioning, the relevant physical examination, an unhurried urodynamic investigation and practical advice. The importance of the urodynamic physical examination is discussed in detail in Chapter 4. Urine examination should be performed in all patients, and radiology and endoscopy have their indications, as will be discussed in Chapter 4. Urodynamic studies should follow only when careful investigations have been performed to exclude other pathologies that might mimic lower urinary tract dysfunction.

The Aims of Urodynamics

The objectives of any test can be achieved if the appropriate questions that the test is designed to address are posed. Therefore, at the outset, it is important to ask the following question:

"What do I want to know about this patient?"

Urodynamic studies have their limitations. It may be useful for the clinician to answer this question in terms of the filling and voiding phases of the micturition cycle and in terms of the bladder and the urethra. In this way the urodynamicist can ask the next relevant question, which is:

"Which urodynamic investigations need to be performed to define this patient's problems?"

This question will concentrate the clinician's thought processes on eliminating those investigations which cannot help to make the diagnosis or indicate the line of management. For example, if a young male patient has had a urethral stricture and restricturing has to be excluded, then urine flow measurement will be the only required test.

Once the questions that need to be answered have been defined and the appropriate urodynamic tests made, the next question should be:

"Is the investigation likely to be of benefit for the patient?"

This question, again, can be answered by an analysis of the possible benefits to the patient, in terms of the increased knowledge generated by the test, and the influence this knowledge will have on his or her clinical management. Even when knowledge does not appear likely to improve the quality of life of that patient there may still be an overall benefit to them if knowledge in a difficult area without effective treatment techniques can be increased: an increase in knowledge is at a future date likely to result in effective treatment being introduced. A good example would be in a young woman who cannot void adequately, when often normal voiding cannot be re-established; here intermittent self-catheterisation is a good treatment, although it is resented by many patients. However, routine investigations usually contribute little to effective management, although neurophysiological testing may show abnormal sphincter activity. Hence investigations may show the cause, although at this stage we do not have the means to reverse these abnormalities.

The benefits of the investigations must be set against the potential harm the tests could do. Fortunately, urodynamics are a relatively harmless investigation, although there is a small incidence of urinary tract infection (1 to 2%) and some discomfort. Further, there is the question of whether the information gained by the tests can offset their financial cost. Also important in deciding the benefit–risk analysis of the investigations will be the answers given to the following further questions.

"Is urodynamics able to make a reliable diagnosis?"

This is a complex question within which the fundamental query is whether or not the tests themselves are reliable and reproducible. Three factors greatly influence the value of urodynamics:

- The urodynamic technique should be free of technical artifacts.
- The results of investigations should be reproducible.
- The clinician should be properly trained and able to interpret the results of urodynamics.

It is clear that, from a technical point of view, the tests must be carried out in a careful way, eliminating all possible artifacts. This aspect of urodynamic studies is discussed extensively in Chapter 3. The patient's own bioconsistency is another problem. We know that symptoms vary considerably with time but we do not have much information as to whether or not urodynamic findings vary. This problem is best dealt with at the end of the urodynamic tests by asking:

"Did the urodynamic studies reproduce the patient's complaints and did the complaints correlate with known urodynamic features?"

In the Bristol unit we have always laid great emphasis on the clinician, who is aware of the therapeutic possibilities of subsequent treatment, being present during urodynamics. The clinician can then be sure whether or not the sensations felt by the patient and the findings demonstrated by urodynamics are typical of the patient's everyday symptoms or whether or not any urodynamic abnormalities can account for these. Occasionally during urodynamic studies either the patient complains of an unrepresentative symptom, for example, urgency, or there is a urodynamic abnormality noted which does not correlate with the patient's symptoms. These discrepancies can be detected and interpreted as artifacts, if the clinician is present. However, if the urodynamics is delegated to a technician they may be reported on their face value, leading to a possible bias in the report that may influence subsequent patient management.

In some instances more than one abnormality can be seen, therefore it is important to ask:

"Can urodynamics decide which is the most significant abnormality if more than one is detected?"

Multiple abnormalities are commonly seen in patients with neuropathic vesicourethral dysfunction. They are also often seen in non-neurological patients such as in women with mixed incontinence. Treatment should be directed to the most significant or troublesome abnormality. Hence, once again, the correlation between the patient's symptomatic complaint and the urodynamic findings are most important. This correlation allows the clinician to advise on which abnormality is the most significant and should therefore receive management priority.

As well as seeking answers to the above questions the urodynamicist needs to define the indications for urodynamic investigation, and these can be viewed in a slightly different way:

1. To increase diagnostic accuracy above that which can be achieved by non-urodynamic means.
2. To make a diagnosis on which a management plan can be based.
3. If there are coexisting abnormalities to provide evidence to determine which should be treated first.
4. To define the current situation, knowing the likely abnormalities, as a baseline for future surveillance.
5. To predict problems that may follow treatment interventions.
6. To assess the natural history of lower urinary tract dysfunction.
7. To provide evidence that influences the timing of treatment.
8. To exclude abnormalities which might interfere with the management of that patient.
9. To assess the results of treatments designed to affect lower urinary tract function.

The first of the indications is self-explanatory. The urological management of spinal cord trauma patients provides a good example of the second and third indications, where early urodynamics seeks a baseline, and subsequent urodynamic tests monitor any changes in urethral or bladder function: these changes in spinal cord patients can have life-threatening implications (see Chapter 5). The fifth indication is illustrated by the frequent request from orthopaedic surgeons to exclude bladder outlet obstruction in elderly patients undergoing prosthetic surgery, in whom the avoidance of urethral catheterisation is desirable. Knowledge of the natural history of LUTD should form part of our decision-making when advising patients on treatment. However there is little information on the long-term outcome when dysfunctions such as bladder outlet obstruction or detrusor instability are untreated. The need for increased knowledge justifies indicators 6 and 7. Indication 8 covers coexisting urodynamic abnormalities such as the functional outlet obstruction seen in multiple sclerosis patients that results in an increase in residual urine after treatment of detrusor instability with anticholinergic drugs. Indication 9 is most important because there must to be objective evidence of benefit for treatments designed to improve LUTD.

After a brief description of the anatomy and physiology of the lower urinary tract in Chapter 2, subsequent chapters discuss urodynamic techniques (Chapter 3) and their applications (Chapters 5 and 6).

References

Abrams PH, Feneley RCL (1978). The significance of the symptoms associated with bladder outflow obstruction. Urol Int 33:171–174.

Andersen JT, Nordling J, Walter S (1979). Prostatism I. The correlation between symptoms, cystometric and urodynamic findings. Scand J Urol 13:229–236.

Bates CP, Whiteside CG, Turner Warwick R (1970). Synchronous urine pressure flow cystourethrography with special reference to stress and urge incontinence. Br J Urol 42:714–723.

Jarvis GJ, Hall S, Stamp S, Miller DR, Johansson A (1980). An assessment of urodynamic examination in incontinence women. Br J Obstet Gynaecol 87:873–896.

Powell PH, Shepherd AM, Lewis P, Feneley RCL (1980). The accuracy of clinical diagnosis assessed urodynamically. Proceedings 10th meeting ICS Los Angeles pp 3–4.

Chapter 2
Anatomy and Physiology

Introduction

Urodynamic investigations developed because of the dissatisfaction with the assessment of patients and their results from treatment, when management was based on symptom assessment and the definitions of anatomical abnormalities. Urodynamics attempts to relate physiology to anatomy, that is function to structure. A sound knowledge of anatomy and physiology form the basis for the effective assessment and treatment of patients. In addition this knowledge can be used to critically evaluate the role of urodynamic studies in assessing patients with lower urinary tract symptoms (LUTS).

Although the bladder and urethra are described separately below, it should be remembered that they normally act as a reciprocal functional unit.

Urethral Structure and Function

Very often the urethra is considered only as a passive conduit for urine, the bladder being the more important and more active part of the lower urinary tract. One of the reasons for this may have been the observation of Lapides that continence was maintained in the isolated bladder even when most of the urethra had been cut off. Urethral function is here discussed first in an attempt to redress this balance. Indeed it would be possible to argue that the urethra is the controlling agent in the micturition cycle.

The urethral closure mechanism and hence urinary continence depends on active and passive factors. Its function may be classified as normal or incompetent on filling, and normal or obstructive on voiding.

Anatomy and Innervation

It is always tempting to infer function from structure. In general the following comments on anatomy are intended to give more perspective to the functional urodynamic observations. The terminology and general arrangement of the lower urinary tract are shown in Fig. 2.1.

FEMALE

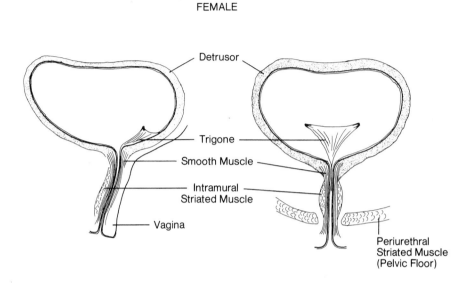

MALE

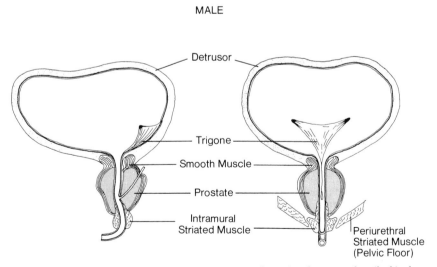

Fig. 2.1 Structural relationships in the lower urinary tract. The various layers are described in the text. (Modified from Gosling 1979)

Mucosa

In both sexes the mucosa is organised in longitudinal folds giving the urethral lumen a stellate appearance when closed. This arrangement allows considerable distensibility. The surface tension may be a factor in urethral closure.

Submucosa

The submucosal layer is a vascular plexus. Zinner discussed the role of this layer in relation to inner urethral wall softness. His suggestion is that the submucosa acts in a passive plastic way to "fill in" between the folds of mucosa as the urethra closes. This is said to occur as the tension increases in the muscular wall of the urethra and its effect is to improve the efficiency of the seal of the urethral lumen.

There is an extensive submucosal vascular plexus which may have more than a passive role. Huisman has suggested that there are myoepithelial cells to be found in association with arteriovenous shunts. This would provide a means of controlling submucosal pressure. Others suggest that the vascular element may be an important factor in the urethral closure in females where it is difficult to attribute all the occlusive forces to urethral muscle. This also explains the presence of urethral pressure changes synchronous with the arterial pulse, and may be the reason for some postural and menstrual pressure changes. Gosling was unable to confirm the anatomical basis for this vascular control. In women after menopause, oestrogen deficiency is thought to lead to a reduction in the turgor of the vascular plexus and hence to be, in part, responsible for the increase in LUTS.

Urethral Muscle in Females

The smooth muscle of the female urethra is arranged longitudinally. Gosling showed from acetylcholinesterase analysis that the dominant innervation is cholinergic. Virtually no noradrenergic nerves are seen. This may appear confusing at first because the majority of the measurable resting urethral pressure depends on the alpha-adrenergic activity, if studies using alpha-blocking drugs are to be believed (Donker et al. 1972). This leads to a choice of conclusions:

- There are alpha-receptors on the smooth muscle but no nerves to produce the transmitter (noradrenaline); this seems illogical.
- The urethral smooth muscle does not produce the urethral pressure. This is not as improbable as it sounds, because the fibres are not circular but longitudinal, and not very prolific.
- The alpha-adrenergic effects occur not on the muscle but at the level of the pelvic ganglia. This is the currently popular explanation.
- Alpha-blocking drugs have effects on the neuromuscular transmission that are not conventionally recognised.

There are two groups of striated muscle fibres in relation to the urethra, called intramural and peri-urethral by Gosling (1979). Intramural striated muscle bundles are found close to the urethral lumen, sometimes interdigitating with smooth muscle. In the female these fibres are found in the greatest frequency anteriorly and laterally in the middle third of the urethra. They do not surround the urethra posteriorly to form a circular sphincter as in the male. The muscle is of a "slow twitch" type, rich in myosin ATPase, and adapted to maintain contraction over a relatively long period of time. No muscle spindles have been seen. There has been controversy over the innervation of the intra-urethral striated sphincter. It has been said that the intramural striated muscle is supplied by myelinated fibres from S2-4 running with the pelvic nerve and therefore not affected by either pudendal block or neurectomy. More recently others have stated that a branch of the pudendal nerve supplies the muscle by fibres also from S2-4.

The pelvic floor is separated from the urethra by a layer of connective tissue and is histochemically and histologically different from the intraurethral striated sphincter. This muscle is a mixture of slow and fast twitch fibres and is supplied by the pudendal nerve and myelinated fibres in the pelvic nerve (S2-4).

Urethral Muscle in Males

The smooth muscle of the preprostatic urethra in males is histochemically distinct from that of the detrusor and from urethral muscle in females. This muscle also forms the prostatic capsule. It is richly provided with noradenergic terminals and little acetylcholinesterase has been found. It is agreed generally that this well-defined muscle represents the "prostatic or genital sphincter" designed to prevent reflux of ejaculate at the time of orgasm. Certainly we have observed changes in pressure in this part of the urethra during penile erection (Fig. 2.2), and these do not seem to occur during any part of the micturition cycle unless there is erection.

The striated muscles in the male can be divided into the same two groups described above for the female. The innervation is similar. The intramural

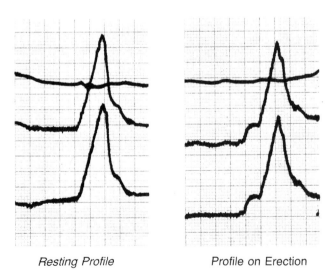

Resting Profile   Profile on Erection

Fig. 2.2 Urethral pressure profile demonstrating the elevation of the pressure in the region of the bladder neck/preprostatic sphincter during penile erection.

striated muscle is orientated circularly around the postprostatic "membranous" urethra as a distinct sphincter.

Receptor Sites and Neurotransmitters

Much recent effort has been directed towards the analysis of receptors in the urinary tract. The distinction between experimentally demonstrable alpha- and beta-adrenergic receptor sites and innervation is not always made clear. Alpha-adrenergic receptors, causing smooth muscle contraction when stimulated, produce their effects mainly in the region of the bladder neck and the proximal 3 cm of urethra in both sexes. Beta-receptor activity is very weak in this area, being present over the bladder dome: beta stimulation encourages bladder relaxation. Appreciation of these functions aids the understanding of the action of drugs on the urinary tract. However the appropriate sympathetic nerves may not even be present anatomically in the areas where receptors have been demonstrated.

The complex interrelation of nerves, transmitter substances and receptor sites has been the subject of controversy for years. Some of the reasons why progress is slow in this field are outlined below:

- Individual nerves may produce more than one neurotransmitter.
- Neurotransmitters may act on more than one type of receptor, producing different actions.
- Neurotransmitters may act in different ways at the same receptor site depending on their concentration.
- Neurotransmitters may interact with one another.
- There are considerable species differences in both neurotransmitters and receptors.

An example of fundamental controversy has been the question of the identity of the principal neurotransmitter to the detrusor muscle. The postganglionic parasympathetic fibres are presumed to be cholinergic in that they are associated with identifiable acetylcholinesterase. However if the transmitter is acetylcholine it should be blocked by atropine. Although some species are atropine-sensitive the majority are not. This has led to the suggestion that another substance may be the principal neurotransmitter. Alternatively the receptor on the bladder muscle may have more nicotinic characteristics than muscarinic. Perhaps some receptors are not accessible to freely circulating atropine. Suggestions for alternative transmitters have included 5-hydroxytryptamine, purine nucleodes such as ATP, and prostaglandins. It is now believed that in normal function acetylcholine is the principal neurotransmitter, although the situation may be different in abnormal conditions such as bladder outlet obstruction and detrusor instability when ATP may be important. A great deal more work needs to be performed on human muscle preparations, so that a better understanding of bladder neuro-pharmacology emerges. Meanwhile the unpredictable response to the phar-macotherapy for detrusor overactivity merely emphasises our incomplete understanding of the pathophysiological processes involved in lower urinary tract dysfunction.

Central Nervous Activity

As can be seen in Fig. 2.3, the organisation of central control is rather a complex business. It can however be reduced to several relatively simple concepts. Sensation from the lower urinary tract must be appreciated centrally and consciously if normal cerebral control is to function. The sensation of bladder fullness and of bladder contraction ascends in the anterior half of the spinal cord and may be affected by damage in that area of the cord, for example in anterior spinal artery thrombosis and bilateral spinothalamic tractotomy, as well as other spinal cord lesions. Sensation of activity in the pelvic floor ascends in the posterior columns.

Sensation must not only reach the conscious level when the subject is awake; it must also, by its collateral effects on the reticular formation perhaps, be able to wake the subject from sleep or otherwise subconsciously to inhibit micturition. This may be the fundamental problem in nocturnal enuresis.

Assuming sensation is normal, the brain acts by balancing the various facilitatory and inhibitory effects suggested in Fig. 2.3 and the final common efferent pathway is through the "bladder centre" in the pontine reticular formation. This centre is essential for normally co-ordinated micturition. It acts on the sacral micturition centre in the conus medullaris, where the final integration of bladder and urethral activity takes place. Since the usual response of a bladder liberated from cerebral control is one of reflex overactivity, it is assumed that the major

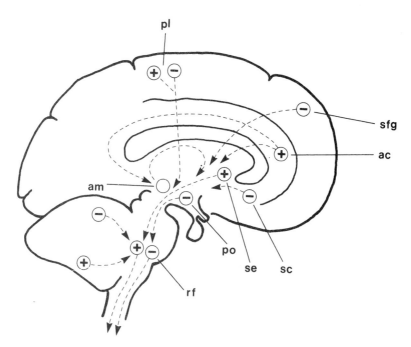

Fig. 2.3 Simplified representation of the cerebral areas involved in micturition. The multiplicity of interactions makes it easy to appreciate why the subject should be left to the research physiologist. +, facilitation; –, inhibition; *ac*, anterior cingulate gyrus; *am*, amygdala; *pl*, paracentral lobule; *po*, preoptic nucleus; *rf*, pontine reticular formation; *sc*, subcallosal cingulate gyrus; *se*, septal area; *sfg*, superior frontal gyrus. (Torrens 1982)

cerebral output is one of tonic inhibition, hence the old term "uninhibited bladder". However this is only an assumption, and prejudging the activity of the nervous system can only slow down the understanding of it. We suggest that terms which imply specific pathophysiolgy should be avoided as much as possible. The detailed neurological control of the bladder has been reviewed elsewhere (Nathan 1976; Fletcher and Bradley 1978; Torrens 1982).

Normal Urethral Function

The normal urethral closure mechanism maintains a positive urethral closure pressure during bladder filling, even in the presence of increased abdominal pressure. Continence can be seen to be maintained at the bladder neck in normal persons. This can be regarded as the proximal urethral closure mechanism. If the vesico-urethral junction (bladder neck) is incompetent then continence may still be maintained at the high-pressure zone in the urethra, about 2 to 3 cm distally. This zone corresponds to the maximum condensation of muscle, both smooth and striated, and may be regarded as the distal urethral closure mechanism. Whether it is really valid to separate two parts of the urethra in this way from the physiological point of view is debatable; the normal urethra probably works as one unit. However from a practical standpoint it is useful because the urethral areas may not be abnormal simultaneously.

Many factors have been thought to contribute to urethral closure; some are obvious, others less so. They are as follows:

- Muscular occlusion by the intraurethral striated muscle.
- Transmission of abdominal pressure to the proximal urethra.
- Mucosal surface tension.
- Anatomical configuration at the bladder neck, including ligamentous support.
- Submucosal softness or vascularity.
- Inherent elasticity, particularly at the bladder neck.
- Urethral length.

While the relative importance of these various factors remains unknown, it is better to consider and describe only those that can be observed objectively: urethral closure pressure, electromyography (EMG) and videoscopic appearance of the urethra. Mechanical and hydrodynamic analogues, such as those quoted by Zinner et al. (1976), serve only to demonstrate how complicated the situation is. However the work of Delancey has helped us to understand the way in which the ligamentous structures and fascial sheets around the urethra and bladder neck are important in normal function. The attachments of the vagina to the pelvic floor provide a hammock under the proximal urethra and bladder base against which the bladder neck can be compressed when intra-abdominal pressure rises.

Typically the urethral closure pressure decreases at or before the onset of micturition and is synchronous with bladder base descent seen by imaging and with the reduction of EMG activity from striated muscle of the intraurethral sphincter of the urethra, the pelvic floor or the external anal sphincter (Fig. 2.4, *overleaf*). It is a fallacy to consider that the urethra is forced open by a head of detrusor pressure. Micturition usually occurs at a voiding pressure less than the maximum resting intraurethral pressure: the decrease in urethral closure

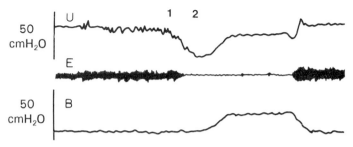

Fig. 2.4 Intravesical (*B*) and urethral (*U*) pressure and striated sphincter EMG (*E*) during volitional voiding. At the initiation of voiding (*1*) the urethral pressure falls to a minimum before the intravesical pressure starts to rise. Flow is initiated at (*2*), before an appreciable intravesical pressure has been generated. Flow is therefore a consequence of urethral relaxation in this female subject. At cessation of flow EMG activity returns after a period of silence, and the urethral pressure transiently rises while the proximal urethra is emptied back into the bladder. (McGuire 1978)

pressure represents an active relaxation process. Part of the pressure decrease can be attributed to the relaxation of the mainly circular orientated striated muscle of the pelvic floor, but part seems to be due to active inhibition of the intraurethral striated sphincter. This can be reproduced by stimulation of the sacral nerves, especially S4 (Torrens 1978). Many women appear to void by relaxation and urethral opening only, no detrusor pressure rise being necessary. Undoubtedly urethral resistance in women is low, and the inner longitudinal smooth muscle may help reduce resistance by contracting and thereby making the urethra shorter and wider, thus facilitating micturition.

Detrusor Function

The urinary bladder is not a sphere even when contracting, and calculations of tension based on that premise must be to some extent erroneous. Its shape is more that of a three-sided pyramid, base posterior and apex at the urachus. The superior surface is covered by peritoneum and is pressed upon by the other viscera. The two inferior surfaces are supported by the pelvic floor and connected to the pelvic fascia by various condensations of fibroareolar tissue. Also important are the pubourethral ligaments. The functional adequacy of the bladder does depend on its correct anatomical position, so heavy viscera or inadequate pelvic support cause functional problems such as incontinence and prolapse. The detrusor is composed of an interlacing network of smooth muscle bundles. These are not layered, as has sometimes been described and as is the case in the intestine. It is not clear whether or not the detrusor around the bladder neck is involved in the mechanisms of closure and opening of the bladder neck and the various mechanical theories of function that have been elaborated are presumptive and should be interpreted with great caution.

The golf enthusiast will readily understand the muscle fibre arrangement of the detrusor, because it is similar to the structure of a golfball beneath its white coating: muscle fibres run in all directions and change depth in the bladder wall. The detrusor muscle is relatively rich in acetylcholinesterase. As discussed previously this is evidence for a dominant cholinergic innervation and very little noradrenergic activity can be demonstrated histochemically.

Innervation

Efferent motor nerves to the detrusor arise from the parasympathetic (cholinergic) ganglion cells in the pelvic plexus. The preganglionic fibres run in the sacral roots 2–4. The third root is the dominant nerve in most cases. The parasympathetic supply is excitatory. Preganglionic parasympathetic fibres and postganglionic sympathetic fibres both synapse with ganglion cells close to and within the bladder wall: it is believed that the sympathetic fibres act to inhibit the parasympathetic before being "switched off" at the onset of micturition.

Nerve-mediated detrusor inhibition has been described, occurring after stimulation of the pelvic floor or perianal area, and may be the mechanism by which new methods of nerve stimulation are effective in treating detrusor overactivity. It is suggested that such inhibition may be mediated by the sympathetic nervous system (Sundin and Dahlstrom 1973). Bladder relaxation evoked by

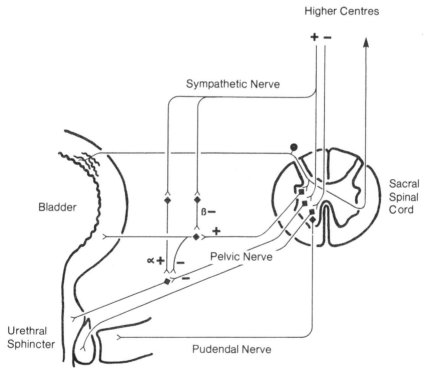

Fig. 2.5 Summary of the possible organisation of the peripheral nervous supply to the lower urinary tract. Preganglionic parasympathetic fibres and postganglionic sympathetic fibres both synapse with ganglion cells close to, and within, the bladder wall. The arrangement in relation to the urethra may be morphologically similar but functionally different. The periurethral striated muscle (pelvic floor) is supplied by the pudendal nerve. The somatic nerve supply to the intramural urethral striated muscle runs with the pelvic nerve and is vulnerable during pelvic surgery. (Torrens 1982)

bladder wall stretch (accommodation) may be similarly mediated. Gosling (1979) has shown that little significant sympathetic innervation reaches the bladder dome in humans, and so it is suggested that this inhibition occurs at the neurones in the pelvic ganglia where noradrenergic axosomatic terminals have been observed. The sympathetic supply to the pelvic ganglia arises at the T10–12 level and runs in the presacral nerves and hypogastric plexus. The muscle around the bladder neck in both sexes is similar to that of the rest of the bladder. Most nerve terminals are acetylcholinesterase-positive and almost no noradrenergic terminals are seen. (This is in contradistinction to certain species of animals.)

The sensory nerves from the bladder run with the motor supply. In general the proprioceptive afferents related to tension enter the sacral segments, as do the greater proportion of enteroceptive afferents related to pain and temperature. Poorly localised sensations of pain and distension enter with the sympathetic fibres at a high level. The innervation of the bladder and urethra is summarised in Fig. 2.5 on the preceding page.

References

Andersson KE (1996). Prostatic and extraprostatic adrenoceptors – contributions to the lower urinary tract symptoms in benign prostatic hyperplasia. Scand J Urol Nephrol 30 suppl. 179.

Andersson KE, Persson K (1993). The L-arginine nitric oxide pathway and non-adrenergic, non-cholinergic relaxation of the lower urinary tract. Gen Pharmacol 24:833–839.

Chapple C R (1995). Selective α1-adrenoceptor antagonists in benign prostatic hyperplasia. Br J Urol 75:265–270.

Delancey JOL (1990). Anatomy and physiology of urinary continence. Clin Obstet Gynaecol 33:298–307.

Donker PJ, Ivanovici F, Noach EL (1972). Analysis of the urethral pressure profile by means of electromyography and the administration of drugs. Br J Urol 44:180–193.

Fletcher TF, Bradley WB (1978). Neuroanatomy of the bladder/urethra. J Urol 119:153–160.

Gosling JA (1979). The structure of the bladder and urethra in relation to function. Urol Clin N Am 6:31–38.

Gosling JA, Dixon JS, Critchley HOD, Thomson SA (1981). A comparative study of the human external sphincter and periurethral levator ani muscles. Br J Urol 53:35.

Huisman AB (1979). Morfologie van de vrouwelijke urethra. Thesis, Groningen, The Netherlands.

Lapides J, Freind CR, Ajemian EP, Reus WS (1962). Denervation supersensitivity as a test for neurogenic bladder. Surg Gynecol Obstet 114:241.

McGuire EJ (1978) Reflex urethral instability. Br J Urol 50:200–204.

Moriyama N, Kurimoto S, Horie S, Kameyama S, Nasu K, Tanaka T, Yano J, Sagehashi Y, Yamaguchi T, Tsujmoto G, Kawabe K (1996). Quantification of a 1-adrenoceptor subtype mRNAs in hypertrophic and non-hypertrophic prostates. J Urol 155–331A (abstract 82).

Muramatsu I, Oshita M, Ohmura T, Kigoshi S, Akino H, Okada K (1994) . Pharmacological characterisation of α1 adrenoceptor subtypes in the human prostate: functional and binding studies. Br J Urol 74:572–578.

Nathan PW (1976). The central nervous connections of the bladder. In: Williams DI, Chisholm GD (eds). Scientific foundations of urology. London, Heineman pp 51–58.

Nilvebrant L, Sundquist S, Gilberg PG (1996). Neurourology and Urodynamics. Athens abstract 34 p 310.

Sundin T, Dahlstrom A (1973). The sympathetic innervation of the urinary bladder and urethra in the normal state and after parasympathetic denervation at the spinal root level. Scand J Urol Nephrol 7:131–149.

Torrens MJ (1978). Urethral sphincteric responses to stimulation of the sacral nerves in the human female. Urol Int 33:22–26.

Torrens MJ (1982). Neurophysiology. In: Stanton SL (ed.) Gynaecological urology. St Louis, Mosby.

Torrens M, Morrison JFB (1987). The physiology of the lower urinary tract. London, Springer-Verlag .

Zinner NR, Ritter RC, Sterling AM (1976). The mechanism of micturition. In: Williams DI, Chisholm GD (eds). Scientific foundations of urology. London: Heinemann pp 39–50.

Chapter 3
Urodynamic Techniques

Introduction

The evolution of urodynamic units may be traced to the interest in the hydrodynamics of micturition which had been simmering since the early cystometric
studies of the nineteenth century, but it was the advent of electronics that acted as
the catalyst for modern urodynamic studies. In 1956 von Garrelts described a
simple practical apparatus, using a pressure transducer, to record the volume of
urine voided as a function of time and thus, by derivation, urine flow rates could
be calculated. His work stimulated a revival of interest in cystometry, because it
was then possible to record the bladder pressure and the urine flow rate simultaneously during voiding. As a result, normal and obstructed micturition could
be defined in terms of these measurements (Claridge 1966) and a formula was
applied to express urethral resistance (Smith 1968). Enhorning (1961) measured
bladder and urethral pressures simultaneously with a specially designed catheter
and he termed the pressure difference between them the urethral closure pressure. He demonstrated that a reduction of intraurethral pressure occurred several
seconds prior to detrusor contraction at the initiation of voiding. This appeared
to be related to the relaxation of the pelvic floor, thus confirming the EMG studies
of Franksson and Peterson (1955).

These original research studies led rapidly to the application of urodynamic
investigations in the clinical field. Radiological studies of the lower urinary tract,
using the image intensifier and cine or videotape recordings, were already established and their value in the assessment of micturition disorders had been
described (Turner Warwick and Whiteside 1970). Thus it was a relatively simple
step to combine cystourethrography with pressure flow measurements (Bates
et al. 1970) Later, more sophisticated techniques, using EMG recordings of the
pelvic floor, were employed, particularly for neuropathic bladder problems
(Thomas et al. 1975). These clinical studies during the 1970s emphasised the need
to investigate the function as well as the anatomical structure of the lower urinary

tract, when evaluating micturition disorders. Urodynamics was established as a necessary service commitment, rather than a research tool.

At the same time as these technical developments were arising, an increasing awareness of the clinical problem of urinary incontinence was becoming apparent. From Exeter, the work of Caldwell (1967) had initiated considerable interest in the subject, as a result of his approach to the treatment of incontinent patients with electronic implants. In his sphincter research unit a small receiver was developed, which could be placed subcutaneously in the abdominal wall and activated by a small external radio-frequency transmitter. Platinum iridium electrodes led down to the pelvic floor muscles, which could be stimulated. Other new techniques were also being advocated at this time, such as pelvic floor faradism applied under general anaesthetic (Moore and Schofield 1967) and a variety of external electronic devices which could be placed in the anal canal or vagina to stimulate pelvic floor contraction (Hopkinson and Lightwood 1967; Alexander and Rowan 1968)

Through the 1980s and 1990s the principles of urodynamics have remained unchanged. As microchip technology has advanced, so has urodynamic equipment become computerised, although this has not always been for the best, as we discuss below. New techniques have become available, such as the measurement of bladder neck electrical conductance, a technique devised by Plevnick. Computerisation has allowed the development of more complex and sophisticated neurological investigations such as cortical evoked responses, although these techniques are used only in specialist centres. James has used long-term (ambulatory) techniques to study bladder and urethral function. His work became the focus of increased attention in the early 1990s, and, with computerisation, the patient has been set free from the fixed urodynamic recording apparatus. It remains to be seen whether ambulatory studies, which represent a more physiological approach, become established as a primary method of investigation.

In this chapter the technical aspects of urodynamics are discussed. The indications of urodynamics are mentioned here only briefly, as their clinical role is discussed fully in Chapter 5.

Principles of Urodynamic Technique

Investigations must be carried out in a safe and scientific manner. The investigator is responsible for ensuring the privacy and comfort of the patient. Micturition is a private matter, and unless this is respected, urodynamics will be less than satisfactory. Proper care must be applied to the infection control aspects of investigation and the principles of sterility followed.

The investigations themselves must be free of technical errors, and, just as the grand prix driver must be familiar with the mechanics of his car, the urodynamacist must be familiar with the technical aspects of the tests they are using. This applies particularly to the measurement of pressure. The investigator must also be satisfied as to the reproducibility of urodynamic results, so that, at the end of the investigation, the patient can be offered explanations for their symptoms and the clinician can be given advice as to how the patient should be managed.

Standardisation of Techniques

Both technique and terminology should be standardised. Of course, techniques must evolve, but not on an unplanned basis. For any department, their individual technique should be standard to allow for interpretation of findings. In order that others may understand and interpret the results from any urodynamic unit, it is essential to use standardised terminology to describe the technique and the results obtained. To facilitate this the International Continence Society in 1973 set up a standardisation committee, which has produced ten reports on the terminology of lower urinary tract function. The first six reports were collated in 1988, the seventh report appeared in 1992 and reports 8 to 10 are in the press. The subjects covered are:

- Procedures related to the evaluation of urine storage.
- Procedures related to the evaluation of micturition.
- Procedures related to the neurological investigations of the urinary tract during filling and voiding.
- A classification of lower urinary tract dysfunction.
- Pelvic floor assessment.
- Intestinal urinary reservoirs: assessment of functional characteristics.
- Pressure–flow studies of voiding, urethral resistance and urethral obstruction.

These standards are proposed to facilitate comparison of results by investigators who use urodynamic methods. It has been recommended that the acknowledgement of these standards in written publications be indicated by a footnote stating: "Methods, definitions and units conform to the standards proposed by the International Continence Society except where specifically noted." The author has accepted these standards, and used them in this book. They are repeated and explained in the relevant chapters, and the reports are published in full in Appendix 1.

This chapter forms the core of the book. Urodynamic studies are described at three levels: uroflowmetry, basic urodynamics (inflow cystometry, pressure–flow studies and pad testing) and complex urodynamics (urethral pressure profilometry, videourodynamics, ambulatory studies and various aspects of neurophysiological testing).

References

Alexander S, Rowan D (1968). An electric pessary for stress incontinence. Lancet I:728.

Bates CP, Whiteside CG, Turner Warwick R (1970). Synchronous urine pressure flow cystourethrography with special reference to stress and urge incontinence. Br J Urol 42:714–723.

Caldwell KPS (1967). The treatment of incontinence by electronic implants. Ann R Coll Surg 41:447–459.

Claridge M (1966). Analyses of obstructed micturition. Ann R Coll Surg 39:30–53.

Enhorning G (1961). Simultaneous recording of intravesical and intra-urethral pressure. Acta Chir Scand [Suppl] 276:1–68.

Franksson C, Petersen I (1955). Electromyographic investigation of disturbances in the striated muscle of the urethral sphincter. Br J Urol 27:154–161.

Hopkinson BR, Lightwood R (1967). Electrical treatment of incontinence. Br J Surg 54:802–805.

Moore T, Schofield PF (1997). Treatment of stress incontinence by maximum perineal electrical stimulation. Br Med J iii:150–151.

Smith JC (1968). Urethral resistance to micturition. Br J Urol 40:125–156.

Thomas DG, Smallwood R, Graham D (1975). Urodynamic observations following spinal trauma. Br J Urol 47:161–175.

Turner Warwick R, Whiteside CG (1970). Investigation and management of bladder neck dysfunction. In: Riches Sir Eric (ed) Modern trends in urology 3. London: Butterworth pp 295–311.

Urethral Function Studies

Abrams P, Torrens MJ (1977). Urethral closure pressure profiles in the male. Urol Int 32:137–145.

Asmussen M, Ulmsten U (1976). Simultaneous urethrocystometry with a new technique. Scand J Urol Nephrol 10:7–11.

Brown M, Wickham JEA (1969). The urethral pressure profile. Br J Urol 41:211–217.

Bump RC, Elser DM, Theofrastous JP, McClish DK (1995). The continence program for women research group. Am J Obstet Gynaecol 173/2:551–7.

Edwards LE (1973). Investigation and management of incontinence in women. Ann Roy Coll Surg 52:69–85.

Hilton P (1983). The urethral pressure profile under stress: a comparison of profiles on coughing and straining. Neurourol Urodyn 2:55.

Kulseng-Hanssen S, Stien R, Fønstelien E (1987). Urethral pressure variations in women with neurological symptoms. In relationship to urethral and pelvic floor striated muscle. Neurourol Urodyn 6:71–78.

Kulseng-Hanssen S (1983). Prevalence and pattern of unstable urethral pressure in 174 gynaecologic patients referred for urodynamic investigation. Am J Obstet Gynaecol 146:895

Lose G (1992). Simultaneous recording of pressure and cross-sectional area in the female urethra: a study of urethral closure function in healthy and stress incontinent women. Neurourol Urodyn 11:55–89.

McGuire EJ, Fitzpatrick CC, Wan J et al. (1993). Clinical assessment of urethral sphincter function. J Urol 150:1452–1454.

Tanagho EA (1979). Urodynamics of female urinary incontinence with emphasis on stress incontinence. J Urol 122:200–204.

Thind P, Lose G, Jørgensen L et al. (1991). Urethral pressure increment preceding and following bladder pressure elevation during stress episodes in healthy and stress incontinent women. Neurourol Urodyn 10:177.

Ulmsten U, Henriksson L, Iosif S (1982). The unstable female urethra. Am J Obstet Gynaecol 144:93.

Yalla SV, Sharma GVRK, Barsamian EM (1980). Micturitional static urethral pressure profile. A method of recording urethral pressure profile during voiding and the implications. J Urol 124:649.

Uroflowmetry

Urine flow studies are the simplest of urodynamic techniques, being non-invasive. Furthermore the equipment needed is simple and relatively inexpensive. Before reliable recording apparatus was commercially available some clinicians made a habit of watching the patient void. Any such semi-objective observation is valuable. However, for any flow rate assessment to be meaningful the bladder should be reasonably full, an uncommon event in the outpatient clinic, while futhermore the patient may find it embarrassing to have the voiding observed, and in women it is not practical in most circumstances. The advantage of modern urine flowmeters is that a permanent graphic recording is obtained. Flowmeters have been available for fifty years, but not until von Garrelts developed his flowmeter in 1956 was equipment sufficiently accurate for the recordings to be clinically useful. If, despite the availability of commercially produced apparatus, the clinician has no flowmeter, the patient can be asked to time his urinary stream with a stopwatch and to record the voided volume by calculating the average flow. In the normal patient, average flow is approximately half the maximum flow, although in patients with obstruction the average flow may almost equal the maximum flow. We found it impractical to obtain adequate urine flow measurements in the routine urological clinic and have therefore established the urine flow clinic (see below).

Definitions

Urine flow may be described in terms of flow rate and flow pattern, and may be continuous or intermittent.

- *Flow rate* is defined as the volume of fluid expelled via the urethra per unit time and is expressed in millilitres per second (ml/s). Certain basic information is necessary in interpreting the flow trace and this includes the volume voided, the environment in which the patient passed urine and the position, that is lying, sitting or standing. It should also be stated whether the bladder filled naturally or if diuresis was stimulated by fluid or diuretics, or whether the bladder was filled by a catheter (either urethral or suprapubic). If filling was by a catheter then the type of fluid used should be stated, as should whether or not the flow study was part of another investigation, e.g. a pressure–flow study.
- *Maximum flow rate* (Q_{max}) is the maximum measured value of the flow rate.
- *Voided volume* (*VV*) is the total volume expelled via the urethra.
- *Flow time* is the time over which measurable flow occurs (Fig. 3.1).
- *Average flow rate* (Q_{ave}) is voided volume divided by flow time.
- *Time to maximum flow* is the elapsed time from onset of flow to maximum flow.

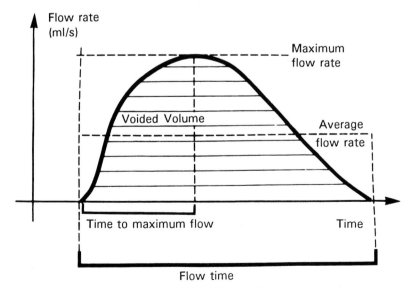

Fig. 3.1 Terminology relating to the description of urinary flow (International Continence Society report (1988) Standardisation of terminology of lower urinary tract function; see Appendix 1, Part 2).

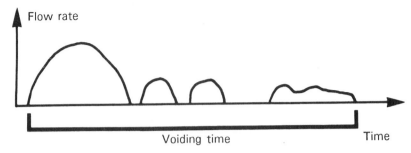

Fig. 3.2 Terminology relating to an intermittent flow rate tracing (see Appendix 1, Part 2).

- *Intermittent flow*   The same measurements are used as when describing a continuous flow curve. However, flow time must be measured carefully: the time intervals between flow episodes are disregarded. Voiding time is the total duration of micturition, including the interruptions (Fig. 3.2). Where flow is continuous, voiding time is equal to flow time. The area beneath the curve or curves represents the volume voided.

Urine Flow Clinic

Urine flow studies should be performed when the patient has a normal desire to void, in a condition of privacy and when they are relaxed. In our experience it is difficult to get an adequate flow study in the routine outpatient clinic, as it is essential that the bladder is adequately full. Furthermore a sterile urine sample is often required for bacteriology, necessitating a second void.

In order to facilitate good-quality flow studies we established a flow clinic in 1981. Following this Carter showed that the proportion of patients who failed to void 150 ml fell from 59% to 21%. The principal objective of the urine flow clinic is to screen for bladder outlet obstruction. With their flow clinic appointment each patient is sent a seven-day frequency–volume chart to complete prior to their attendance. They are also asked to drink approximately 1 litre before they leave home on the day of their appointment. On arrival, each patient is seen by the clinic nurse, who checks that they have had adequate intake. If for any reason the patient has not been able to hydrate themselves adequately they are given additional fluid. Occasionally the patient is given a 20 mg tablet of frusemide. Every patient is asked to drink 1 litre of fluid on arrival in the clinic. In their clinic letter they have been told that the clinic stay is likely to last two to three hours, during which time they will be asked to pass urine on at least three occasions. The patients are asked to hold their water until comfortably full. At that point they find the nurse and are led into the flow room, having already been made familiar with the equipment. The door is then closed and they are left to pass their urine in privacy. The flow room contains a couch and after voiding the patient's bladder is scanned ultrasonically to assess residual urine (see Fig. 3.3). When the patient has performed three flow rates and three ultrasound estimates of residual urine have been made the results are presented on a flow rate nomogram (see the following sections). A variety of nomograms are available and these relate maximum flow rate to voided volume taking sex and age into account.

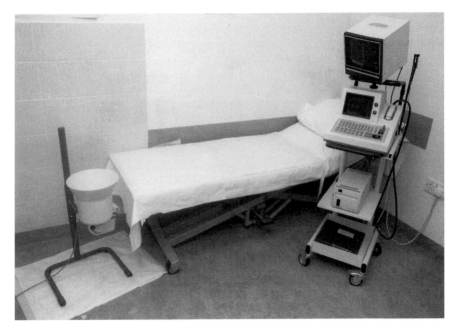

Fig. 3.3 Urine flow clinic: room layout. The flowmeter and commode are at the foot of the couch with the ultrasound machine at the head of the bed.

Various authorities have produced such nomograms: Von Garrelts (1958); Backman (1965); Gierup (1970); Siroky et al. (1979); Kadow et al. (1985) and Haylen (1990). In children and in older subjects the voided volume may not reach 150 ml. In these patients the shape of the flow trace may be helpful in deciding whether or not outlet obstruction is present. Marshal et al. (1983) suggested that by measuring the initial slope of the flow trace when the voided volume was less than 150 ml., it was possible to make a reliable diagnosis of obstruction or no obstruction. In contrast, Gleason suggested that studying the stream velocity in the last 30 ml of the void would allow similar deductions to be made. The work of the above authors, together with that of Rollema (1981), shows that there is more information in flow traces than is appreciated. However, it would be true to say that most investigators use only the maximum flow rate values, together with a subjective evaluation of the shape of the trace, in association with a flow rate nomogram, to make a clinical diagnosis. Based on the results from the flow clinic the patient may be referred on for pressure–flow studies of micturition or videourodynamics.

Equipment

The available flowmeters (Fig. 3.4, *overleaf*) use several different principles, as follows:

- The weight transducer flowmeter involves weighing the urine voided, thereby measuring the volume of urine voided. It also calculates the urine flow rate by differentiation with respect to time.

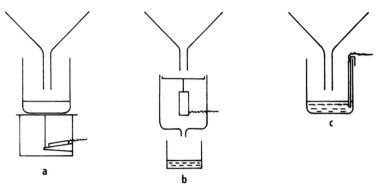

Fig. 3.4 Urine flowmeters: using the weight transducer (**a**), spinning disc (**b**) and capacitance methods (**c**).

- The rotating-disc flow meter has a spinning disc on which the urine falls. The disc is kept rotating at the same speed by servomotor, in spite of changes in the urine flow rate: the weight of the urine tends to slow the rotation of the disc. The differing power needed to keep disc rotation constant is proportional to the urine flow rate. The flow signal is electronically integrated to record the volume voided.

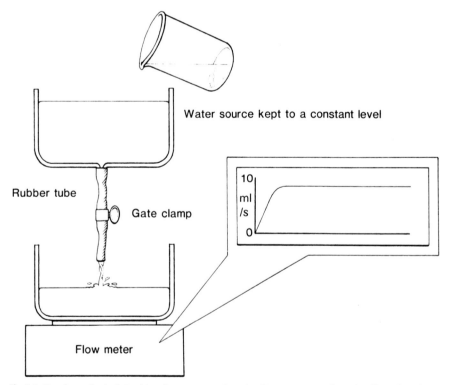

Fig. 3.5 Simple method of checking the accuracy of a urine flowmeter: gateclamp is adjusted to give a constant flow of a given volume of 100 ml in 10 s.

- The dipstick (capacitance) flow meter has a metal strip capacitor attached to a plastic dipstick, which is inserted into the urine collection vessel. This dipstick is held vertically in the straight-sided container. The solutes in urine conduct electricity across the capacitor and as the urine level rises the effective area of the capacitor decreases and the capacitance falls. The changing capacitance gives the volume voided. This signal is electronically differentiated and the rate of change of volume gives the urine flow rate.
- It is also possible to "weigh" urine by measuring the hydrostatic pressure exerted by a column of urine, using an ordinary pressure transducer.

Most commercially available flowmeters have acceptable accuracy. However, the buyer should always seek independent information on the machine's performance and, in particular, the accuracy (errors should be less than 5%), the linearity of response over the range 0 to 50 ml per second, the reliability of the apparatus, the compatibility with any existing equipment, the safety of the flowmeter, and its ease of cleaning. It is wise to check the performance of the flowmeter at regular intervals and a simple flowmeter tester has been described (Fig. 3.5). Most manufacturers also produce a chart recorder, which is marketed as a package with the flowmeter. Because changes in flow rate are relatively slow in electronic terms, an inexpensive pen recorder is adequate for uroflowmetry. In the last five years the flowmeter package has included an automatic printout of the major measurements listed above. This development is the cause of many problems, however. The software within these flowmeters is not adequately intelligent to distinguish physiological flow changes from flow changes produced by artefact (Fig. 3.6, *overleaf*). Hence the flowmeter will often record an artifactually high maximum flow rate, and if the nurse or doctor interpreting the trace is not sufficiently trained then a falsely high maximum flow rate will be recorded, and this may influence the patient's management. In a recent study 23 857 flow curves were reviewed and the machine readout compared with a manual assessment: there was a difference of more than 1 ml/s in 62% and a difference of more than 3 ml/s in 9% (Grino 1993). There has been one recent innovation in flowmeters. There are now commercially available flowmeters for use in the home (Fig. 3.7, *overleaf*). They are battery-operated and have a microprocessor which will record multiple individual voids. After the study period, the patient returns to the hospital and the flow rates can be printed out with computer-derived flow parameters. Whether this method of uroflowmetry is superior to that carried out in a properly established flow clinic remains to be seen.

Normal Flow Patterns

When considering the normality of flow rates the patient's age and sex and the voided volume should be taken into account. As well as the numerical data derived from any flow trace, the shape of the trace is also important.

In *normal flow*, the flow curve has a "bell" shape. Maximum flow is reached in the first 30% of any trace and within 5 seconds from the start of flow. The flow curve varies according to the volume voided (Fig. 3.8, *overleaf*). Figure 3.9 (*overleaf*) shows how different traces can look quite different in the same unobstructed individual voiding different volumes. Although the traces look superficially different, they all have similar first and final phases. The final phase

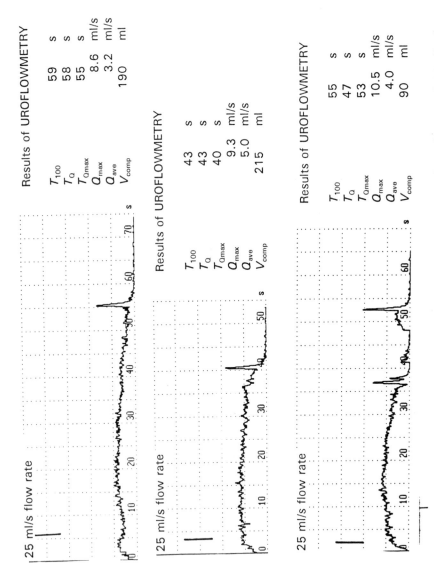

Results of UROFLOWMETRY

T_{100}	59	s
T_Q	58	s
T_{Qmax}	55	s
Q_{max}	8.6	ml/s
Q_{ave}	3.2	ml/s
V_{comp}	190	ml

Results of UROFLOWMETRY

T_{100}	43	s
T_Q	43	s
T_{Qmax}	40	s
Q_{max}	9.3	ml/s
Q_{ave}	5.0	ml/s
V_{comp}	215	ml

Results of UROFLOWMETRY

T_{100}	55	s
T_Q	47	s
T_{Qmax}	53	s
Q_{max}	10.5	ml/s
Q_{ave}	4.0	ml/s
V_{comp}	90	ml

Fig. 3.6 Traces from the flow rate clinic showing spike artefacts that result in the machine giving Q_{max} values of 8.6, 9.3 and 10.5 ml/s, whereas the three Q_{max} values are 4.5, 6 and 6 ml/s respectively.

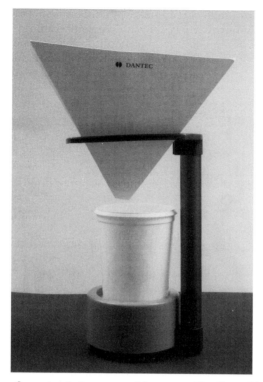

Fig. 3.7 Home flowmeters: battery-powered flowmeter with a disposable paper funnel.

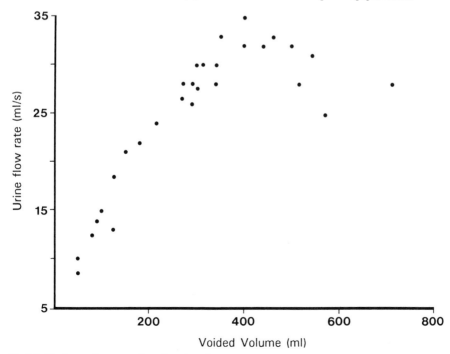

Fig. 3.8 Maximum flow rate plotted against the volume voided for a large number of voids in one individual normal case.

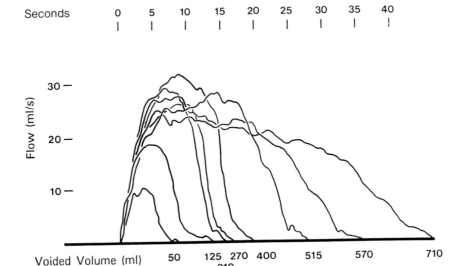

Fig. 3.9 Superimposition of various flow rate tracings; the examples are taken from the same case as in Fig 3.8. This is a very useful way to display multiple flow rate tracings.

of a normal flow trace shows a rapid fall from high flow, together with a sharp cutoff at the termination of flow (two similar Q_{max} readings in different patients can give quite different flow curve shapes owing to the different voided volumes (Fig. 3.10). The appearance of the trace also depends on the paper speed of the recorder. If this is very slow then flow will appear as a vertical line; if it is faster

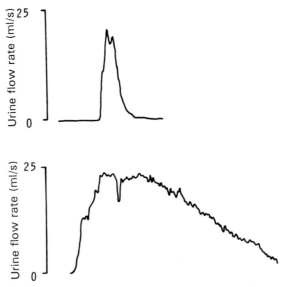

Fig. 3.10 Similar Q_{max} readings of 21 and 23 ml/s giving very different flow curve shapes due to different voided volumes of 80 ml and 550 ml respectively.

Table 3.1. Lowest acceptable maximum urine flow rates according to age and sex for minimum voided volumes[a]

Age years	Minimum volume ml	Male ml/s	Female ml/s
4–7	100	10	10
8–13	100	12	15
14–45	200	21	18
46–65	200	12	15
66–80	200	9	10

[a]Values given are taken from personal experience and relevant literature. In general the values are one standard deviation below the mean for the maximum flow. Values below those given may not be abnormal, but need further consideration.

then the flow curve will be elongated. A paper speed of 0.25 cm/s is practical and allows easy interpretation of the shape of the curve. Urine flow rate is highly dependent on the volume voided. Detrusor muscle when stretched achieves an optimal performance, but if stretched further it becomes inefficient: at above 400 ml the efficiency of the detrusor begins to decrease and Q_{max} is lower (Fig. 3.8). Flow rates are highest and most predictable in the volume range between 200 and 400 ml and through this range the maximum flow tends to be constant. In practice the definition of normality can be considered in two ways. The simplest way is to have a minimum acceptable flow rate for any sex and age group. Because of the dependence on volume voided this is relatively inaccurate, but may be acceptable provided that the volume voided is in the range 200 to 500 ml. Such values are given in Table 3.1.

Much work has been devoted to the construction of flow rate nomograms. Nomograms have been described for boys, girls, men under 55, men over 55 and women. In our unit we use the Siroky nomogram for men under 55 (Fig. 3.11, *overleaf*) and the Bristol nomogram for men over 55 (Fig. 3.12, *overleaf*).

Abnormal Flow Patterns – Classification and Interpretation

Urine flow is a product of the interaction between the expressive forces (detrusor contraction plus any abdominal straining) and urethral resistance. Hence urine flow rates have limitations which must be appreciated.

Table 3.2. Flow and pressure combinations giving different diagnoses

Flow	Pressure	Diagnosis
NORMAL	normal/low	UNOBSTRUCTED
Normal	high	obstructed
LOW	high	OBSTRUCTED
Low	normal	equivocal
low	low	unobstructed

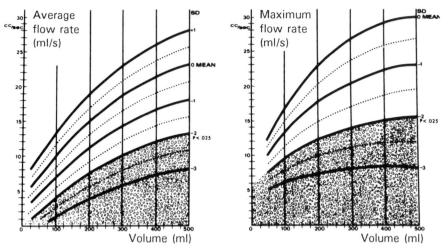

Fig. 3.11 Nomogram for flow rate in male subjects, allowing an estimate for the probability of normality. Three standard deviations below the mean are plotted. The *stippled zone* indicates flow rates that occur in less than 2.5% of the normal male population. (Siroky et al. 1979).

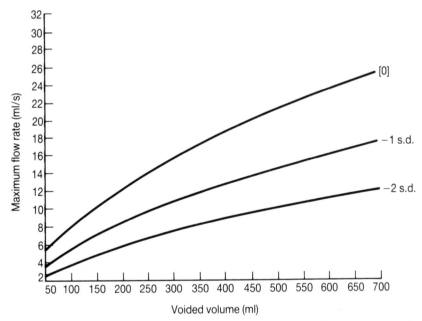

Fig. 3.12 Bristol uroflow nomogram for men over 55. Constructed from 286 flow measurements from 123 asymptomatic men.

Although patients fit into two main patterns, normal flow and normal pressure, and low flow and high pressure (obstructed, as in Fig. 3.6), the information from urine flow traces, without simultaneous pressure recording, must be interpreted with care. Two examples of misleading situations are shown in Table 3.2: patients

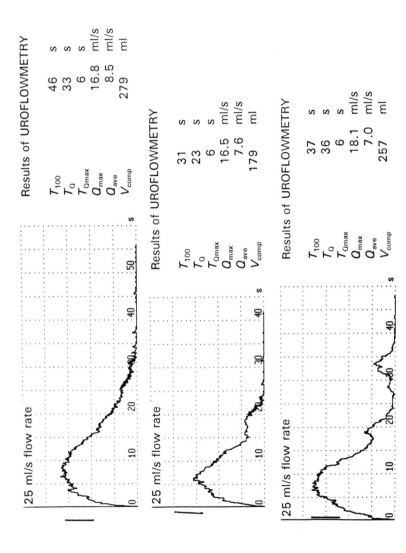

Fig. 3.13 Flow clinic data from a man of 80 with normal Q_{max} readings but who on pressure flow studies was shown to be obstructed.

with normal flow can have bladder outlet obstruction when a normal maximum flow rate is maintained by abnormally high voiding pressures (Fig. 3.13, *previous page*). The other misleading group comprises patients whose low flow rates are due to detrusor underactivity rather than to bladder outlet obstruction.

Continuous Flow Curves

Normal. As already described, the normal flow curve is bell-shaped but its appearance will differ quite markedly according to the volume of urine voided (Fig. 3.9). Maximum flow is normally reached within 3 to 10 seconds from the onset of micturition.

Detrusor Instability. Strictly speaking, the pattern sometimes seen in detrusor instability is not abnormal, but is supranormal (Fig. 3.14). Very high maximum flow rates may be achieved by such patients who have detrusor muscle that has high contraction velocities, giving a flow trace that shows a very rapid increase in flow to a high maximum reached in an abnormally short time (1 to 3 s). The reduction in time to maximum flow is achieved because the detrusor contraction has already opened the bladder neck widely, hence reducing the urethral resistance. Thus when the patient starts to void he or she has only to relax the distal sphincter which has previously prevented the unstable contraction from producing incontinence.

Bladder Outlet Obstruction (BOO). Flow curves in obstructed patients are characterised by a low maximum and reduced average flow, with the average flow greater than half the maximum flow rate. Maximum flow is usually obtained relatively quickly (3 to 10 s), but the flow rate then decreases slowly (Fig. 3.15). In outlet obstruction the flow rate is expected to be continuous, although it may end in a terminal dribble.

Obstruction may be "compressive", for example in benign prostatic obstruction, or "constrictive" as in a urethral stricture. The two types of obstruction give different types of trace. The "constrictive" obstruction gives a "plateau"-shaped

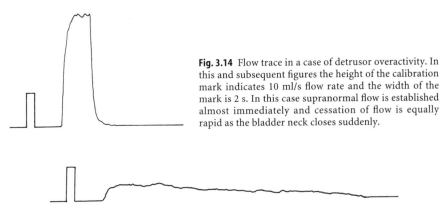

Fig. 3.14 Flow trace in a case of detrusor overactivity. In this and subsequent figures the height of the calibration mark indicates 10 ml/s flow rate and the width of the mark is 2 s. In this case supranormal flow is established almost immediately and cessation of flow is equally rapid as the bladder neck closes suddenly.

Fig. 3.15 Flow trace in a case of outlet tract obstruction. Maximum flow is established soon after the onset of voiding.

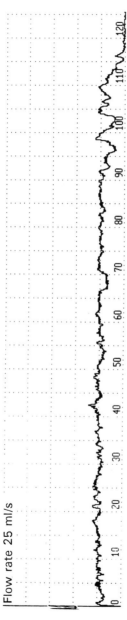

Fig. 3.16 Flow trace from a man of 50 with a 10 year history of bulbar urethral stricture: the characteristic "plateau"-shaped trace is shown ($Q_{max} = 5$ ml/s).

trace with little change in flow rate, and little difference between Q_{max} and Q_{ave} (Fig. 3.16). In compressive obstruction the first third of the flow trace may appear relatively normal, although the Q_{max} will be reduced, but the latter part of the trace usually is elongated into a pronounced "tail" of reducing flow rate (Figs 3.13 part 1 and 3.15).

Detrusor Underactivity (DUA). This diagnosis is discussed later in this chapter under "Cystometry". However, it can be suspected if a symmetrical trace with a low maximum flow rate is seen (Fig. 3.17). The characteristic in detrusor under-activity is that the time to reach maximum flow is very variable, and the maximum flow may occur in the second half of the trace. However, there is con-siderable overlap between the flow traces of the obstructed and the underactive detrusor group, and therefore the diagnosis can only be suspected: proof comes from a pressure–flow study.

Interrupted Flow Patterns

Irregular Trace Secondary to Straining. Some patients are in the habit of using, or need to use, their diaphragmatic and abdominal muscles to increase urine flow. Straining makes the flow trace irregular (Fig. 3.18). With straining the changes in flow tend to be relatively slow and the stream is usually continuous. Straining flow traces are very variable in appearance, because they may occur in the pres-ence or absence of obstruction and in the presence or absence of a detrusor con-traction. The situation often needs further elucidation by a pressure–flow study that includes detrusor pressure recording.

Irregular Trace Secondary to Urethral Overactivity. In neurologically abnormal patients involuntary contraction of the distal urethral sphincter mechanism is termed detrusor sphincter dyssynergia. It is also seen in patients without neuro-logical abnormality, where it may merely be due to anxiety in unfamiliar sur-roundings. However, an abnormal trace found on repeat investigation in neurologically normal patients is due to a pattern termed dysfunctional voiding.

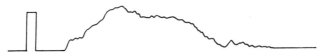

Fig. 3.17 Flow trace in a case of detrusor underactivity. Maximum flow is established near the middle of the voiding time.

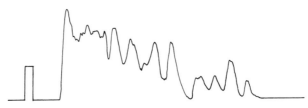

Fig. 3.18 Straining producing an irregular tracing.

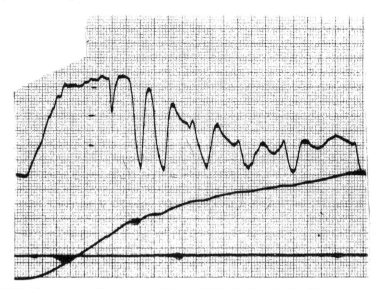

Fig. 3.19 Dysfunctional voiding in a man of 63 with LUTS. The irregularity of flow was due to anxiety resulting in pelvic floor overactivity: subsequent flows had a smooth pattern (Q_{max} is 17 ml/s and VV 360 ml).

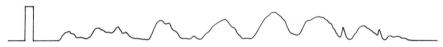

Fig. 3.20 Intermittent flow due to fluctuating detrusor contraction. The changes in flow rate are relatively slow.

As with straining, the appearances are variable, but in general flow rate changes are faster than those due to straining (Fig. 3.19).

Irregular Trace Due to Poor Sustained or Fluctuating Detrusor Contractions. This abnormality is generally seen in patients who have a neurological problem, and most commonly in multiple sclerosis. The detrusor contraction, instead of producing an approximately constant pressure throughout voiding, fluctuates. This produces either a continuous but varying flow or, more commonly, an interrupted flow (Fig. 3.20).

Irregular Trace Secondary to Artifacts

There are a number of artefacts that may trick the urodynamicist.

"Cruising". The most potent is caused by the patient, usually a man, moving their stream in relation to the central exit from the collecting funnel; Fig. 3.21 (*overleaf*) is a good example. The "peaks" occur when the point of impact of the stream is moving down the side of the funnel towards the central exit; that is, the urine being passed is catching up with the urine passed immediately before. The "valleys" occur when the impact point is moving away from the exit. Usually the

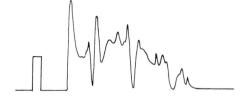

Fig. 3.21 "Cruising": the irregular trace resulting from a male patient moving his stream backwards and forwards across the neck of the collecting funnel. The changes in flow are rapid and biphasic in type.

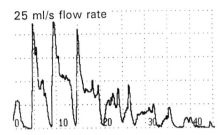

Results of UROFLOWMETRY

T_{100}	65	s
T_Q	49	s
T_{Qmax}	10	s
Q_{max}	25.0	ml/s
Q_{ave}	4.9	ml/s
V_{comp}	240	ml

Fig. 3.22 "Squeezing" artefact due to the patient intermittently compressing the end of the penis during voids. The peaks of flow are due to urine building up in the penile urethra to give spurts as the man releases his grip.

"peaks" will fit into the "valleys" in this type of tracing. Manufacturers have attempted to minimise this phenomenon by complex baffles in the funnel, although a better solution might be to paint a target onto the funnel for the patient to aim at! Whereas this artefact is almost exclusive to men, the next one described is entirely so.

"*Squeezing*". Perhaps in an effort to deny the onset of age (and reducing urine flow) some men have the habit of squeezing the tip of their penis or foreskin during voiding (Fig. 3.22). This leads to a series of peaks, as shown in the upper diagram (Fig. 3.23). When the patient is asked to stop this practice the flow trace becomes classically obstructed and the flow rate is no longer within the normal range (lower trace). These artefacts are not detected by the computerised analysis of flow, which potentially misleads the clinician.

Uroflowmetry and the Recording of Residual Urine

In our flow clinic we routinely measure the residual urine after voiding by ultrasound. The formula, $D_1 \times D_2 \times D_3 \times 0.7$ gives an approximation of the residual volume in millilitres. D_1, D_2 and D_3 are three different diameters (of the bladder). The diameters D_1 and D_2 are measured in the coronal plane (D_1 is bladder neck to fundus and D_2 is anterior to posterior wall) and D_3 is measured in the sagittal plane (D_3 is right side to left side). Such measurements are subject to considerable observer error in particular because the bladder assumes an irregular shape at the end of voiding; sometimes it looks rather more like a squashed football, being much wider in the transverse plane than it is from the bladder neck to the fundus. Nevertheless, from the clinical point of view an adequate degree of accuracy can be obtained from relatively inexpensive ultrasound machines, one of which is

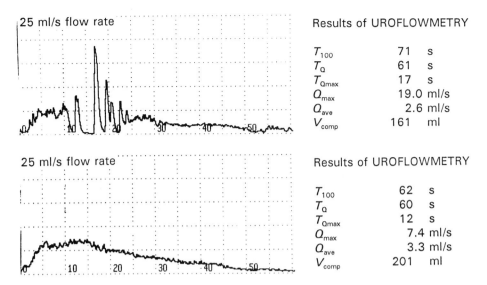

25 ml/s flow rate	Results of UROFLOWMETRY		
	T_{100}	71	s
	T_Q	61	s
	T_{Qmax}	17	s
	Q_{max}	19.0	ml/s
	Q_{ave}	2.6	ml/s
	V_{comp}	161	ml

25 ml/s flow rate	Results of UROFLOWMETRY		
	T_{100}	62	s
	T_Q	60	s
	T_{Qmax}	12	s
	Q_{max}	7.4	ml/s
	Q_{ave}	3.3	ml/s
	V_{comp}	201	ml

Fig. 3.23 A "squeezing" artefact is shown in the upper trace. The lower trace shows a smooth "obstructed" curve after the patient has been asked not to hold the penis during voiding.

hand-held (Fig. 3.24). However, it should be noted that there is some conflict as to the significance of increased residual urine. It had been assumed to be indicative of obstruction, but from the work of Abrams and Griffiths (1979) and others it has been suggested that an increase in residual urine may represent detrusor

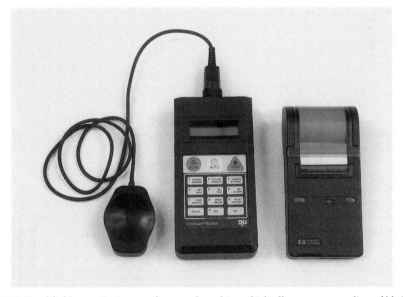

Fig. 3.24 Hand-held or patient-worn ultrasound machine which allows easy recording of bladder volume/post void residual, in clinic, on the ward or in the patient's home. The photo shows the ultrasound head, the microprocessor with display and a small printer.

underactivity rather than outflow obstruction. Despite this, many or perhaps most clinicians allow the quantity of residual urine to influence their management of patients. In our urodynamic unit the residual urine is stated both on the results from the flow clinic and after pressure–flow studies.

Indications for Uroflowmetry

Urine flow studies are an excellent screening study in a wide variety of patients, but frequently must be followed up by pressure–flow studies which allow more precise definition of bladder and urethral function. Uroflow is used to investigate possible bladder outlet obstruction and can also give a guide to detrusor contractility. It should be used in all ages and for both sexes:

Children

Uroflow is the screening test for all neurologically normal children with possible functional outlet obstruction (dysfunctional voiding, see "Voiding Cystometry", p. 83).

Women

When surgery for stress incontinence is planned, uroflow provides evidence of normal detrusor voiding function if flow rates are excellent. Reduced flows may lead to post-operative voiding problems as they are indicative of abnormal voiding function. In elderly women, uroflow is useful in excluding relative outlet obstruction resulting in residual urine, which may be the cause of recurrent urinary tract infections.

Men

Uroflow is the screening test of choice in men of all ages with symptoms suggestive of outlet obstruction. This applies to those men who have less classic symptoms such as recurrent infections, as well as those with the classic symptoms of poor stream and hesitancy.

Uroflow should be measured before and after any procedure designed to modify the function of the outflow tract, e.g. for urethral stricture, bladder neck obstruction and benign prostatic obstruction.

Note: All urine flow curves should be evaluated by the clinician, so that artefacts can be eliminated and a true value of Q_{max} derived.

The indications for uroflowmetry are further dealt with in Chapter 5 under patient groups.

References

Abrams P (1991). The Urine flow clinic. In Fitzpatrick JN (ed) Conservative treatment of BPH Edinburgh: Churchill Livingstone pp 33–43.

Abrams P (1977). Prostatism and prostatectomy: The value of urine flow rate measurement in the preoperative assessment for operation. J Urol 117:70–71.

Backman KA (1965). Urinary flow during micturition in normal women. Acta Chir Scand 130:357–370.

Backman KA, von Garrelts B, Sundblad R (1966). Micturition in normal women. Studies of pressure and flow. Acta Chir Scand 132:403–412.

Chancellor MB, Blaivas JG, Kaplan SA, Axelrod S (1991). Bladder outlet obstruction versus impaired detrusor contractility: the role of uroflow. J Urol 145:810–812.

Drach GW, Steinbronn DV (1986). Clinical evaluation of patients with prostatic obstruction; correlation of flow rates with voided, residual or total bladder volume. J Urol 135:737–740.

Garrelts B von (1956). Analysis of micturition. A new method of recording the voiding of the bladder. Acta Chir Scand 112:326–340.

Garrelts B von (1958). Micturition in the normal male. Acta Chir Scand 114:197–210.

Gierup T (1970) Micturition studies in infants and children. Scand J Urol Nephrol 4:217–230.

Gleason DM, Bottaccini MR, Perling D, Lattimer JK (1967). A challenge to current urodynamic thought. J Urol 97:935.

Golomb J, Linder A, Siegel Y, Korezah D (1992). Variability and circadian changes in home uroflowmetry in patients with benign prostatic hyperplasia compared to normal controls. J Urol 147:1044–1047.

Griffiths CJ, Murray A, Ramsden PD (1983). A simple uroflowmeter tester. Br J Urol 55:21–24.

Griffiths DJ, Scholtmeijer RJ (1984). Place of the free flow curve in the urodynamic investigation of children. Br J Urol 56:474–477.

Grino PB, Bruskewitz R, Blaivas JG, Siroky MB, Andersen JT, Cook T, Stower E (1993). Maximum urinary flow rate by uroflowmetry: Automatic or visual interpretation. J Urol 149:339–341.

Haylen BT, Parys BT, Anyaegbunam WI, Ashby D, West CR (1990). Urine flow rates in male and female urodynamic patients compared with Liverpool nomograms. Br J Urol 65:483–487.

Jensen KM-E, Jørgensen JB, Mogensen P (1985). Reproducibility of uroflowmetry variable in elderly males. Urol Res. 13:237–239.

Jørgensen JB, Jensen KM-E, Bille-Brahe NE, Morgensen P (1986). Uroflowmetry in asymptomatic elderly males. Br J Urol 58:390–395.

Jørgensen JB, Jensen KM-E, Morgensen P (1993). Longitudinal observations on normal and abnormal voiding in men over the age of 50 years. Uroflowmetry and symptoms of prostatism. Br J Urol 72:413–420.

Kadow C, Howells S, Lewis P, Abrams P (1985). A flow rate nomogram for normal males over the age of 50. Proc. ICS 15th Annual meeting, London 138–139.

Rollema HJ (1981). Uroflowmetry in males. Reference values and clinical application in benign prostatic hypertrophy. Rijksuniveriteit te Groningen, Druk-kerij van Denderen BV, Groningen.

Ryall RR, Marshall VR (1982). Normal peak urinary flow rates obtained from small voided volumes can provide a reliable assessment of bladder function. J Urol 127:484–488.

Siroky MB, Olsson CA, Krane RJ (1979). The flow rate nomogram. 1. Development. J Urol122:665–668.

Szabo L, Fegyverneki S (1995). Maximum and average urine flow rates in normal children – the miskolc nomograms. Br J Urol 76:16–20.

Cystometry

Introduction

In the previous section, "Uroflowmetry", we examined the role of urine flow studies in defining bladder and urethral function and concluded that its role is limited because flow is a product of the forces of expulsion against the resistance given by the urethra. Whilst urine flow rate gives an idea as to whether or not voiding is normal, it tells us little about the storage phase of micturition and cannot offer a precise diagnosis as to the cause of abnormal flow.

Cystometry is used to study both the storage and the voiding phase of micturition in order to make a diagnosis which enables effective treatment to be given. Cystometry is the method by which the pressure–volume relationship of the bladder is measured. Cystometrograms have been performed for many years

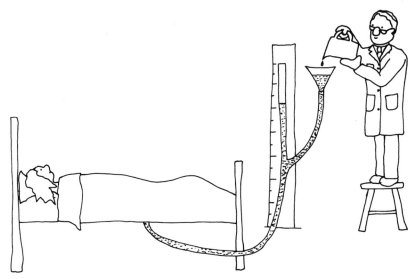

Fig. 3.25 Simple cystometry using a water manometer.

using incremental filling and intermittent pressure measurement by water manometer (Fig. 3.25). However, since the introduction of reliable pressure transducers, which have allowed the continuous measurement of pressure during bladder filling, new cystometric patterns have been recognised.

When thinking about the diagnosis and treatment of micturition disorders, it is useful to think of bladder and urethral function separately, defining the behaviour of each during the storage phase and during the voiding phase. Hence, in normal micturition, during the storage phase the bladder is relaxed and the urethra is contracted, whereas during voiding the bladder contracts and the urethra relaxes (Table 3.3).

It therefore follows that abnormal function must be a failure of either the bladder or the urethra to behave normally during either storage or voiding (Table 3.3). During storage the bladder cannot be described as underactive, because in normal function it should be relaxed; and during voiding it cannot be described as overactive, because its function is to contract with maximal efficiency in order to empty the bladder.

Table 3.3. Normal and abnormal lower urinary tract function described in terms of bladder and urethral behaviour during the storage and voiding phases

Normal function			Abnormal function	
	STORAGE	VOIDING	STORAGE	VOIDING
BLADDER	Relaxed	Contracts	Overactive	Underactive
				Acontractile
URETHRA	Contracted	Relaxes	Incompetent under stress	Functional obstruction
			Inappropriate relaxation	Anatomic obstruction

Similarly, the urethra cannot be described as overactive during storage or as underactive during voiding, because its function is to give total continence during storage and total "incontinence" during voiding. Newcomers to urodynamics find the subject easier to understand if bladder and urethral function is viewed in this way and by asking themselves four simple questions:

- Is the bladder relaxed during storage?
- Is the urethra contracted during storage?
- Does the bladder contract adequately during voiding?
- Does the urethra open properly during voiding?

Although cystometry seems a simple technique, there are a number of areas where its difficulties and limitations must be appreciated. First, the measurement of pressure is subject to numerous artefacts, so precise scientific method is vital in ensuring that valid data is obtained. Second, there is increasing evidence that the technique used for cystometry will have a bearing on the results obtained. Both these points are discussed in full below.

Principles of Cystometry

Cystometry is used to study bladder and urethral function during the micturition cycle, that is during bladder filling and during voiding. During standard cystometry the pressure within the bladder (intravesical pressure) is measured together with the pressure within the abdominal cavity (intra-abdominal pressure: almost always by measuring the pressure in the rectum). Intravesical pressure measurement reflects detrusor activity and intra-abdominal pressure measures the intra-abdominal pressure, which may be affected by contraction of the diaphragmatic and abdominal wall muscles.

The measuring of both bladder and abdominal pressure allows the investigator to assess whether changes seen in intravesical pressure are due to contraction of the bladder alone or whether they are due to abdominal straining.

Bladder pressure (p_{ves}) and rectal pressure (p_{abd}) are measured by catheters, and by electronically subtracting intra-abdominal pressure from intravesical pressure the detrusor pressure (p_{det}) can be calculated: $p_{det} = p_{ves} - p_{abd}$. In Fig. 3.26 (*overleaf*), a series of changes can be seen during the measurement of bladder pressure. Without the measurement of abdominal pressure it is very difficult to know what has produced these changes. However, when p_{abd} is also measured then the changes can readily be defined as due to detrusor activity, raised intra-abdominal pressure or a combination of both.

The pressure changes seen on the p_{ves} trace of Fig. 3.26 allow simple rules to be devised:

- If a change is seen in both p_{ves} and p_{abd} but not in p_{det} then it is due to raised intra-abdominal pressure (event S).
- If a pressure change is seen on p_{ves} and p_{det} but not on p_{abd} then it is due to a detrusor contraction (event U).
- If a pressure change is seen on p_{ves}, p_{abd} and p_{det} then there is both a detrusor contraction and increased abdominal pressure (event C + U).
- Whilst detrusor function can be assessed directly by observation of the pressure changes, urethral function must be inferred from the pressure changes

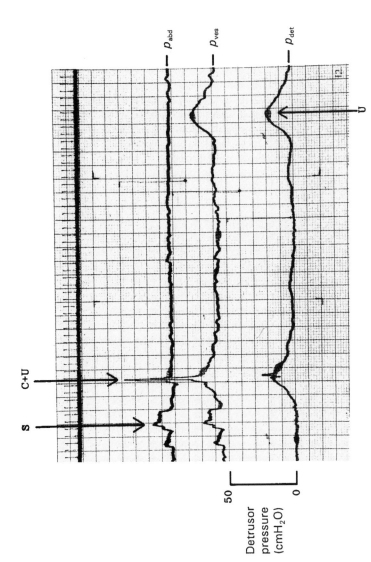

Fig. 3.26 Cystometry trace showing the patient straining (*S*), a cough superimposed on an unstable detrusor contraction (*C + U*) and an unstable contraction (*U*).

within the bladder and by measuring any urine leakage during filling, and by measuring urine flow during voiding.

Aims of Cystometry

The aims of cystometry are to define detrusor function and urethral function during both filling and voiding. This will give four possible diagnoses during cystometry, for example: on filling, detrusor function normal, urethra incompetent (patient leaked); on voiding, detrusor underactive (low flow rate, patient strained to void), and urethra normal. Having reached these diagnoses it is essential that the clinician relates these to the symptomatic complaints of the patient and any abnormal physical findings. In this way the relevance of the results can be assessed and, should the clinical problems not have been answered, then further investigations can be planned.

Measurement of Pressure

The principles and practice discussed below apply to the measurement of pressure at any site, be it the bladder, the urethra, or the rectum. There are certain key elements to the process of pressure measurement and the investigator needs to

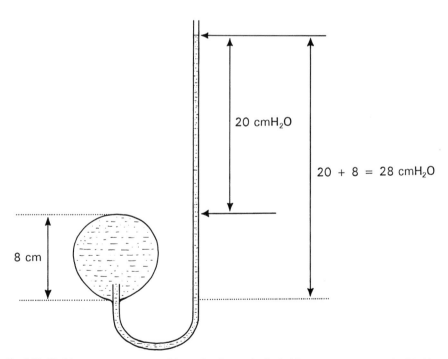

20 cmH$_2$O

20 + 8 = 28 cmH$_2$O

8 cm

Fig. 3.27 Bladder pressure measured by a simple, vertically held water manometer: the bladder pressure equals the height of the bladder plus the height of the water column above the bladder (8 + 20 cm) or the height from the bladder outlet to the top of the column.

understand the principles of pressure measurement. Pressure can be measured simply by a water column (Fig. 3.27, *previous page*) with a catheter placed in the bladder. The height of the water column in centimetres above the bottom of the bladder gives the pressure within the bladder, measured in centimetres of water. However, modern urodynamic systems utilise transducers for the accurate measurement of pressure.

Pressure Transducers

A pressure transducer is a device which converts (transduces) a change in pressure, occurring, for example in the bladder, into a change in electrical voltage. The change in electrical voltage can then be magnified (amplified) until it is large enough for a recorder to register the change on a paper trace. Pressure transducers used in urodynamics are of two main types, the first being the conventional external strain gauge transducer, mounted on a stand and connected to the patient by a water-filled tube (Fig. 3.28) down which passes a pressure wave which moves a thin metal diaphragm (Fig. 3.29). Attached to the back of the diaphragm is a strain gauge manufactured from a metal alloy which when bent generates an electrical charge. A "large" pressure change will produce a "large" movement of the transducer diaphragm, and will produce a "large" degree of

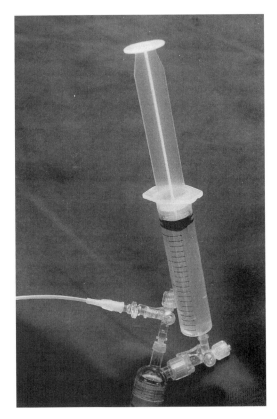

Fig. 3.28 External stand-mounted pressure transducer showing the syringe used to flush the transducer and tubing.

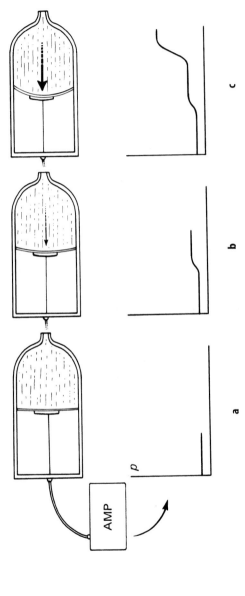

Fig. 3.29 External pressure transducer showing the resting state (**a**) and the effect of increasing pressure (**b** and **c**) producing greater deformity of the diaphragm and the strain gauge mounted behind the diaphragm. The resultant increased electrical charge is amplified (AMP) and recorded as increased pressure (*p*) on graphs **b** and **c**.

bend in the strain gauge, producing a "large" electrical voltage (Fig. 3.29c). This type of transducer is relatively cheap, robust and easy to handle. However, the tube by which it is linked to the patient can itself introduce artefacts (see below).

More recently a second type of transducer has been developed, namely the catheter tip (catheter-mounted) transducer. The principle of measurement is identical to that employed in the previous device, but the diaphragm and strain gauge are sited on the catheter (Fig. 3.30) and therefore within the bladder or rectum. By using slightly larger catheters, additional transducers can be used, and even a filling channel built into the catheter. The advantages of catheter-mounted transducers are the elimination of the artefacts arising from the fluid-filled connecting line which links the patient to a transducer of the external type. Their disadvantages include the relatively high cost, their greater fragility and the fact that they are more difficult to handle. However, they are especially useful if rapid changes in pressure need to be measured, for example during stress urethral profilometry (see p. 109).

It has to be remembered that transducers of these two types measure pressure differently. The actual measurement of p_{ves} by an external transducer depends on the level of the transducer in relation to the bladder (Fig. 3.31). On the other hand

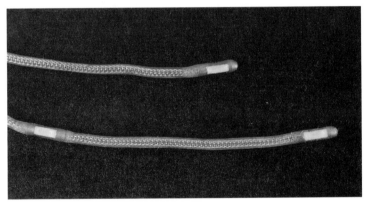

Fig. 3.30 Catheter tip transducers: in these solid-state devices the transducer (strain gauge type) is mounted on a catheter; dual and single transducers are shown.

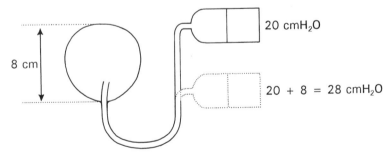

8 cm

20 cmH$_2$O

20 + 8 = 28 cmH$_2$O

Fig. 3.31 External pressure transducers measure pressure according to their position (outside the body) in relation to the bladder: the lower position (dotted lines) also records the 8 cm pressure head of the bladder itself. The position of the catheter in the bladder does not change the pressure measurement.

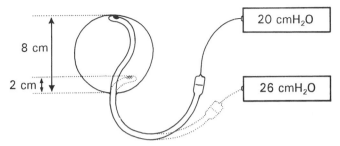

Fig. 3.32 Catheter tip transducers measure pressure according to the position of the transducer within the bladder. When the transducer is high in the bladder (solid lines) the pressure is lower (20 cmH$_2$O); when the transducer is lower in the bladder the pressure is higher (26 cmH$_2$O = 20 cm H$_2$O *plus* the 6 cm column of urine on top of the transducer).

the pressure measured by a catheter tip transducer depends on the position of the transducer *within* the bladder (Fig. 3.32).

Measuring Pressure Correctly

There are three fundamental and vital steps:

- Set zero.
- Calibrate the transducers.
- Establish the pressure reference level.

Step 1: Setting Zero. The International Continence Society (ICS) has published a technical report which established the convention that *zero pressure is atmospheric pressure*. The zero is *never* set with the transducer exposed to intravesical pressure after the catheter is passed into the bladder. Figure 3.33, (*overleaf*) shows a typical arrangement of a transducer (T) linked by two three-way taps to the manometer tubing that connects the transducers to the bladder and rectal catheters and to a syringe (S) used to flush saline through the system in order to eliminate bubbles and check for leaks. The transducer can either be held vertically, or horizontally as shown in Fig. 3.34, *overleaf.* In both systems the zero level is taken as the open end of the manometer tubing (connected to the three-way tap B) when the open end is held at the same horizontal level as the transducer (Fig. 3.34, *overleaf*). Before zero is set the manometer tubing connected to the two transducers should be flushed.

Step 2: Calibrating the Transducer. Most urodynamic systems have the facility for the electronic calibration of the pressure transducers, but it is wise to check this manually, from time to time. This is easiest with a machine which supplies a stand with transducers attached and two identified points 100 cm apart. If no such system is available then a 100 cm ruler is required, to be employed as follows:

- With the open end of the manometer tubing at the 0 cm mark the machine should read zero and the trace on the paper should be at the zero point (see above).

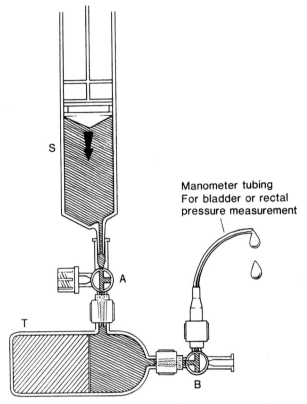

Fig. 3.33 External pressure transducer connected by three-way tap to a syringe used to flush the transducer and manometer connected to the transducer via tap B.

- The open end of the catheter is now raised to the 100 cm mark, whereupon the machine should read 100 and the trace should have moved up the paper from 0 cm to the 100 cm H$_2$O level (Fig. 3.35, *overleaf*).

Catheter tip transducers can be calibrated by submerging them in a water column of measured depth.

Step 3: Establishing a Reference Level for Pressure. The ICS has defined the reference level for external traducers and fluid-filled catheters as the superior edge of the symphysis pubis. Hence it is essential to level the transducers to this horizontal plane. Catheter tip transducers do not need a reference level in this way.

Sterility of Transducers and Tubing

AIDS has changed our sterilisation practices. It has become necessary to change the tubing linking the infusion pump to the patient, as well as the tubing linking the patient to the external transducers, and this must be done after each patient.

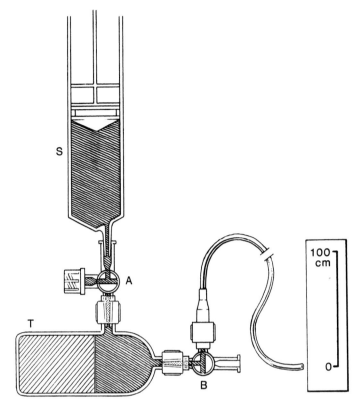

Fig. 3.34 Setting zero: with tap A selected to isolate the syringe, the end of the manometer tube is positioned at the same horizontal level as the transducer.

The external transducers need not be sterilised, but are flushed through with chlorhexidine solution (0.2%). If the transducers are not being used regularly then the domes should be removed and sterilised with Cidex (gluteraldehyde). Catheter tip transducers must be kept sterile using Cidex. At present controversy surrounds the use of gluteraldehyde and staff have to be protected as far as possible from exposure to it; it must not get into the transducer connection and the transducer must be washed well before use, for which sterile water or saline is suitable.

Recording Equipment

The previous edition of this book dealt at length with the various types of recorders, but such an exposition is now redundant because all manufacturers of urodynamic equipment supply a recorder as part of their system. However, certain principles remain, as follows, and unfortunately some of these have come under threat from so-called "developments":

- The printout must be clear. Some of the modern recorders have a much narrower paper width, which necessitates the traces crossing each other on

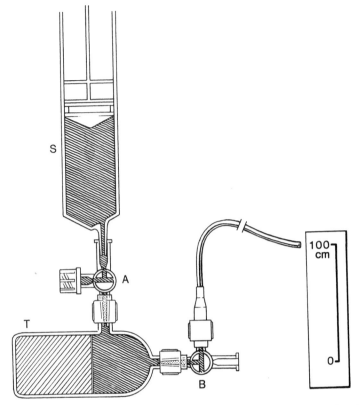

Fig. 3.35 Calibrating the transducer: the open end of the manometer tubing is levated to the 100 cm mark on the vertical scale.

occasions during investigation. This can make a trace very difficult to read (Fig. 3.36), and it can only be hoped that the manufacturers will learn from this mistake and produce better printers in the future.

- The printout must be based on an adequate sampling rate. In each of the new computerised systems the data is sampled at rates unique to that urodynamic system. A minimum sampling rate of 10 data points per second is necessary for a good-quality trace (10 Hz). Failure to sample at this rate may mean the loss of important data when fast changes are seen particularly in pressure recording, for example when the patient coughs (Fig. 3.36).

- The recorder must have an adequate frequency response for the intended use. Hence in more sophisticated electrophysiological testing, such as single-fibre electromyography, a very rapid response is needed. This can only be met by systems such as UV recorders or oscilloscopes that use light to record the signals.

The paper speed should be such that the clinician can identify important events during filling and voiding. In computerised systems, to minimise the use of paper, different paper speeds may be used according to the phase of urodynamic measurement. Hence the paper speed for the filling phase tends to be slower than

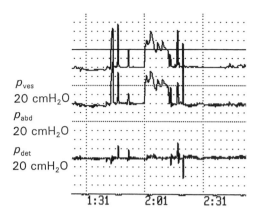

p_{ves}
20 cmH$_2$O

p_{abd}
20 cmH$_2$O

p_{det}
20 cmH$_2$O

1:31   2:01   2:31

Fig. 3.36 Recording artefacts: the figure shows a series of 3 coughs before the patient was asked to perform a Valsalva manoeuvre (strain) and 2 coughs afterwards. There are positive deflections on p_{det} for coughs 2 and 3 indicating defective electronic subtraction due to infrequent measurement sampling. The strain shows perfect subtraction because the changes are slower and the machine can record them; coughs 1 and 5 are difficult to interpret as the p_{ves} and p_{det} traces overlap.

that used during voiding. For urethral pressure measurements the paper speed of some recorders is matched to the rate of withdrawal of the urethral profile catheter during profilometry (see below). Where the intent is to "custom build" a system then expert medical physics advice should be sought. Expense, reliability and the appropriateness of design will be important factors in the choice of equipment. Whilst most companies are extremely helpful in ensuring that pieces of equipment will connect to each other, local medical physics advice can be invaluable.

Technique of Filling Cystometry

Performing Filling Cystometry

To evaluate the storage phase of filling cystometry, four essential measurements must be made throughout filling:

- Intravesical pressure (p_{ves}).
- Intra-abdominal pressure (p_{abd}).
- Detrusor pressure ($p_{det} = p_{ves} - p_{abd}$) – calculated electronically.
- Urine flow rate to detect leaks.

   Other optional measurements may be made during cystometry:

- Bladder volume.
- Simultaneous video cystography.
- Electromyography.
- Urethral pressure measurement.

Intravesical Pressure (p_{ves}) Measurement

p_{ves} is the pressure measured within the bladder. Usually it is measured continuously, although sometimes in children the technique needs to be changed so that only intermittent pressure measurement is performed (see "Urodynamics in Children" in Chapter 5).

Unfortunately it is essential to pass a catheter into the bladder in order to measure p_{ves}, and access may be via the perurethral or percutaneous (suprapubic) route. In the adult patient the bladder rises to the upper border of the pubis when the bladder volume is approximately 300 ml, and only becomes easily palpable in a thin patient when the bladder volume is approximately 500 ml, so the routine use of the suprapubic route can present practical difficulties. Further, the suprapubic route is relatively contra-indicated in the presence of lower abdominal scars, which may tether intraperitoneal contents to the lower part of the abdominal wall. It is also more difficult in obese patients. However, the suprapubic route for intravesical pressure measurement remains the ideal, because it avoids the unphysiological effects of a catheter in the urethra and the possible effects of urethral anaesthesia. The recent availability of portable ultrasound machines allows a suprapubic catheter to be introduced with more confidence than before. Some workers put in a urethral catheter in order to fill the bladder prior to insertion of a suprapubic catheter, but this in some part compromises the advantages of a suprapubic catheter as outlined above.

If p_{ves} is measured using external strain gauge transducers then the transducer must be linked to the patient by a fluid-filled tube. The fluid in the tube is usually water, because the use of solutions (such as saline) may lead to the deposition of crystals in the transducer, affecting its performance. James has pioneered the use of air-filled tubes, although these are still not commercially available. When a water-filled tube (known as manometer tubing) is used to conduct pressure changes from the bladder to the transducer then certain physical characteristics of the tubing are important:

- The tubing must be flexible, yet the walls must not be elastic. If the tubing was to be elastic then the pressure measured would be lower than the true pressure, because part of the energy of the pressure wave would be used to stretch the elastic walls of the connecting tube.
- The manometer tubing should not be excessively long, narrow or wide.
- There should be no marked changes in the calibre of the tubing where the tubing joins the catheter or the transducer.

Anaesthesia for Urethral Catheterisation. In a female patient who has a short, straight urethra, local anaesthetic is probably unnecessary, adequate lubrication being all that is needed to ensure patient comfort. Occasionally the urethra may be extremely sensitive, and here it is better to use local anaesthetic rather than upset the patient and risk unusual stimulation of the bladder. Some would state that male patients also require only adequate lubrication, although it is the current practice of the author to use local anaesthetic gel. Investigations in our unit have shown that urethral anaesthesia has no effect on the measurements recorded during filling cystometry or pressure–flow studies. In most men the anaesthetic jelly does not pass through the pelvic floor region into the prostatic urethra.

Introducing the Catheter(s). The system we have used for twenty years to measure p_{ves} works well. An epidural catheter is used to measure pressure and is passed *per urethram* into the bladder together with an 8 Fr filling catheter. In women this is quite straightforward, but in men the epidural catheter needs to be "railroaded" into the bladder on the filling catheter.

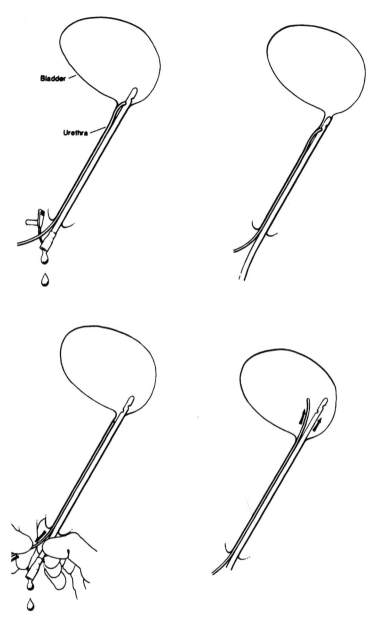

Fig. 3.37 Introducing the bladder catheters: the railroading technique.

- First the epidural catheter is introduced into the eyehole of the filling catheter.
- Both catheters are then passed into the bladder, until the urine drips from the filling catheter (Fig. 3.37, *top left*).
- Both catheters are then withdrawn until the urine flow just stops. The catheters will then be just inside the bladder neck (Fig. 3.37, *top right*).

- The catheters are then advanced by 1 to 2 cm until urine drips again. The catheters will now be lying in the bladder just above the bladder neck. Whilst the filling catheter is gripped so it cannot move, the epidural catheter is pulled gently until it is felt to disengage from the eyehole of the filling catheter, which is possible with a little experience (Fig. 3.37, *bottom left*).
- Both catheters are now advanced together so that the epidural passes into the bladder with the filling catheter (Fig. 3.37, *bottom right*).
- The epidural catheter is next held and the filling catheter partly withdrawn (approximately 10 cm), so that the epidural is left within the lumen of the bladder (Fig. 3.37, *top left*).
- Both catheters are now advanced together so that the epidural is railroaded into the bladder and begins to curl up. The epidural catheter has convenient markings on the side to show the length that has been introduced into the bladder (Fig. 3.38, *top right*).
- The process is repeated until the epidural catheter has been fully advanced into the bladder, leaving only 15 cm outside the urethra (Fig. 3.38). This precise technique prevents the annoyance (for both the patient and the doctor) of the pressure-measuring catheter being inadvertently withdrawn when the filling catheter is removed prior to voiding, which may occur if the epidural catheter has not been dislodged from the eyehole of the filling catheter (Fig. 3.39, *overleaf*).

Fixing the Catheters. We have used a two-catheter technique for many years. It is cheap, and after the filling catheter is removed the epidural catheter will not cause obstruction during voiding.

In the male patient the epidural catheter should be taped back over the shaft of the penis, ensuring that the tape does not compress the urethra on the underside of the penis (Fig. 3.40, *overleaf*). The filling catheter should be passed well into the bladder, so that at least 10 cm protrudes into the lumen. The filling catheter should also be taped to the penis, leaving no gap between the external urinary meatus and the point at which the catheter is attached to the tape. The tape should be folded back over the dorsum of the glans penis and the shaft of the penis, as shown (Fig. 3.41, *overleaf*).

In the female patient the epidural catheter should be taped, as close as possible to the external urethral meatus, on the inside of the thigh.

An alternative technique is to use a single catheter which has two channels, one for the measurement of p_{ves} and the other for bladder-filling. Catheters are now available in size 6 Fr and allow a filling speed of 50 ml/min using a peristatic pump. A 6 Fr catheter does not cause obstruction in adults except in exceptional circumstances (for example, a very tight urethral stricture). The catheter should be secured by tying a silk thread around the catheter junction box and sandwiching the silk ties between two layers of tape attached to the shaft of the penis (Fig. 3.42, *overleaf*). As in the two-catheter technique, the tape must not obstruct the urethra on the underside of the penis. In women, the single-catheter technique can be used: the catheter must be taped as close to the urethral meatus as possible on the inside of the thigh.

The key to success in fixing the urethral catheters is to be sure that there is not a loop of catheter between the external meatus and the point of tape fixation. If the above technique is used then there should be only minimal problems with

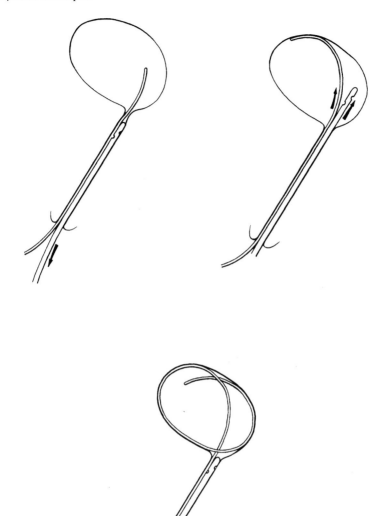

Fig. 3.38 Advancing the bladder catheter.

catheters being voided during micturition or being displaced or falling out during bladder-filling.

Measurement of Abdominal Pressure (p_{abd})

Intra-abdominal pressure (p_{abd}) is taken to be the pressure surrounding the bladder. In current practice it is estimated from rectal pressure or less commonly

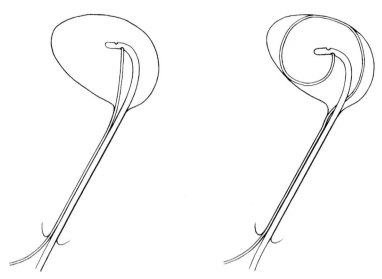

Fig. 3.39 If the technique described in Figs 3.37 and 3.38 is not followed then the epidural catheter may fail to disengage. It will then be pulled out when the filling catheter is removed at the end of the filling phase.

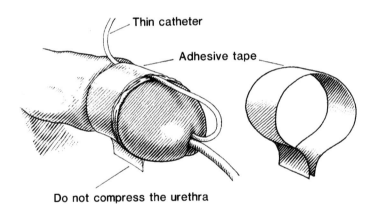

Do not compress the urethra

Fig. 3.40 Fixing the epidural catheter.

by intraperitoneal pressure. It is also possible to measure intra-abdominal pressure vaginally, from the stomach or from the pre-peritoneal space: only vaginal measurement of p_{abd} is a widely used alternative to rectal pressure measurement.

The purpose of measuring p_{abd} simultaneously during bladder or urethral pressure recordings is to aid interpretation of the observed pressure changes. If pressure rises in the bladder then the increase may be due to contraction of the detrusor or to changes in extravesical pressure (p_{abd}) transmitted to the bladder. In the normal person changes in p_{abd} are transmitted to the whole of the bladder and that part of the proximal urethra that lies above the pelvic floor. Figure 3.43 (*overleaf*) illustrates the importance of measuring p_{ves} and p_{abd}. If only p_{ves} were to

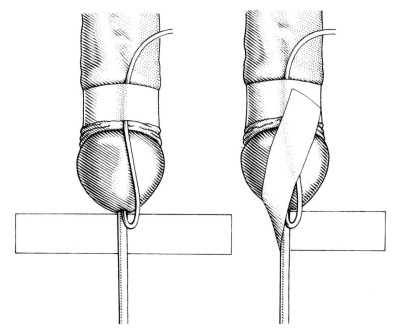

Fig. 3.41 Fixing the filling catheter.

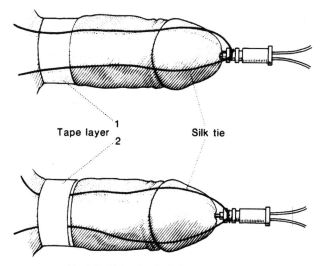

Tape layer 1
             2   Silk tie

Fig. 3.42 Fixing the dual-channel catheter.

be measured then the changes seen on the trace would be very difficult to interpret. However the addition of the p_{abd} pressure trace, together with the electronic
subtraction to produce detrusor pressure, will clarify the traces enormously.
Certain artefacts may arise as a direct result of using the rectal pressure as an
approximation of p_{abd}, and these must be appreciated. Rectal contractions may be
recorded in the rectum particularly if there is faecal loading (Fig. 3.44, *overleaf*),

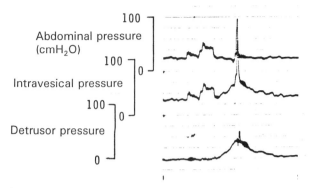

Fig. 3.43 Multi-channel trace showing, from the left, a short period of straining (pressure increases on the p_{abd} and p_{ves} traces but *not* on the p_{det} trace) followed by an unstable contraction during which the patient has coughed (the unstable wave is recorded on p_{ves} and p_{det} but *not* on p_{abd}; the coughs record only on p_{abd} and p_{ves}).

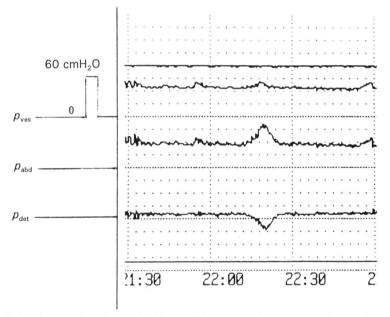

Fig. 3.44 Rectal contraction: characterised by a positive wave on the p_{abd} trace and a negative artefact on the p_{det} trace.

and a patient noted to have a full rectum should be asked to empty his or her bowels.

The rectal recording line can be made cheaply from manometer tubing protected at its rectal end by a finger cot cut from a thin disposable plastic glove (Fig. 3.45). The finger cot is used to avoid blockage of the line with faeces. Prior to recording, the tubing needs to be flushed from the transducer end. So that the finger cot is not distended, it is wise to make a small cut in it to allow excess air or

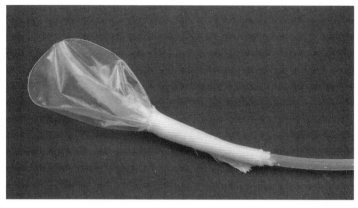

Fig. 3.45 "Home-made" rectal catheter constructed from the manometer tubing protected at its end by a plastic glove finger.

fluid to escape. If a commercially supplied rectal catheter is used then it is wise to make a small hole in the balloon for the same reason.

The rectal catheter is introduced using lubricant through the anus so that the tip is positioned 10 to 15 cm above the anal verge. The perianal area should be dried and the catheter taped as close as possible to the anal verge (Fig. 3.46).

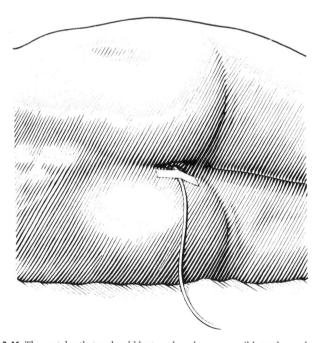

Fig. 3.46 The rectal catheter should be taped as close as possible to the anal verge.

Detrusor Pressure (p_{det}) Measurement

Detrusor pressure (p_{det}) is that component of intravesical pressure that is created by forces in the bladder wall (passive and active). It is estimated by the electronic subtraction of p_{abd} from p_{ves} ($p_{det} = p_{ves} - p_{abd}$). The simultaneous measurement of p_{abd} is essential in allowing the continuous calculation of p_{det}, and all modern urodynamic systems have the electronic equipment which allows this calculation.

The accurate measurement of p_{det} is entirely dependent on the accuracy with which p_{abd} and p_{ves} are measured. These can be readily assessed during urodynamics. In Fig. 3.47 the patient has been asked to cough. The cough should be identical on the p_{ves} and p_{abd} traces (*upper traces*), however if the p_{abd} line has not been flushed properly then the cough is not properly transmitted (*lower traces*). After flushing, the p_{abd} trace should show equal cough transmission and the resultant p_{det} trace no significant deflection. In order to get equal transmission the

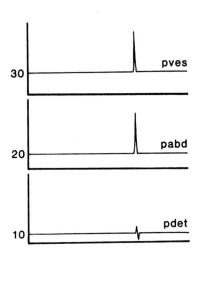

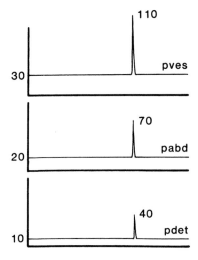

Fig. 3.47 Quality control: upper traces show good subtraction of a single cough with a small (acceptable) artefact on the p_{det} trace; lower traces show inadequate subtraction with a large cough artefact on p_{det}, which necessitates a check of the transducers and recording lines.

tubing used for the p_{abd} and p_{ves} lines should be similar. However, transmission can never be identical if fluid-filled lines are used and therefore the small biphasic deflection seen on the p_{det} trace (Fig. 3.47, *upper traces*) is acceptable. If transmission of pressure reading is not similar then adjustments should be made during cystometry to ensure accurate pressure recording, for example, to tighten a joint if a leak of fluid has developed.

Media Used for Bladder Filling

Water or physiological saline are the most commonly used media in urodynamics, together with radiographic contrast material if video urodynamics is being performed. Following the introduction of gas cystometry (Merrill 1971) there was a vogue for the use of carbon dioxide as a filling medium. While water or saline can have the obvious advantage that they mimic urine, carbon dioxide can have no such pretension.

Gas Cystometry. Gas cystometry has been evaluated objectively (Torrens 1977; Wein et al. 1978). CO_2 cystometry underestimates the maximum cystometric capacity, when compared with filling using saline, by an average of 20%. The variability of maximum cystometric capacity on repeated testing with gas infusion is about 30%. Similarly the measurement of pressure on repeated testing varies by a similar degree. Detrusor overactivity (instability – see pages 65–66), is quite easily seen during CO_2 cystometry, but high CO_2 infusion rates may inhibit detrusor instability rather than provoke it. Also, carbon dioxide causes pain in hypersensitive bladders, by combining with water to form carbonic acid which irritates the mucosa. In summary, there are several reasons why gas cystometry should not be used:

- CO_2 is a gas and an unphysiological medium.
- Measurement of capacity is inaccurate because CO_2 is compressible and dissolves in urine; CO_2 in solution (carbonic acid) is an irritant and may cause inflammation of the mucosa, as can be seen on subsequent cystoscopy.
- Following gas cystometry, no pressure–flow analysis of micturition can be obtained.
- Although gases are negative contrast media, it is not possible to obtain adequate synchronous video cystourethrography
- When filled with gas, there is no increase in bladder weight during distension. The increase in bladder weight during filling may have some physiological importance.

On the other hand, CO_2 cystometry does have certain advantages which accounted for its temporary popularity. These advantages apply particularly in the "office" environment: it is quick, simple and free of mess. There are no puddles on the floor, no sterilisation is required and the filling catheter and connecting link are disposable; also, only one catheter is required. However, because of the various limitations of the technique it is now no longer popular and is rarely practised.

Temperature of Filling Fluid

Formerly, we heated our infusion fluid to body temperature (37 °C). However we have slipped from this practice and now use fluid at room temperature (70 °F or

22 °C). There has been no perceptible change in the results we obtain, although this has not been analysed scientifically. It is important not to use cold fluid, because as it has been shown that the use of ice-cold infusion fluid stimulates bladder contractility at low bladder volumes. The ice water test remains a research investigation, and is used only as a routine at one or two centres.

Patient Position During Cystometry

Having catheterised the patient when they are supine, it is our practice to fill them either sitting (in the case of women) or standing (in the case of male patients), because the supine position does not reflect the everyday stresses to which the bladder is subjected, and most patients complain of bladder symptoms only when they are active (erect). Some patients complain of symptoms when they change posture, for example when rising from a sitting position, and if the patient has symptoms related to change of posture then this should be tested during the urodynamic studies. Investigators who use video urodynamics as their investigation of choice tend to fill the patient in the supine position and then tilt the X-ray table so they stand to void. Again this practice seems to us to fail to adequately mimic the stresses on the bladder imposed by the vertical position. The sitting and standing positions result in an increase in intravesical pressure compared with when the patient is lying. Therefore changing the patient's position during investigation may cause an artefact if pressure transmission to the bladder or rectum is affected. If the patient's position is changed then the transducer's position must be readjusted to the pressure reference level of the upper border of the symphysis pubis.

- In some circumstances it is may be impossible to fill the bladder with the patient in any position but supine. Patients who are severely disabled by neurological disease may have to be investigated in the lying position. In this situation it is desirable to attempt to measure their flow rate. In men this can be done by the use of a plastic drain pipe (D. Thomas, personal communication), though in women this is clearly not practical.
- If there is gross detrusor instability preventing proper filling then slow filling in the supine position may help.

Rate of Bladder Filling

The ICS defines three categories of filling rate:

- *Slow-fill cystometry* up to 10 ml per minute.
- *Medium-fill cystometry* between 10 ml and 100 ml per minute.
- *Fast-fill cystometry* when the rate is greater than 100 ml per minute.

The rate of bladder filling has considerable influence on the resulting measurements. The faster the bladder is filled, the lower the bladder compliance, as defined below (see p. 68). A series of cystometrograms repeated one after the other with a medium or rapid filling rate will show a gradually increasing capacity – the phenomenon of hysteresis. This has been shown not to occur at more physiological rates of filling (Klevmark 1974). The rate of filling chosen depends on whether the investigator is attempting to reproduce normal physiological events or to provoke the bladder into involuntary contraction whenever possible. Often the filling rate chosen will be a compromise between these two extremes, and a convenient rate, which does not prolong the test unduly, is 50 to 60 ml per minute. In children and patients with neurological abnormalities and in particular patients with reflex bladders secondary to spinal trauma the bladder should be filled very slowly (less than 10 ml per minute) because faster flow rates may produce artefactual bladder activity (Thomas 1979). This is discussed further in Chapter 5.

What to Do About Residual Urine?

Prior to catheterisation the patient is asked to empty the bladder as fully as possible. If they self-catheterise then they are asked to do this before urodynamics commences and to empty the bladder. However if the patient has neurological disease and does not self-catheterise then the bladder should *not* be emptied: in these patients the post-void residual (PVR) can be measured by passing a catheter after the voiding phase of urodynamic studies. If a patient without neurological abnormalities has evidence of hydronephrosis, which could be secondary to elevated bladder pressure, then the bladder should not be drained at the beginning of the filling phase of urodynamic studies. Removing the PVR and/or filling too quickly can fundamentally change the results, particularly in respect of bladder compliance, detrusor overactivity and cystometric capacity. In patients with neurological disease and/or upper tract dilatation, the artefacts of low compliance and reduced capacity are likely to be produced if a standard technique is used.

Ensuring a High-Quality Recording from the Patient

Before starting recording and after the patient is catheterised, both the bladder and rectal lines should be flushed once more to ensure that all bubbles and leaks have been removed. Once the catheters are in place and connected to the transducers then the tubing must be flushed to ensure that all bubbles are removed. As well as bubbles in the tubing, bubbles close to the transducer diaphragm must be removed. Failure to remove bubbles will lead to errors in measurement. Similarly the connections between the catheters and the manometer tubing and the tubing and the transducer should be tight: any leak will cause errors in the pressure measurement. Leaks, bubbles or elastic-sided tubing will tend to lead to the recording of lower values of pressure.

Quality control is ensured by asking the patient to cough at regular intervals during the investigation. Before recording starts, the patient should be asked to cough and the p_{ves} and p_{abd} traces observed. There should be an equal rise in pressure when the patient coughs (Fig. 3.47, *upper traces*). The patient should be asked to give a cough that produces a deflection of approximately 100 cmH$_2$O. The deflection should show a rapid increase to the peak, and then a rapid fall, as shown in the diagram. On the p_{det} line there may well be a small biphasic blip, but this does not matter: what is crucial is that the height of the spikes on the p_{ves} and the p_{abd} lines are identical.

If the spikes are not identical, as shown in Fig. 3.47, *lower traces*, then the explanation may be that there are bubbles or leaks, or that the catheters are

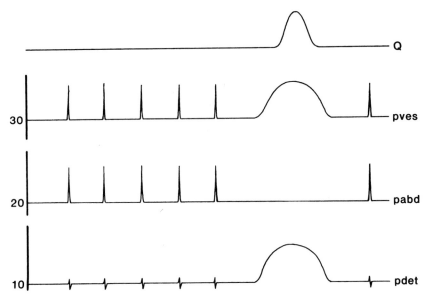

Fig. 3.48 Quality control: the patient is asked to cough every minute during filling *and* after voiding to ensure that the catheters have not become displaced during micturition.

malpositioned, or that there is interference with the measurement of p_{abd} due to faecal loading. All these points must be checked and the cough repeated until the proper pattern is observed.

Once the initial cough gives a good-quality signal then the bladder filling can commence. Throughout bladder filling, the patient should be asked to cough every minute (Fig. 3.48). If at any stage the quality deteriorates, then the investigation must be stopped and the cause of the poor pressure transmission investigated. Once the fault is corrected then the filling can recommence.

After filling, the patient must be asked to cough again, in order to ensure that the catheters have not moved during micturition. Failure to show an equal transmission of pressure after voiding means that the results of voiding cannot be confidently interpreted, and the investigation needs to be repeated if the voiding phase is vital for patient diagnosis.

Performing Filling Cystometry

The investigator should approach cystometry with one of the principles of urodynamics at the front of their mind, namely that "The role of urodynamics is to provide a pathophysiological explanation for the patient's complaints."

This means there should be a continuous dialogue between the investigator and the patient *throughout* the investigation. It is particularly important in assessing the sensations the patient experiences during cystometry.

During bladder filling the following should be assessed:

● Bladder sensation
● Detrusor activity

- Bladder compliance
- Urethral function
- Bladder capacity

Bladder Sensation

Certain terms have been accepted, but it should be emphasised that relating a precise bladder volume to one of them is subjective and is likely to vary considerably. These terms are:

First desire to void (FDV). This sensation is often difficult to interpret during cystometry, because the mere presence of the urethral catheter is often interpreted as a desire to void. It occurs at approximately 50% of cystometric capacity.

Normal desire to void (NDV). This is defined as the feeling that leads the patient to pass urine at the next convenient moment, but voiding can be delayed if necessary. It is felt at about 75% of cystometric capacity.

Strong desire to void (SDV). This is defined as a persistent desire to void without the fear of leakage; it is felt at approximately 90% capacity.

Urgency. This is defined as a persistent desire to void accompanied by a fear of leakage or fear of pain.

Pain. The site and character should be specified. Pain during bladder filling or micturition is abnormal.

A person with normal bladder function may occasionally feel urgency: bladder pain would only be felt in exceptional circumstances, for example if prevented from passing urine when trapped in a lift (elevator).

Abnormal sensation. Sensation can be said to be abnormal if it is one of the following:

- *Increased (hypersensitive).* If urgency or bladder pain are frequent and troublesome symptoms then these sensations are likely to represent disordered function. *Bladder hypersensitivity* is a term we have used and found useful. We define it as the condition of a bladder in which there is an early FDV at less than 100 ml which instead of passing away until a normal NDV occurs, persists and increases, limiting the cystometric capacity to less than 250 ml.
- *Reduced.* Reduced sensation is characterised by a later FDV and NDV, with the patient never experiencing an SDV, urgency or bladder pain.
- *Absent.* Absent sensation necessitates the patient passing urine "by the clock" and is usually indicative of a neurological condition such as spinal cord trauma or meningomyelocele.

Detrusor Activity

During bladder filling this can be either normal or increased (overactivity).

The normal bladder may also be termed "stable" in contradistinction to "unstable" (see below). This means that detrusor overactivity does not occur

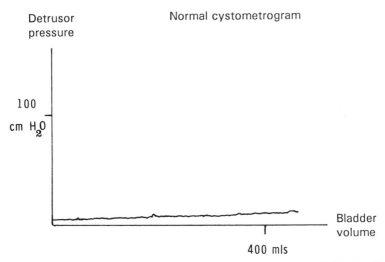

Fig. 3.49 Normal filling cystometrogram with almost no increase in p_{det} as the bladder fills.

under any circumstances, for example during the provocation tests used in an effort to uncover detrusor instability (DI). In normal function the detrusor relaxes and stretches to allow the bladder to increase in size without any change in pressure (accommodation) (Fig. 3.49). This ability is essential for two reasons. The first of these is to allow normal urine transport from the kidneys; ureteric muscle is relatively weak, being capable of generating pressure of approximately 30 cmH$_2$O. The second is that increased bladder pressures during filling would be likely to compromise continence.

Detrusor overactivity exists when, during the filling phase, there are involuntary detrusor contractions that the person cannot suppress. These contractions may be spontaneous or else may occur only on provocation as described above. Detrusor overactivity during voiding may be indicated by an involuntary voiding contraction, or by the inability to suppress a voluntary contraction. At present this last category, impaired suppression, is not commonly recognised. Various special terms have been used to describe these features and they are defined as follows.

- *The unstable detrusor* is one that is shown objectively to contract spontaneously or on provocation, during the filling phase while the patient is attempting to inhibit micturition. The unstable detrusor may be asymptomatic, and its presence does not necessarily imply a neurological disorder. DI is the commonest form of detrusor overactivity.

- *Detrusor hyperreflexia (DHR)* is defined as overactivity due to disturbance of the nervous control mechanisms. It must be confirmed by objective evidence of a neurological disorder. DHR occurs frequently in neurological conditions such as multiple sclerosis and cerebrovascular disease, as well as in conditions such as meningomyelocele and after spinal cord trauma. The cystometric trace in DHR is very variable and highly dependent on urodynamic technique. It is in the neuropathic patient that the difference between detrusor overactivity and low bladder compliance can become blurred (see below). Other conceptual and undefined terms should be avoided; these include hypertonic, systolic, spastic, automatic and uninhibited.

There has been considerable confusion over the applied definition of DI, with some investigators labelling patients as having DI if there is an increase of p_{det} greater than 15 cmH$_2$O during filling. However the ICS standardisation document of 1988 makes it clear that DI is characterised by phasic contractions in which the pressure rises and then falls. The ICS definition does not specify a minimum change in p_{det}, although waves of an amplitude of less than 5 cmH$_2$O are difficult to detect using most modern urodynamic equipment. However it is undoubtedly true that low-pressure DI waves (5 to 15 cmH$_2$O) can and do produce troublesome symptoms of urgency and urge incontinence, particularly in women with poor urethral function.

Is DI Normal or Abnormal? The answer is that probably it is not abnormal and that most of us will have an occasional unstable wave. DI is abnormal when it produces troublesome symptoms: this illustrates the fundamental principle of urodynamics, i.e. the need to relate urodynamic findings to the patient's symptoms.

If an unstable wave is seen then the investigator should ask the patient a series of questions as follows:

"Do you feel anything now?"
If an unstable wave is present but the patient either is unaware of the wave or feels the wave as a normal desire to void, then the DI is probably not clinically significant. If the patient answers "yes" and feels the wave as an urgency or discomfort then a follow-up question should be asked:

"Is this the feeling that gives you trouble in your everyday life?"
If the patient answers "no" then the DI may be an artefact of the investigation. Artefactual waves usually occur at the beginning of filling, after which the bladder settles down. If the patient answers "yes" then the association between symptoms and the urodynamic finding of DI has been made and the diagnosis confirmed.

DI occurs in different patterns. In general, unstable waves become more frequent and of greater amplitude as bladder filling proceeds (Fig. 3.50, *overleaf*). DI during cystometry may or may not be accompanied by leakage (urge incontinence), as in Fig. 3.51, *overleaf*. DI is often described as spontaneous or provoked.

Spontaneous DI means that the instability had no particular trigger (Fig. 3.51, *overleaf*), whereas provocation instability is usually qualified by the provoking factor, the commonest of which are:

● Changing position, for example, rising from sitting or lying to standing.
● Coughing; Fig. 3.52 (page 70) shows cough-induced DI.
● Hand-washing or putting the hands in cold water, for example whilst gardening on a cold day.
● "Latchkey incontinence" where a patient wishing to pass urine reaches their front door but before they can turn the key has extreme urgency and leaks.

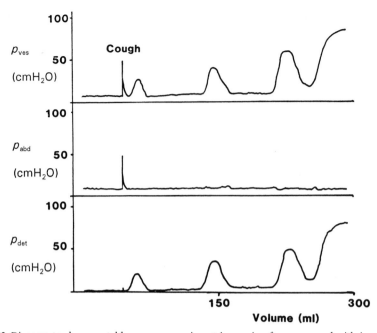

Fig. 3.50 Diagram to show unstable waves occurring at increasing frequency and with increasing pressure as the bladder fills.

- "Telephone urgency" – a terrifying disease of the post-industrial world where telephone conversations lead to urgency and even, in the case of one of the author's children, the need to attempt to interrupt the conversation in order to pass urine.

The recognition that DI may develop in response to certain triggers has led some urodynamicists to advocate "provocative cystometry" in an effort to uncover "latent DI". In the author's view, provocation should be used if the patient gives a history suggestive of provoked DI. If not then the patient should only be asked to cough during bladder filling. Coughing is of course also useful for quality control purposes and in women as a means of demonstrating genuine stress incontinence (GSI). There has been considerable work attempting to quantify DI, and Fig. 3.53 (*overleaf*) shows a DI index based on the number and height of the DI waves; other indices have measured the area under the p_{det} curve.

Bladder Compliance

In normal bladder function there should be little change in intravesical pressure from empty to full. Bladder compliance describes the relationship between bladder volume and bladder pressure ($\triangle V/\triangle p$) and is expressed as: increase in bladder volume per centimetre of water increase in pressure (ml/cmH$_2$O).

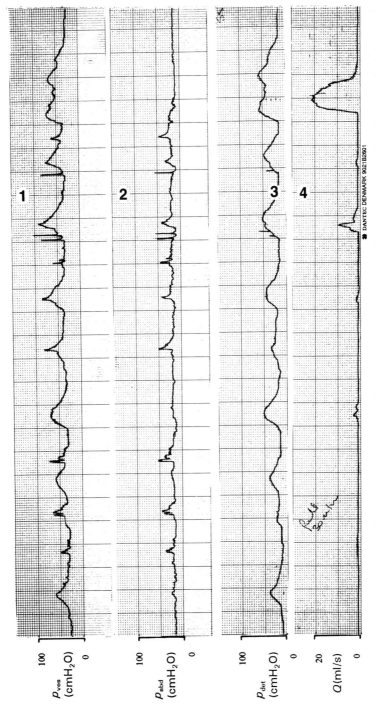

Fig. 3.51 Multi-channel trace showing multiple unstable waves, four of which cause leakage detected on the flow rate trace (bottom trace, Q (ml/s)). A normal void occurs at the extreme right-hand end of the recording.

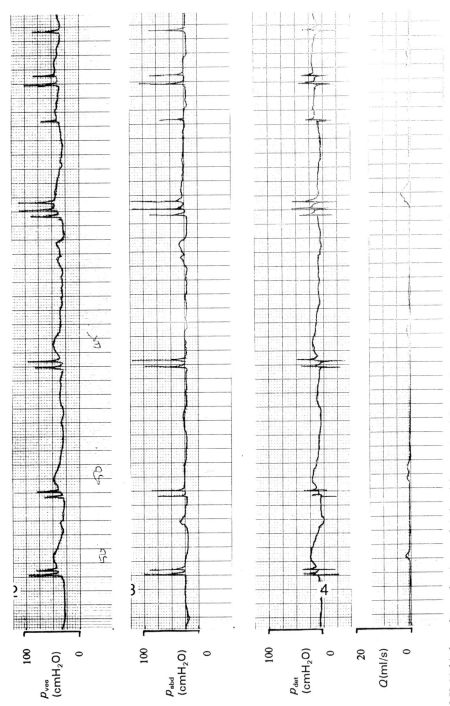

Fig. 3.52 Multi-channel trace showing cough-induced detrusor instability. On the p_{det} trace there are acceptable biphasic artefacts reflecting the coughs seen in p_{ves} and p_{det}. The flow trace detects leaks with most of the DI waves.

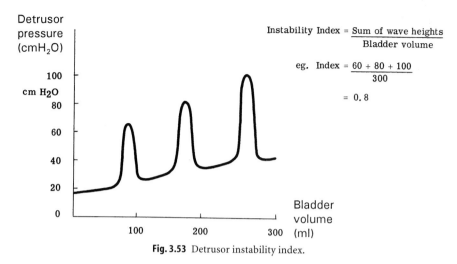

Fig. 3.53 Detrusor instability index.

In the normal bladder with a capacity of 400 ml the change in pressure from empty to full should be less than 10 cmH$_2$O, giving a figure for normal compliance of greater than 40 ml/cmH$_2$O. Bladder compliance is dependent on the rate of bladder filling, on bladder function, and on the neurological state of the patient. Klevmark showed that if bladders are filled at physiological rates then there is little or no change in bladder pressure on filling. Figure 3.54 demonstrates how to determine whether or not low compliance is due to fast filling.

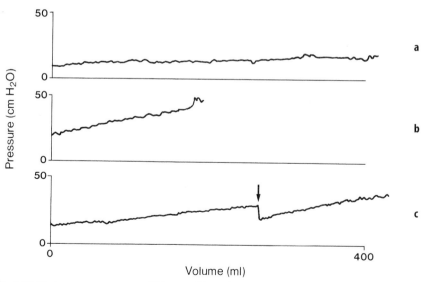

Fig. 3.54 Various responses to filling. a Normal cystometrogram. b Constantly reduced compliance. c Reduced compliance due to fast filling. When infusion is stopped (at the arrow) the pressure falls immediately, to increase again when infusion is restarted.

When there is evidence of low compliance with a gradual increase in p_{ves}, then bladder filling should stop for at least two minutes. If the intravesical pressure falls as in Fig. 3.54c then the reduced compliance was, at least in part, due to filling too fast. Once the pressure has stabilised then filling should be restarted, but at a significantly slower rate: if initial filling was at 50 ml/min then it should be reduced to 10 ml/min.

In theory, bladder compliance has a passive and an active component. The passive component is dependent on bladder wall composition, and if there are significant quantities of fibrous tissue within the bladder wall, then compliance may be reduced. In fact, even in interstitial cystitis or after radiotherapy it is unusual to see compliance changes. This may be because pain limits the degree to which the bladder can be filled. As we have said, the normal bladder distends without significant change in pressure; hence if the pressure rises gradually throughout bladder filling then this can be assumed to be an active process, at least in so far as the detrusor muscle is not relaxing normally. This view is supported by the fact that reduced compliance can be partly abolished by the use of intravenous anticholinergic agents.

In a small number of male patients with benign prostatic obstruction, chronic retention may lead to upper tract dilatation. This has been termed "high-pressure

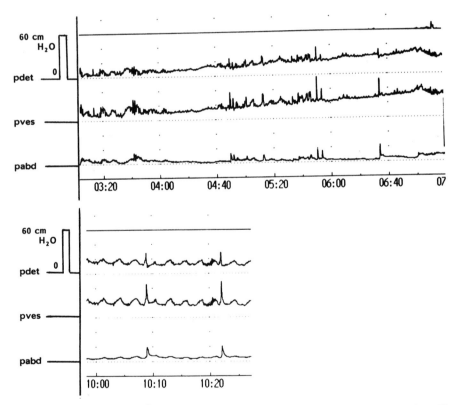

Fig. 3.55 Effect of filling rate on bladder compliance; the upper trace shows a conventional medium fill CMG in a man with prostatic obstruction and demonstrating reduced compliance; the lower trace is recorded during natural-fill cystometry and now demonstrates DI, masked during faster filling.

chronic retention" and it had been shown that these men have reduced bladder compliance. However it was later demonstrated that low compliance in this group of patients was largely artefactual and that, if filled at physiological rates, low compliance was replaced with phasic detrusor instability, albeit with a related underlying increased pressure (Fig. 3.55). In this author's view detrusor instability and low compliance, in most cases, should both be viewed as part of the spectrum of detrusor overactivity on filling.

The previous edition of this book (1983) discussed detrusor underactivity in the section on filling cystometry. Since then the ICS collected report of 1988, reprinted as Appendix 1 Part 1, has been published and reasonably states that the detrusor can only be normal or overactive during filling. *Detrusor underactivity can only be diagnosed during the voiding phase.* Patients with detrusor underactivity during voiding will often have a large cystometric capacity, although this is by no means the rule (see p. 78).

Urethral Function During Filling

During the storage phase the urethral closure mechanism function is either normal or incompetent:

- The *normal urethral closure mechanism* maintains a positive urethral closure pressure during filling, even in the presence of increased abdominal pressure. Immediately prior to micturition the normal closure pressure decreases to allow flow.
- *Incompetent urethral closure mechanism.* An incompetent urethral closure mechanism is defined as one which allows leakage of urine in the absence of a detrusor contraction. Leakage may occur whenever intravesical pressure exceeds intraurethral pressure (genuine stress incontinence) or when there is an involuntary fall in urethral pressure (urethral instability).

Incontinence has several causes and incompetence of the urethral sphincter mechanism leading to genuine stress incontinence is an important one. However if incontinence occurs due to an unstable detrusor contraction then the urethral closure mechanism is not thought of as incompetent, because urethral relaxation is a reflex action occurring as part of normal micturition. This begs the question, "Can an unstable contraction be viewed as the premature activation of the micturition reflex?" During an unstable detrusor contraction, with urethral relaxation, continence can be maintained by voluntary pelvic floor contractions until the individual can inhibit the unstable wave. But urge incontinence due to DI is seen more frequently in women because urethral function and pelvic floor function, particularly after childbirth, is less powerful.

Genuine stress incontinence (GSI) is defined as leakage occurring when the intravesical pressure (p_{ves}) exceeds the intraurethral pressure (p_{ura}) in the absence of a detrusor contraction. The demonstration of GSI is straightforward in most patients. The standard procedure is to ask the patient to cough to perform the Valsalva test. GSI is easier to show with the patient in the vertical position, either sitting or standing, and with a full bladder. If the patient has the symptom of stress incontinence and no leakage has been demonstrated by the time the bladder is full then two of the following manoeuvres can be tried. First, remove

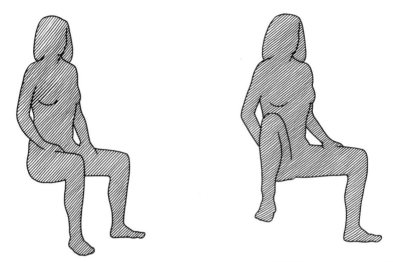

Fig. 3.56 Testing for GSI: ask the woman to flex and abduct one hip if GSI is not demonstrated in the usual more dignified position!

the filling catheter and repeat the provocative tests. Second, GSI is more easily provoked in women, if they are asked to separate their legs widely, presumably because leg abduction weakens pelvic floor support to the sphincter mechanism (Fig. 3.56). If standard urodynamics are being used without simultaneous lower urinary tract imaging then it is necessary to view the external meatus when the patient coughs. Women in particular may become embarrassed and must be reassured and put at their ease.

Urethral Instability. The unstable urethra was the urodynamic diagnosis of the 1980s. It has been defined as a change in maximum urethral closure pressure of greater than 15 cmH$_2$O measured on urethral pressure profilometry (p. 100). Urethral instability alone is an unusual cause of incontinence and when seen in its pure form it is easier to understand if termed "inappropriate urethral relaxation". However what is not clear is whether or not it is a variant of a prematurely activated micturition reflex in which the rise in detrusor pressure due to an unstable wave is too small to see. This may be the case, because the phenomenon is seen only in women, and as many continent women void normally merely by relaxing their urethra, without a measurable detrusor contraction unless a "stop test" is done (see "Voiding Cystometry" below).

Bladder Capacity

In describing bladder capacity the ICS has recommended the following terms:

- *Maximum cystometric capacity (MCC)* is the volume at which the patient feels that they can no longer delay micturition. MCC is difficult to define if the patient's sensation is absent or reduced. In deciding how far to fill the bladder in these circumstances the urodynamicist should be guided by evidence of the functional bladder capacity from the frequency–volume chart.

- The *functional bladder capacity* or voided volume is assessed from the frequency–volume chart completed by all patients before urodynamic studies (see "Analysis of Symptoms" in Chapter 4). If the urodynamicist is using functional capacity to determine how full to fill the bladder then any residual urine should be added to the average voided volume taken from the frequency volume chart.

- *Maximum bladder capacity* is defined as the volume measured during anaesthesia (either deep general or general/epidural) and may often be very different from the functional bladder capacity, particularly in conditions such as DI.

Artefacts During Cystometry

The urodynamicist is aware that urodynamics even with natural filling rates is not physiological. This is due not only to the need for catheters for bladder filling and for measuring pressure but also because, even with ambulatory UDS, the patient is being observed. These limitations must be accepted and appreciated but not ignored. We have already discussed how technique must be adapted in the light of particular findings such as low compliance; further adaptations aimed at minimising artefacts are discussed in later chapters.

The artefacts seen during cystometry can be divided into measurement and "physiological" artefacts.

Measurement Artefacts. This book tries to give sufficient practical detail to enable the urodynamicist to generate high-quality traces and avoid measurement artefacts. Measurement artefacts are produced by problems in the equipment: somewhere between the tip of the catheters and the writing mechanism of the recorder. Setting up the equipment will uncover and deal with most of these problems. Modern electronic equipment is reliable, but if there are problems with the transducers or the urodynamic equipment, after proper calibration and setting zero procedures have been followed, then the agent or manufacturer will have to help. As filling cystometry is largely concerned with pressure measurement, it is this area that produces most artefacts. Bubbles and leaks will alter the transmission of pressure from the patient to the transducer. The cough test is designed to eliminate this problem: hence the importance of asking the patient to cough *every minute*. If there is unequal transmission of pressure on the p_{ves} and p_{abd} traces then the catheters and lines should be flushed from the syringes attached to the transducer as described above and the connections between catheter, tubing and transducer checked for leaks (see pages 58–59).

If there continues to be unequal transmission of coughs then catheter positions must be checked. Either the bladder or the rectal catheter may have slipped down into the sphincter region causing a pressure transmission problem. This is rather more common with the rectal catheter, which in patients with poor anal function can be difficult to keep in position. A gradual slippage of the rectal catheter can produce a confusing picture, with p_{abd} falling gradually, leading to an apparent increase in p_{det}. However examination of the p_{ves} line shows that intravesical pressure is constant and uncovers the cause of the artefact.

"Physiological" Artefacts. Rectal contractions are a cause of problems in interpretation and may lead to the misdiagnosis of DI. Rectal contractions are seen relatively frequently during urodynamic studies, and may be single or multiple. If single they should not create confusion, because there is then a single fall in p_{det} at the time of the rectal contraction (Fig. 3.44). However when they are repetitive then the effect on the p_{det} trace can give the illusion of rhythmic DI. Rectal contractions cannot be prevented other than in patients who come for urodynamics with a loaded rectum. Such patients should be asked to visit the toilet before the start of urodynamic studies, because this can avoid a lot of trouble (and mess)!

Voiding Cystometry

Introduction

The improvements in electronic equipment that led to the increased acceptance and practice of cystometry were essential in the development of techniques for the accurate measurement of intravesical pressure and urine flow rate during voiding. These studies represent a natural progression from urine flow studies. As discussed above, urine flow studies can only provide limited information. Flow rate is dependent both on the outlet resistance and on the contractile properties of the detrusor. A low flow rate may be associated with a high voiding pressure, or with a voiding pressure that is below normal. Similarly, the finding of a normal flow rate does not exclude bladder outlet obstruction (BOO), because normal flow may be maintained by a high voiding pressure in the presence of BOO. In the female normal flow may occur despite there being no increase in intravesical pressure. Pressure–flow studies (*pQS*) are essential for a complete functional classification of lower urinary tract disorders, although personal experience of *pQS* allows greatly improved interpretation of isolated urine flow rate tracings.

Definitions. During a pressure–flow study of voiding, intravesical pressure and flow rate are measured continuously.

- *Premicturition pressure* is the pressure recorded immediately before the initial isovolumetric contraction. It will be the same as the full resting pressure if the patient has not moved following the filling cystometrogram (Appendix 1, Part 1, Fig. A.1.1.4).
- *Opening time* is the time elapsed from the initial rise in detrusor pressure to the onset of flow. This is the initial isovolumetric contraction period of micturition.
- *Opening pressure* is the pressure recorded at the onset of measured flow. It should be remembered that there is a delay in the recording of flow because of the time taken for urine to reach the flowmeter. The delay is of the order of 0.5 to 1.0 second and must be allowed for when interpreting the *pQ* relationship.
- *Maximum voiding pressure* is the maximum value of the measured pressure during voiding.

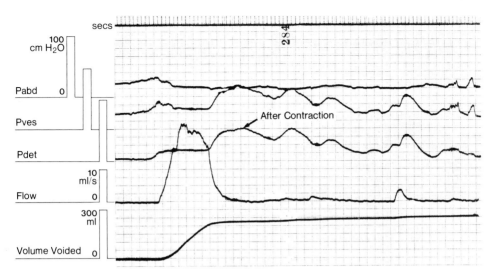

Fig. 3.57 Pressure–flow study of micturition demonstrating the phenomenon known as an after-contraction. This is sometimes associated with detrusor overactivity but has not been shown to be abnormal.

- *Pressure at maximum flow* is the pressure recorded at the time of maximum flow rate. Again, any delay in the recording of flow rate must be allowed for.
- *Contraction pressure at maximum flow* is the difference between the pressure at maximum flow and the premicturition pressure.
- *After-contraction* describes the common findings of a pressure increase after flow ceases at the end of micturition. The significance of this event is not understood (Fig. 3.57).

The Concept of Urethral Resistance

The bladder and urethra have independent functional properties and in combination these characteristics determine the pressure–flow relationships of micturition. By knowing both factors and relating them to the normal values of each it is possible to ascertain whether voiding function itself is normal. This can be done more accurately than from either measurement alone. To formalise the relationship of pressure and flow, various urethral resistance factors have been elaborated. At one stage urethral resistance (UR) was defined according to the equation $UR = p_{ves}/Q_{max}^2$. However this calculation of resistance fell into disrepute largely because it was based on the hydrodynamics of laminar flow through rigid straight tubes: the urethra is neither rigid nor straight and flow is often turbulent and not laminar. In 1987 the ICS recommended that pressure–flow data should be presented graphically plotting one quantity against the other (Appendix 1, Part 1, Fig. A.1.1.5). From this basic idea have developed the nomograms used in the diagnosis of bladder outlet obstruction (see Chapter 5).

Performing Voiding Cystometry

In most patients it is quite clear when bladder filling should be stopped. But if the patient has little sensation it is important to use the functional bladder capacity from the frequency–volume chart as a guide to cystometric capacity, remembering to add on the patient's residual volume if present. Once filling has stopped the filling catheter is removed with care being taken not to dislodge the strapping holding the epidural catheter in place. Prior to allowing the patient to void they should be asked to cough to ensure that proper pressure transmission is occurring. The patient is then instructed to void to completion if possible.

It is even more important during the voiding phase to respect the patient's privacy. Few women have ever voided in the presence of others and therefore it may be necessary to leave the room in order that patients can initiate voiding. It is also important to allow the patient to void in a position that is natural for them: for women sitting and for most men standing.

Interpretation of Voiding Cystometry

Detrusor activity and urethral function should be qualified separately whilst remembering that urethral characteristics will define the precise voiding pressure.

Detrusor Activity. This can be classified as follows:

- Normal when the detrusor contracts to empty the bladder with a normal flow rate (Fig. 3.57).
- Underactive when either the detrusor contraction is unable to empty the bladder or the bladder empties at a lower than normal speed (Fig. 3.58).

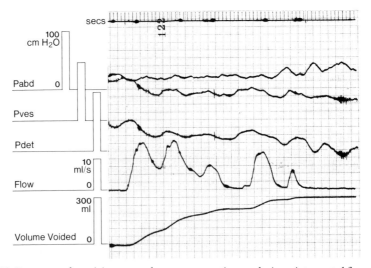

Fig. 3.58 Detrusor underactivity: a poor detrusor contraction results in an interrupted flow wave.

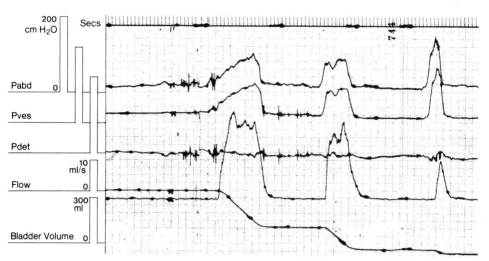

Fig. 3.59 Acontractile detrusor: *pQS* in a male patient who voids by straining without any sign of detrusor contraction.

- Acontractile when no measured detrusor pressure change occurs during voiding (Fig. 3.59).

These categories are easy to understand and use if there is no increase in outlet resistance, but become more difficult to use if there is a coexisting bladder outlet obstruction. For example, in benign prostatic obstruction (BPO) then failure of the detrusor contraction to fully empty the bladder does not mean that contractility is abnormal: in BPO voiding pressures are higher than would be expected if no bladder outlet obstruction existed, and most patients will show

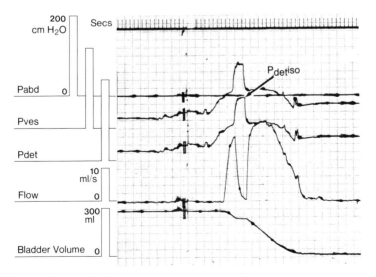

Fig. 3.60 Pressure–flow study of interrupted micturition showing the isovolumetric pressure increase generated by a normal bladder on cessation of flow. In this case the pressure increase is 66 cmH₂O.

normal detrusor activity, with complete bladder emptying, after the BPO has been surgically resected.

It is not the intention of the author to enter into the complexities and controversies of measuring detrusor contractility. However the urodynamicist can make a simple assessment of detrusor contractility by using the "stop test" (Fig. 3.60, *previous page*). Once the patient is voiding and when the observer judges that Q_{max} has been reached the patient is asked to stop voiding. The patient achieves this by contracting the pelvic floor muscles and possibly the intrinsic striated muscle of the urethra. However the detrusor is not immediately inhibited and continues to contract. As the contraction is now against a closed outlet it becomes an isometric (isovolumetric) contraction and the intravesical pressure increases sharply to a new maximum. After 2 to 5 seconds the patient is asked to continue voiding and the p_{ves} falls to its previous level. The height of the increase in p_{det} is known as the $p_{det, iso}$ and gives some idea of detrusor contractility. This test can be performed only if the patient is able to interrupt flow instantaneously. However in many patients in whom an assessment of detrusor contractility would be useful, for example in women prior to stress incontinence surgery, where post-operative voiding difficulty is common, it is not possible. This is because many older women have lost the ability to interrupt their urine flow. This inability can be circumvented if a Foley balloon catheter is left *in situ* during voiding and when Q_{max} is achieved the catheter is pulled down so that the bladder outlet is blocked: this variant of the stop test has not found favour in the urodynamic community! Figure 3.61 shows the stop test in a woman where a much lower $p_{det, iso}$ results than the one seen in the male patient (Fig 3.60). This does not mean that the woman has detrusor underactivity, but it may be indicative of the fact that women have less powerful bladders than men.

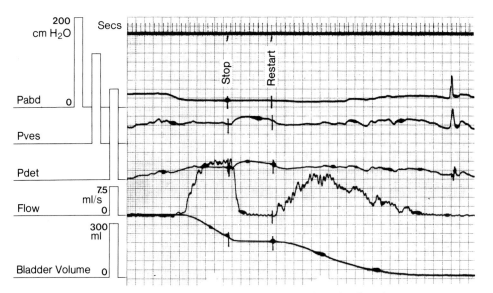

Fig. 3.61 Stop test: small increase in $p_{det,iso}$ (20 cmH$_2$O) in a female patient.

Detrusor Underactivity. This cannot be diagnosed from a filling cystometrogram; a voiding study is necessary. Problems arise when the patient cannot initiate micturition and it is unclear whether this inhibition is psychogenic or neurogenic. If synchronous urethral pressure or sphincter EMG is being recorded then it may be evident that the urethra cannot, or will not, relax. In such a case the inability to void is either psychogenic or, if neurogenic, due to a lesion above the sacral spinal cord. Psychogenic suppression of detrusor contraction is less common if the patient is put at ease by the investigator and the investigation environment.

In other cases it may be difficult to distinguish between neuropathic and myopathic causes for detrusor underactivity. If the urethral function is quite normal then neuropathy is unlikely; if urethral function is abnormal then the sacral reflex arc can be tested using an evoked response and a denervation supersensitivity test may be performed.

Urethral Function During Voiding

During voiding the urethra may be either normal or obstructive. A *normal* urethra is relaxed throughout voiding. An *obstructive* urethra is most commonly due to *mechanical obstruction*. If there is a mechanical obstruction such as an enlarged prostate then sphincter relaxation is likely to be normal but prostatic enlargement will interfere, resulting in limited opening of the proximal urethra. Mechanical obstruction may occur at any site from the bladder neck to the external urinary meatus. Urethral obstruction for whatever reason leads to increased voiding pressures. In mechanical obstruction, the voiding pressures are constantly elevated (Fig. 3.61) whereas if the obstruction is due to urethral overactivity then the voiding pressures may fluctuate as in detrusor–sphincter dyssynergia (Fig. 3.62).

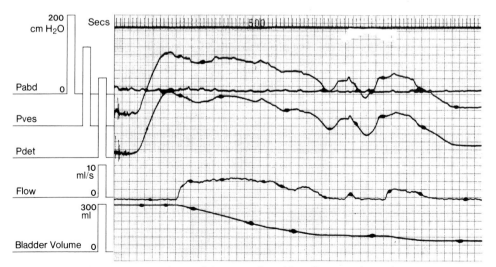

Fig. 3.62 Pressure–flow study in a man of 62 with outflow tract obstruction.

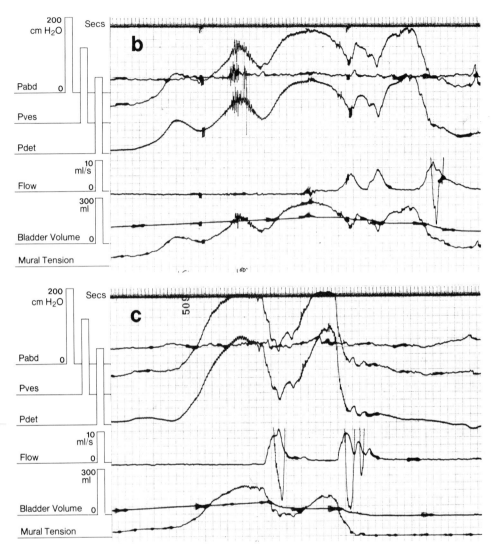

Fig. 3.63 Detrusor–sphincter dyssynergia: two examples both showing a high pre-voiding pressure (greater than 200 cmH₂O) which falls as voiding spurts but increases rapidly as the urethra closes between urine spurts.

Urethral obstruction due to *urethral overactivity* is characterised by the urethra contracting during voiding or the urethra failing to relax. Urethral overactivity can be divided into:

- *Detrusor–sphincter dyssynergia (DSD)* is seen only in patients with neurological disease and most classically in high-level (cervical) spinal cord injury. It is characterised by phasic contractions of the intrinsic urethral striated muscle during detrusor contraction (Fig. 3.63). This produces a very high voiding pressure and an interrupted flow. The urodynamic characteristic of

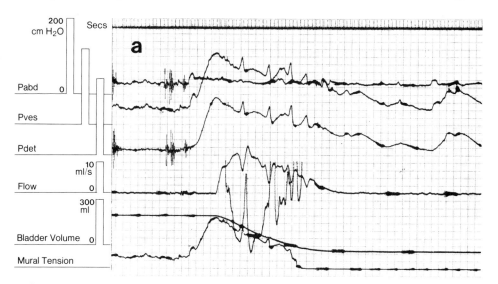

Fig. 3.64 Dysfunctional voiding: the flow curve shows dips which correspond to spikes on the p_{det} trace. This indicates that the patient is not properly relaxed and that the pelvic floor is partially contracted at intervals.

this type of urethral overactivity is a falling flow rate accompanied by a rising detrusor pressure which then falls when the urethra relaxes, leading to resumption of urine flow.

- *Dysfunctional voiding (DFV)* produces the same urodynamic pattern as DSD but occurs in a different group of patients and has a different cause. DFV occurs, most characteristically, in children who are neurologically normal but present with urinary incontinence and/or infections. The interrupted flow in these children is due to pelvic floor overactivity rather than to intrinsic striated muscle as in DSD. Figure 3.64 is from a man who showed some inhibition in the urodynamic room.

Isolated distal sphincter obstruction (IDSO) is seen in classical form in meningomyelocele patients. In this condition there is a failure of urethral relaxation rather than urethral contractions during attempted micturition. The urethra opens except for the area of the internal striated sphincter, at pelvic floor level. IDSO produces a continuous obstruction with reduced flow rates. Patients with ISDO often suffer from genuine stress incontinence owing to sphincter incompetence during bladder filling.

Artefacts During Voiding Cystometry

It is important that the limitations of voiding cystometry are understood and that any differences between the patient's performance during urodynamics and his or her normal voiding are appreciated. This is best judged by asking the patient and also by comparing the free urine flow rate with the flow rate during *pQS*.

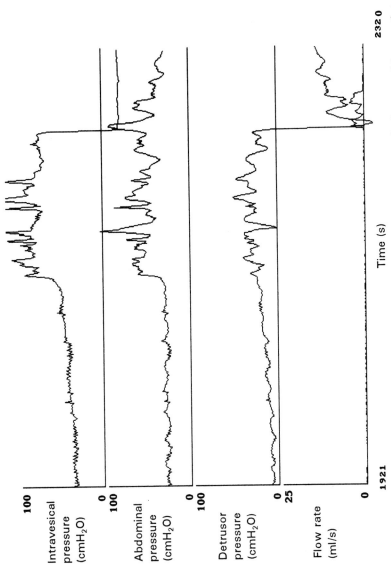

Fig. 3.65 Multi-channel recording showing a sharp decrease in p_{ves} and p_{det} at the start of voiding due to displacement of the p_{ves} catheter.

Mechanical Artefacts. If p_{ves} is measured by an epidermal catheter, by a 6 Fr dual channel catheter or by a suprapubic catheter, there should be no obstructive effect due to the catheter itself. However catheter problems can make the interpretation of the voiding phase difficult or impossible. Even when the catheter is attached, as described above, either the urethral or the rectal catheter may move during voiding. The urethral catheter may slip down into the sphincter area or it may be voided with the urine stream. If it is voided then a characteristic trace results (Fig. 3.65). If it has slipped down into the sphincter area, when the patient coughs after voiding in order for a check to be made of pressure-measuring quality, then unequal transmission will be seen, with p_{abd} being greater than p_{ves}. If on the other hand the rectal catheter falls out or slips into the anal sphincter area then the p_{abd} cough spike will be absent or reduced. If the urethral catheter is voided at the beginning of voiding then the test will have to be repeated, whereas if the catheter moves after the maximum flow rate is achieved, then a repeat test is probably not necessary. If problems occur with the rectal catheter then careful inspection of the p_{ves} trace is needed to assess whether a repeat test is required: if the cough spike on the p_{ves} trace, after voiding, is similar to that preceding voiding then it is likely that p_{ves} has been accurately measured. However if the p_{abd} recording is unreliable, it will not be possible to exclude straining as a significant part of the expressive force used by that individual patient to void. Indeed if the rectal catheter has slipped down or come out this is quite likely to be due in part, at least, to the patient straining: it may be necessary to repeat the *pQS*.

"Physiological" Artefacts. Voiding in the urodynamic laboratory is likely to be affected by a variety of factors:

- The *environment* may result in a patient who voids without problems at home finding it very difficult to void in the test situation. It has been estimated that 30% of women asked to void during video urodynamics carried out in the X-ray department cannot do so. This is hardly surprising if they are surrounded by complex equipment, and asked to void in an unnatural position, watched by strangers!

- *Technique* used may also be important. Overfilling of the bladder generally makes normal voiding difficult. The effect of relatively fast filling may also be significant, because most studies which compare ambulatory urodynamics (with natural bladder filling) and conventional urodynamics show that voiding pressures are higher with natural filling, suggesting that the detrusor may be incompletely stimulated, partially inhibited or mechanically less efficient after being filled at a supraphysiological rate.

- *Abdominal straining* during voiding may be either a habit or a necessity for the patient. The effect of straining on the voiding trace needs to be understood. The patient should always be asked to void normally and in as relaxed a way as possible. If the patient has an acontractile detrusor then voiding can only be achieved by straining as in Fig. 3.59. If the detrusor contracts during voiding but the patient also strains then the trace can be difficult to interpret. It is also difficult to know precisely what effect straining has on urine flow: in patients without obstruction straining increases flow, but it does not produce the same increase in flow as that achieved by a detrusor pressure rise of the same magnitude (Fig. 3.66, *overleaf*). In obstructed patients straining does not increase flow. This may be because the narrow, obstructed urethra is squeezed from outside by the

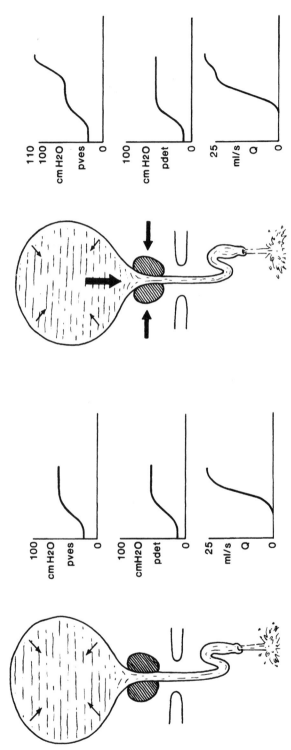

Fig. 3.66 Effect of straining in unobstructed voiding: flow is increased when intra-abdominal pressure increases (heavy arrows indicate straining forces).

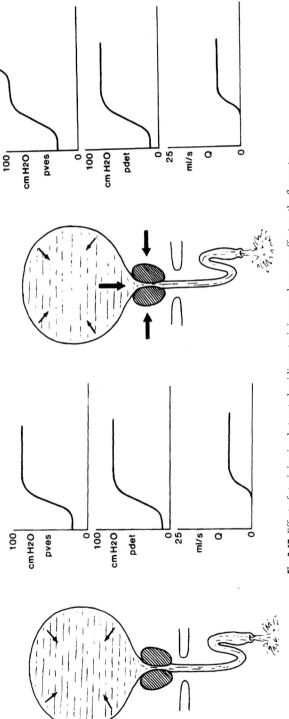

Fig. 3.67 Effect of straining in obstructed voiding: straining produces no effect on the flow rate.

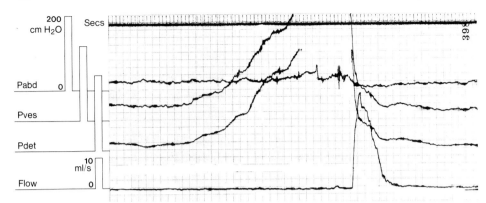

Fig. 3.68 Pressure–flow study in a case of bladder instability in a man of 28. Involuntary contraction of the bladder is producing a pressure of more than 260 cmH$_2$O; this pressure falls suddenly as soon as flow starts. The voided volume on this occasion was only 150 ml; the flow rate being achieved was 33 ml/s.

same force that is raising the intravesical pressure and trying to open the bladder neck: hence there is no effect of straining on flow in this situation (Fig. 3.67, *previous page*).

● *Detrusor instability* may produce a misleading trace. Because premicturition pressure may be very high, the patient may appear to be obstructed. Careful inspection reveals a normal voiding pressure and Q_{max} (Fig. 3.68).

The indications for cystometry are dealt with in Chapter 5 under patient groups.

References

Abrams P, Breskewitz R, de la Rossette J, Griffiths D, Koyanagi T, Nordling J, Park YC, Schafer W, Zimmern P (1995). The diagnosis of bladder outlet obstruction: Urodynamics. The 3rd International Consultation on BPH p 297.

Abrams P, Griffiths DJ (1979). The assessment of prostatic obstruction from urodynamic measurements and from residual urine. Br J Urol 51:129–134.

Cannon A, Tamnela T, Barrett D, Abrams P, Schafer W, Malice MP and the UDS study group (1996). Repeat pressure flow studies (pQS) in patients with benign prostatic obstruction (BPO). Neurourol Urodyn 15:387–390.

Coolsaet BL (1985). Bladder compliance and detrusor activity during collection phase. Neurourol Urodyn 4:263.

Coolsaet BL, Van Duyl WA, Van Mastright R, van der Zwart (1973). Stepwise cystometry of the urinary bladder. Urology II:255.

Griffiths DJ (1973). The mechanics of the urethra and micturition. Br J Urol 45:497–507.

Griffiths DJ, Van Mastrigt R, Bosch R (1989). Quantification of urethral resistance and bladder function during voiding, with special reference to the effects of prostate size reduction on urethral obstruction due to benign prostatic hyperplasia. Neurourol Urodyn 8:17–27.

Hellstrom PA, Tammela TLJ (1993). The bladder cooling test. Int Urogynaecol J 4:116.

Hellstrom PA, Tammela TLJ, Kontturi MJ et al. (1991). The bladder cooling test for urodynamic assessment: Analysis of 400 examinations. Br J Urol 67:275.

Hofner K, Kramer AEJL, Tan HK, Krah H, Jonas U (1995). CHESS classification of bladder outflow obstruction. A consequence in the discussion of current concepts. World J Urol 13:59–63.

James ED, Niblett PG, MacNaughton JA, Sheldon C (1987). The vagina as an alternative to the rectum in measuring abdominal pressure during urodynamic investigations. Br J Urol 60:212.

Klevmark B (1974). Motility of the urinary bladder in cats during filling at physiological rates. 1. Intravesical pressure patterns studied by a new method of cystometry. Acta Physiol Scand 90:565–577.

Lim CS, Abrams P (1995). The Abrams-Griffiths nomogram. World J Urol 13:34–39.

Merrill DC (1971). The air cystometer, a new instrument for evaluating bladder function. J Urol 106:865–866.

Reynard J, Lim CS, Abrams P (1995). Pressure flow studies in men: the obstructive effect of a urethral catheter. J Urol in press.

Ryall RL, Marshall VR (1982). The effect of a urethral catheter on the measurement of maximum urinary flow rate. J Urol 128:429–432.

Schäfer W (1990). Basic principles and clinical application of advanced analysis of bladder voiding function. Urol Clin N Am 17:553–566.

Sethia KK, Smith JC (1987). The effect of ph and lignocaine on detrusor instability. Br J Urol 60:516.

Sørensen S, Jonler M, Knudson UB, Djurhuus JC (1989). The influence of a urethral catheter and age on recorded urinary flow rates in healthy women. Scand J Urol Nephrol 23:261–266.

Spangberg A, Terio H, Engberg A, Ask P (1989). Quantification of urethral function based on Griffiths' model of flow through elastic tubes. Neurourol Urodyn 8:29–52.

Thomas DG (1979). Clinical urodynamics in neurogenic bladder dysfunction. Urol Clin N Am 6:237–253.

Torrens MJ (1977). A comparative evaluation of carbon dioxide and water cystometry and sphincterometry. Proc Int Cont Soc Portoroz 7:103–104.

Wein AJ, Hanno PM, Dixon DO, Raezer D, Benson GS (1978). The reproducibility and interpretation of carbon dioxide cystometry. J Urol 120:205–206.

Complex Urodynamic Investigations

Videourodynamics

The advent of cinefluoroscopy of the bladder in the early 1950s was a major stimulus to the development of a better understanding of lower urinary tract functionality. In the early 1960s pressure studies were synchronised with cystourethrography (Enhorning et al. 1964), providing further information, and this technique has been developed in certain larger urodynamic centres over the last decade as videourodynamics. However in some of these centres it is used as the routine investigation. The author has never agreed with this approach, arguing that video urodynamics should be reserved for more complicated patients where there is a high chance of anatomical abnormality coexisting with bladder and urethral dysfunction.

Imaging of the urinary tract both at rest and on coughing and straining, during filling and during voiding, allows the following useful information to be obtained:

- *Full, at rest.* Bladder capacity, shape, outline, e.g. diverticulum, trabeculation.
  Vesico-ureteric reflux at rest.
- *Strain/cough.* Assessment of degree of bladder base descent and bladder neck competence.
- *Voiding.* Speed and extent of bladder neck opening.
  Calibre and shape of urethra.
  Site of any urethral narrowing/urethral dilatation/diverticula
  Vesico-ureteric reflux.
- *"Stop test".* Speed and adequacy of voluntary urethral closure mechanism.
  "Milk back" from posterior urethra.
  Trapping of urine in prostatic urethra.
- *Post-voiding.* Residual urine.

For most routine problems conventional urodynamics are sufficient and the additional information given by simultaneous imaging of the urinary tract does not help the patient's management.

Equipment

VUDS requires an image of the urinary tract, given by either a fixed X-ray unit (Fig. 3.69) or an image intensifier (Fig. 3.70). Recently, some units have started to use ultrasound as an alternative, arguing that it gives a better image of the bladder outlet in women and eliminates the risks of irradiation from X-rays. Furthermore, recent data has suggested that the measurement of bladder wall thickness by ultra-

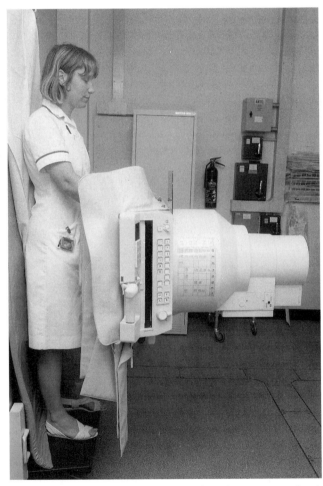

Fig. 3.69 X-ray unit: such apparatus, found only in radiology departments, makes it difficult for a woman to void in "a standing" position.

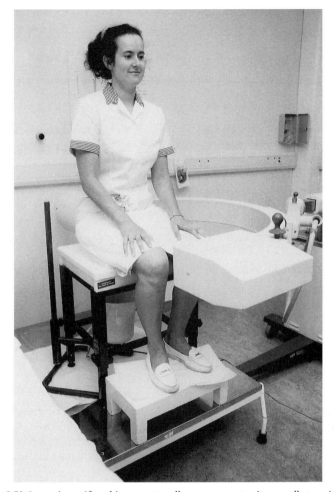

Fig. 3.70 Image intensifier: this apparatus allows a woman to sit normally to void.

sound may be a guide to the diagnosis of detrusor instability (DI): the thicker the wall the more likely there is to be DI. Ultrasound has its limitations:

- Particularly in the male it cannot easily be used to visualise the whole urethra.
- If a vector scanner is used at the introitus in women then there is distortion requiring correction before taking measurements (a linear array scanner cannot be used, because it may alter the vaginal anatomy by its presence).
- The upper tracts cannot be visualised synchronously.
- Apart from bladder wall thickness, other aspects of bladder wall anatomy are not as well seen.

In view of the limitations of ultrasound, X-ray is still used in most urodynamic departments to image the urinary tract. We have chosen to use our image intensifier system for several reasons:

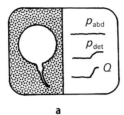 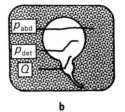

a   **b**

Fig. 3.71 Videourodynamics: **a** screen split with X-ray image and urodynamic data separated; **b** urodynamics superimposed over X-ray image.

- We are independent of the X-ray department and can therefore use the system at any time. In most units VUDS is carried out in the X-ray department during set sessions.
- We have been able to create a more friendly and less hostile atmosphere than in the more utilitarian X-ray department.
- The patient can sit or stand in a natural position, ensuring the least inhibition to voiding.

However there are disadvantages:

- The image quality is not as high as with fixed X-ray units, particularly if the patient is obese and a lateral view is needed to visualise the bladder neck because it is obscured by anterior vaginal wall descent in the AP (anterio-posterior) view.
- We have to pay to replace the X-ray equipment – a not inconsiderable sum!

There are many companies that supply equipment for VUDS. These systems are computerised and convert the analogue urodynamic signals to a digital format; they then mix these with the digitised X-ray image to produce a combined image on the TV or computer screen. The presentation of data may be by either of two main methods:

- On a split screen, with the urodynamic traces on one side and the X-ray picture on the other (Fig. 3.71a).
- By superimposition of urodynamic traces over the X-ray image. The traces can be faded so as not to obscure the X-ray image (Fig. 3.71b).

Alterations in Technique During Videourodynamics

- Certain changes in urodynamic technique are necessary to accommodate to the radiological environment. The first is that the contrast medium used for visualising the bladder is of a density different from that of urine. This means that adjustments may have to be made to the flowmeter, which would otherwise record an artefactually high reading because of the greater weight of the voided fluid.
- If it is necessary for women to void in the standing position then a specially shaped funnel system needs to be used to collect the voided urine and pass it to the flowmeter. This may delay further the registration of the flow tracing on

the polygraph, relative to the pressure. However, as long as this potential problem is recognised it is unlikely to cause any practical difficulties.
- If the patient is to void in the sitting position some further modification of technique may be required. The simplest way to provide a radiotranslucent commode seat is to construct a thick foam cushion, cut to the shape of a toilet seat, and cover it with a hygienic material. Certain X-ray manufacturers have this equipment available.
- It is useful to be able to visualise the bladder neck in the straight lateral projection. This may mean an increase in the radiation exposure, but is facilitated by the use of special high-density contrast (260 mg I/ml). Such contrast has a higher density and viscosity, though this is less significant if the contrast is heated to 37 °C. The effect on flow is not as great as might be expected because the flow is less turbulent.

Interpretation of Videourodynamics

If VUDS is performed with synchronous intraurethral pressure measurement and pelvic floor electromygraphy then a perfect demonstration of the mechanisms of continence (voiding) can be obtained:

Normal Results. Videourodynamics allows the relationships between anatomical events, for example bladder neck opening, to be related to hydrodynamic recordings. The normal sequence of events on voiding is as follows:

- Bladder base descent
  Urethral pressure decrease
  Reduced sphincter EMG activity
- Bladder neck opening
  Detrusor pressure increase
  EMG silent
- Flow in progress
  Detrusor pressure maximal
  EMG silent
- Urethral pressure increased
  Flow ends, no residual urine
  Detrusor pressure usually decreases, but may increase (after contraction)
  EMG transiently increases

If urine flow is voluntarily interrupted in "mid stream" (the stop test), then the stream is interrupted at the level of the pelvic floor. The urine in the proximal part of the urethra is "milked back" into the bladder, the bladder base then elevates and the bladder neck closes. When the pelvic floor and urethral sphincter are strong, which often happens with bladder overactivity, bladder base elevation may appear quite forceful and has been described as a "kick". Under these circumstances the isometric detrusor pressure ($p_{det, iso}$) usually reaches a high level.

During the filling phase of VUDS the bladder neck should be closed, although the bladder neck in up to 50% of continent post-menopausal women opens on

coughing. However in younger women and men, if it is seen to open either spontaneously or during stress or postural change, this is abnormal. Such an opening may
be due to intrinsic incompetence of the bladder neck or because the bladder neck is
being opened in association with an unstable detrusor contraction. On voiding, the
bladder neck should open widely. If it is seen to remain closed this may be because
the detrusor is not contracting strongly enough (low p_{det}) or because the bladder
neck itself is failing to relax (detrusor–bladder neck dysynergia) and so producing
obstruction (high p_{det}). A clue to its existence is the presence of "trapping" of
contrast in the posterior urethra, proximal to the distal urethral sphincter mechanism, owing to failure of retrograde emptying of the urethra. Alternatively the failure
of the bladder neck to open may be due to fibrosis (bladder neck contraction) or to
benign prostatic enlargement "splinting" the bladder neck.

Urethral overactivity during voiding occurs in neuropathic vesico-urethral
dysfunction and is characterised by a narrowing at the level of the distal urethral
sphincter mechanism, proximal to which the posterior urethra is distended by
the force of the detrusor pressure. This subvesical distension may emphasise the
bladder neck, which appears as a bar or ring on X-ray or endoscopy. The bladder
neck may also appear prominent as part of a global detrusor hypertrophy
secondary to detrusor overactivity.

Advantages and Disadvantages of Videourodynamics

VUDS has some advantages over basic urodynamics but there are also
disadvantages:

Advantages

- Combining X-ray and urodynamic investigations, VUDS offers the most
  comprehensive means of assessment. For example radiology is the best way to
  localise the site of urethral obstruction.
- Videotape recording improves case review sessions, and teaching promotes a
  greater interest and understanding of urodynamics by allowing clinicians to
  relate the urodynamic measurements to familiar structural and radiological
  features.
- Sound recording on the tape adds another dimension to assessment, as well as
  allowing more spontaneous recording of incidental observations.

Disadvantages

- Not all patients need radiological imaging; in these patients VUDS will
  lead to unnecessary X-ray exposure. Clinicians should select out such patients.
- Expensive urodynamic equipment may be lying idle in the X-ray department
  for four days a week unless it is portable and is used for basic urodynamics
  elsewhere.
- The unnatural environment for voiding leads to psychological suppression of
  micturition in many patients (up to 30% of women). Women especially dislike
  voiding "in public".
- If VUDS are conducted in the X-ray department the busy atmosphere may
  mean there is less time for the clinician to spend with the patient in history-

taking and discussion. We have found that the overall benefit of assessment depends very much on the time allowed to understand the patient's problem and to set the patient at ease.

Is There a Role for Micturating Cystourethrography (MCUG)?

If VUDS is not readily available in your own hospital or in a nearby centre then MCUG can be of value. Much information can be acquired by asking the radiologist to take the following films or, even better, record the whole investigation on videotape.

- AP films at rest, on straining and on coughing.
- Lateral film during voiding.

Indications for VUDS

The prime indication for VUDS is when anatomical information is required as well as physiological (urodynamic) data.

- Defining the site of bladder outlet obstruction: VUDS is the best method and is important when the level of obstruction cannot be predicted, unlike in the older man when the prostate is overwhelmingly likely to be the culprit.
- In women the main area of anatomical interest is the bladder base when the clinician is looking for information on bladder neck position, bladder base support and the function of the pelvic floor.
- Patients with neurological disease likely to cause vesico-urethral dysfunction are best investigated by VUDS. In this group of patients there are likely to be both anatomical abnormalities (for example vesicoureteric reflux and bladder diverticula) as well as voiding dysfunction such as detrusor and sphincter dyssynergia.
- Patients with post-operative problems, for example, men with post-prostatectomy incontinence, should be investigated by VUDS in order to acquire the maximum amount of information prior to further invasive therapy such as artificial sphincter implantation.

Indications for VUDS – Summary

- Suspected bladder outlet obstruction in younger patients.
- Children with abnormal voiding in whom invasive therapy is contemplated.
- Recurrent female stress incontinence if further surgery is planned.
- Neuropathic vesico-urethral dysfunction.
- Postprostatectomy incontinence prior to artificial sphincter implantation.
- Impaired renal function without intrinsic renal disease where urethral over-activity may be a cause.

Ambulatory Urodynamics (AUDS)

In the previous edition of this book (1983) AUDS did not appear in the index and there was only a passing mention of the pioneering work of Douglas James in Exeter. He was considered idiosyncratic in his decision to investigate patients using natural-fill cystometry and to allow the patient to walk around the uro-dynamic investigation room, something he was able to achieve by using air-filled lines rather than water-filled ones to link the patient to the transducer. The air-filled lines minimised the movement artefacts that prevent fluid-filled lines being used in this situation. Dr James's patients were restricted by the length of the cabling connecting the transducers mounted on a belt around the patient's waist to the urodynamic apparatus.

Little changed until the later 1980s, when workers in Bristol, Maastricht, Newcastle and Oslo developed their own home-made ambulatory systems. Subsequently several companies have developed commercially available systems based on the use of catheter-mounted transducers connected to a microcomputer worn over the shoulder by the patient (Fig. 3.72). This arrangement allows real

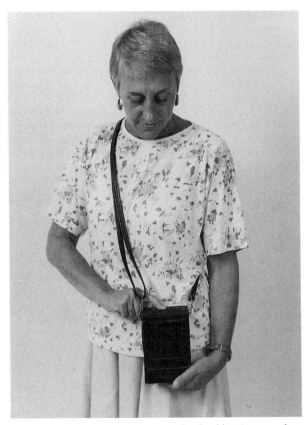

Fig. 3.72 Ambulatory UDS: microcomputer worn over the shoulder. Event marker allows the patient to code events such as urgency or leakage.

freedom of movement to the extent that the patient can reproduce the activities that produce incontinence. In principle these systems are the same as those used for conventional UDS and the same basic methodology applies.

AUDS are used when conventional UDS fail to achieve the prime aim of UDS, which is, as stated on page 1, to "provide a pathophysiological explanation for the patient's symptoms". Our prime indications for AUDS are:

Technique of Ambulatory Urodynamics

We record three micturition cycles during AUDS: a resting cycle when the patient sits in a chair; an ambulent cycle when the patient moves around the hospital, and an exercising cycle which should include any specific incontinence-provoking measures, for example walking downstairs or, in a more extreme way, performing an overhead smash in tennis! Once the three cycles are recorded then the information has to be downloaded onto a personal computer for analysis. The analysis is relatively time-consuming and requires considerable expertise.

The data acquired during AUDS should include voiding data and information on urine leakage. There are problems associated with both these areas.

Urine Leakage. Because one of the prime indications for AUDS is the detection of incontinence, it is important that the episode of leakage is recorded synchronously with the pressure data. However recording urine leak has proved

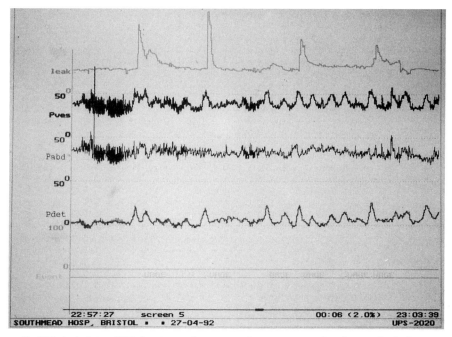

Fig. 3.73 Ambulatory UDS showing on the top trace the temperature rises due to urine leakage.

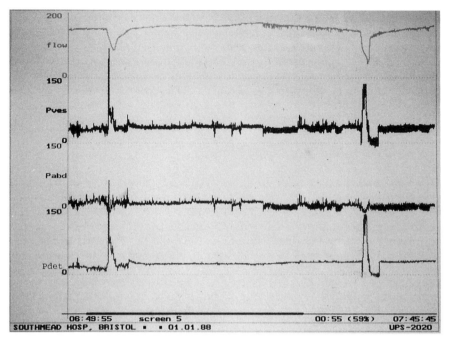

Fig. 3.74 Ambulatory UDS: a normal study; the falls in the temperature trace are due to the pants being removed at normal voids.

problematic: methods have included the Exeter nappy and temperature-sensitive techniques. The Exeter nappy is a body-worn garment in which there is a network of wires in a grid arrangement. A small current is passed through the grid and when leakage occurs, because urine conducts electricity, part of the grid is short-circuited. By measuring the resistance of the grid the occurrence of leakage and to some extent the degree of leakage can be recorded. However, the nappy is rather bulky and somewhat uncomfortable. A temperature-sensitive device has been developed at Bristol in which temperature-sensitive diodes are implanted in a standard incontinence pad, giving a constant reading of perineal temperature of approximately 35 °C. When the patient leaks the temperature of the pad is increased because urine is at body temperature (Fig. 3.73, *previous page*). On the other hand, when the patient undresses to void the pad temperature falls (Fig. 3.74) as the pad is taken away from the body.

Voiding Data. The patient unit should allow the connection of a flowmeter so that the urine flow rate can be recorded synchronously with intravesical and intra-abdominal pressure. Unless this is achieved it is difficult to deduce whether or not bladder outlet obstruction exists.

As well as measuring p_{abd}, p_{ves}, flow and leakage the AUDS equipment should have an event-maker which the patient uses in conjunction with a diary to signal sensations such as first desire to void, urgency or leakage episodes. In the diary the patient is also asked to record their activities so that leakage episodes can be correlated with physical and other activities.

Interpretation of Ambulatory Urodynamics

As well as providing the evidence for, and the cause of, the patient's incontinence, much additional interesting information is being generated by AUDS. Present ideas on detrusor instability, compliance and voiding function are being questioned. AUDS on normal individuals have shown a 30% incidence of detrusor instability, although this is of no significance to the individual unless it is accompanied by urgency and urge incontinence. This provides yet another illustration of the aim of urodynamics "to provide a pathophysiological explanation of the patient's symptoms". In a neurologically normal person, without symptoms, the finding of DI is not significant, particularly if a third of normal individuals can be shown to have such findings. Does DI in these circumstances have any positive significance? There are a number of ways in which these findings might be explained:

- By all people being shown to have DI if studied for long enough.
- By DI being an artefact of investigation due to the presence of an intravesical catheter.
- By the 30% of normal individuals with DI developing symptoms of bladder overactivity in future years.

Klevmark showed that bladder compliance is related to the speed of bladder filling, and AUDS has confirmed this fact. In two groups of patients in whom conventional UDS frequently shows low compliance (namely neuropathic patients and older men with "high-pressure chronic retention"), AUDS has shown that if the bladder is filled naturally then low compliance disappears and is replaced by the finding of phasic detrusor instability. However in both groups there are higher filling pressures than in patients with BOO or neuropathy who have DI (Fig. 3.55).

Voiding pressures during AUDS have been shown to be significantly higher than during conventional UDS (in most females). The explanation for this finding may be common to both higher voiding pressures and the apparent uncovering of DI in patients with low compliance on conventional UDS. Fast filling may prevent the detrusor from showing its full contractile pressures, either because fast fill interferes with the mechanical reorganisation of the muscle or because the biochemical environment of the detrusor is altered. A similar phenomenon can be experienced by any of us if we allow our bladder to overfill with the result that we have hesitancy and poor flow.

Indications for Ambulatory UDS

- To confirm the patient's history of incontinence where conventional UDS has been normal;
- to determine whether detrusor instability or sphincter weakness is the main cause of incontinence if the patient desires further treatment.

AUDS is a valuable method of investigating the lower urinary tract. However the tests are time-consuming and require considerable interpretative skills. AUDS is best used only in the larger units with extensive experience of basic UDS.

Urethral Function Studies

As described in the section earlier in this chapter on cystometry, urethral function can be inferred from the findings during filling and voiding. If the patient is continent, urethral function during filling is satisfactory. If voiding is unobstructed then full urethral relaxation can assume to have taken place. However both criteria are met by few patients attending urodynamic clinics, because there is a high likelihood of urethral dysfunction. There are a number of possible ways in which urethral function can be measured more accurately:

- Urethral pressure profilometry (UPP)
  - Static
  - Dynamic or stress
  - Voiding
- Urethral electrical conductance
- Fluid bridge test
- Leak point pressure estimation

These tests are clinically used as aids in the diagnosis of incontinence with the exception of voiding UPP, which is used in a few centres to diagnose the presence and site of bladder outlet obstruction. The diagnosis of incontinence is best made by seeing urine leave the external urinary meatus, because this is a *direct* means of diagnosing incontinence. Urethral function studies represent an *indirect* method of diagnosis.

Static Urethral Pressure Profilometry

Definitions

- *The urethral pressure profile (UPP)* indicates the intraluminal pressure along the length of the urethra with the bladder at rest. Appendix 1, Part 1, shows the ICS terminology for urethral pressure measurement. The zero pressure reference point is again taken as the superior edge of the symphysis pubis. When describing the method, it is necessary to specify the catheter type and size, the measurement technique, the rate of infusion (if the Brown and Wickham technique (see below) is used), the rate of catheter withdrawal, the bladder volume and the position of the patient.
- *Maximum urethral pressure* is the maximum pressure of the measured profile.
- *Maximum urethral closure pressure* is the difference between the maximum urethral pressure and the intravesical pressure.
- *Functional profile length* is the length of the urethra along which the urethral pressure exceeds intravesical pressure.

Techniques. Three main methods for urethral pressure measurements are currently used. The Brown and Wickham technique is the best-known method of measuring urethral pressures at rest (Fig. 3.75). However catheter tip transducers may be used, although there is a rotational effect depending in which direction the transducer faces: MUP is highest if it is anterior-facing and lowest if posterior-facing, so it is suggested that it should be pointed facing laterally. Balloon catheters have previously been used but require frequent recalibration.

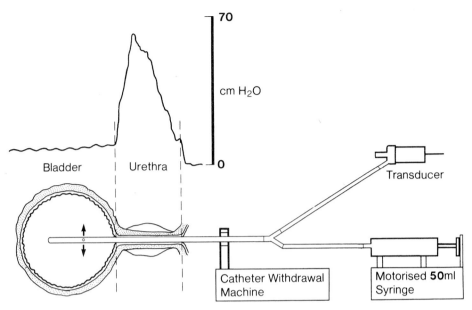

Fig. 3.75 Brown and Wickham technique.

Fluid Perfusion Profilometry

The basis of the Brown and Wickham technique is the measurement of the pressure needed to perfuse a catheter at a constant rate. The catheter is passed into the bladder and withdrawn slowly through the urethra. The catheter has eyeholes 5 cm from its tip through which the perfusion fluid escapes into the bladder or urethra. The constant infusion is maintained by a syringe pump. The technique has been shown experimentally to be measuring the occlusive pressure of the urethral walls. Figure 3.75 illustrates the equipment required for urethral closure pressure profile measurement using this technique.

Catheter Size. There is no appreciable difference in pressure measurements provided the catheter is between sizes 4 and 10 FG. It seems likely that the sizes above 10 FG may record urethral elasticity as well as urethral closure pressure and therefore give falsely high readings. The comparison of pressure between small and much larger catheters may provide a basis for measuring urethral elasticity.

Catheter Eyeholes. A single end-hole or side-hole is known to be inaccurate, the first because of the lack of adequate mucosal contact and the second owing to differences in pressure measurement due to orientation. A catheter with two opposing side-holes set back from the catheter tip is known to be of adequate accuracy. The presence of more than two holes does not improve the accuracy significantly. If the holes are 5 cm from the tip then catheterisation is facilitated.

Rate of Perfusion. It is desirable that the catheter is perfused at a constant rate. This necessitates the use of a motorised syringe pump *or a very accurate peristaltic pump.* A perfusion rate of between 2 and 10 ml/min gives an accurate measurement of closure pressure. Perfusion rates of less than 2 ml/min usually fail to record the true urethral pressure unless an extremely slow withdrawal rate is used. The reason for this is outlined below. Perfusion rates in excess of 10 ml/min are likely to lead to falsely high readings, because at such rate the fluid cannot escape from the catheter eyeholes along the urethra fast enough.

Rate of Catheter Withdrawal. It is most satisfactory to withdraw the catheter mechanically at a constant speed using a motorised system. Speeds of less than 0.7 cm/s are satisfactory when used with perfusion rates of 2 to 10 ml/min.

Response Time. The technique of UPP requires great attention to detail and illustrates most of the general problems that must be appreciated in order to perform good-quality urodynamics. The issue of response time is important for all urodynamic techniques, particularly now that computerised systems with their limited sampling rates have become the most frequently used systems (see "Cystometry"). The attention to technique is vital and the methods discussed above should allow the investigator to measure pressure profiles accurately. However it is still essential to assess each individual measurement system for its recording accuracy. The response time of the system should be calculated. In a Brown and Wickham system this is most easily done by occluding the eyeholes of the perfused catheter during recording. A graph of pressure against time will be obtained (Fig. 3.76). The slope of the line will give the maximum response at that perfusion rate as centimetres of water per second; for example, if the system has a maximum response at a given perfusion rate of 50 cmH$_2$O per second and the urethral pressure rises by 100 cmH$_2$O in the proximal 2 cm of the urethra then it follows that the catheter must not be withdrawn faster than 1 cm/s at the test infusion rate or the pressure will be underestimated. The response time of the system is determined by three factors: the length and diameter of the tubing from

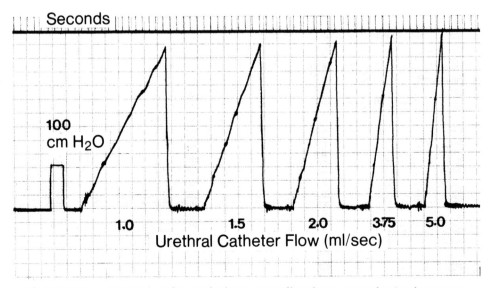

Fig. 3.76 Varying response times for a urethral pressure profile catheter system, showing the pressure response to catheter occlusion at different infusion rates.

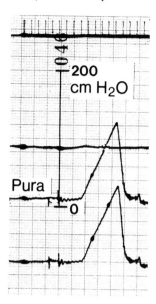

Fig. 3.77 Artifactual "saw tooth" urethral pressure profile, with a straight ascending limb which underestimates the actual urethral pressure. The abbreviations in figures correspond to those suggested by the International Continence Society (Appendix 1, Part 2).

the patient to the external pressure-measuring transducer, the rate of catheter perfusion and the speed of catheter withdrawal. In practice a 100 cm length of manometer tubing is a satisfactory means of connecting the profile catheter to the pressure transducer and to the syringe pump.

By studying the shape of the urethral pressure profile it is relatively easy to decide whether the response time has been adequate to obtain an accurate profile. The tracing we describe as a "sawtooth" profile (Fig. 3.77) is diagnostic of an inaccurately measured maximum urethral pressure. The upstroke of the profile is smooth and straight and looks unphysiological. The downstroke is usually faster than the upstroke and more irregular. If such a profile is recorded then the perfusion rate should be increased or the withdrawal rate decreased. Other factors influencing the response time of the system are air bubbles or fluid leaks.

Reproducibility of the Urethral Pressure Profile

Provided that suitable attention has been paid to detail of technique, the results are highly reproducible. Certain "normal" variations in the urethral pressure profile have been described. The most common reason for pressure fluctuation is voluntary contraction of the urethral or periurethral musculature. It seems likely that most of the maximum urethral pressure of the resting profile is produced by the intramural urethral striated muscle described by Gosling (1979). If the patient is not relaxed during urethral pressure profile measurement then the pelvic floor, which lies in close proximity to the urethra, may by its contraction produce a pressure increment along the urethra. This can be recorded deliberately by asking the patient to contract the pelvic floor voluntarily as if they were holding on when desperate to pass urine. If the urethra is sensitive it is not uncommon for the first urethral profiles to be of a higher pressure because of the failure of the patient to relax. If reproducible profiles cannot be obtained in any particular case then this is an indication for the performance of a profile which records the maximum urethral pressure with a stationary catheter over a longer period of time. Sometimes vascular pulsations are seen on such recordings; this is not abnormal.

Effect of Posture on the Urethral Pressure Profile

From the technical point of view it is easier to perform urethral profiles if the patient is supine. Most tests are performed in this position. The posture of the patient does have a considerable influence on urethral muscle tone. The normal response to the assumption of a more upright posture is an increase in the maximum urethral closure pressure of about 23%. In some abnormal patients this increase may not occur, and in others, some neuropathic, the increase in pressure may be excessive (greater than 100%). The absence of an increase in pressure on standing may be a diagnostic test for genuine stress incontinence (Tanagho 1979).

The Normal Urethral Pressure Profile

The figures for normal urethral pressures in the available literature are all taken from very small series. The figures in Table 3.4 below are taken from a large number of our patients who have been assessed and considered to be both clinically and urodynamically normal. The figures are for patients who are in a supine position with the bladder empty. Adequate information on normal pressures in other postures and for other bladder volumes is not available. This does limit the value of urethral pressure profile measurement, because it is the urethral response to bladder filling and postural change which may be most important in diagnosis.

There are certain sex differences. In the male, the maximum urethral pressure does not decline significantly with age, whereas in the female, particularly after the menopause, the maximum urethral pressure is lower. Similarly, in the male, the prostatic length tends to increase with age while in the female the maximum urethral pressure and the functional urethral length tend to decrease (see Figs 3.78 and 3.79).

Table 3.4. Values for maximum urethral pressure (cmH_2O) in patients in whom no abnormality has been found

| Age | Male | | Female | |
---	Mean	Range	Mean	Range
< 25	75	37 to 126	90	55 to 103
25 to 44	79	35 to 113	82	31 to 115
45 to 64	75	40 to 123	74[a]	40 to 100
> 64	71	35 to 105	65[a]	35 to 75

[a] Edwards (1973) quotes figures for normal urethral pressure in the over-45 age groups that are much lower than this, in the range of 20 to 50 cmH_2O.

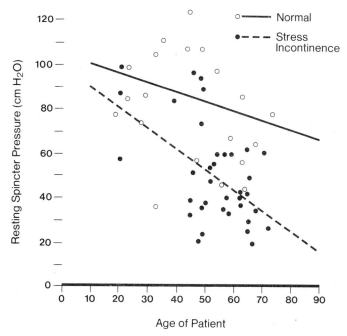

Fig. 3.78 Resting maximum urethral pressure plotted against age in normal and stress-incontinent patients, with regression lines calculated statistically.

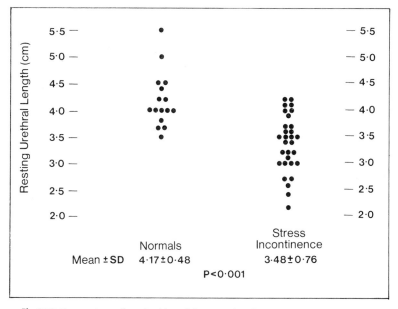

Fig. 3.79 Comparison of urethral length in normal and stress-incontinent females.

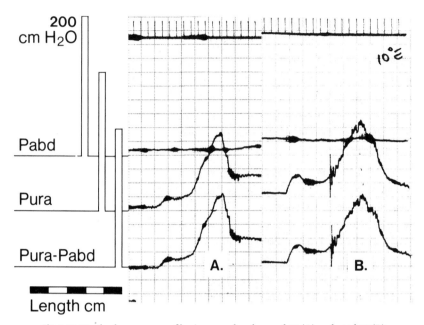

Fig. 3.80 Urethral pressure profiles in normal males aged 14 (A) and aged 50 (B).

It is evident that there is a wide overlap between the range for normal urethral parameters and for abnormal situations, e.g. stress incontinence. There is a better correlation between normality and abnormality if an index is used. This is most commonly some estimate of total urethral muscle function such as maximum urethral closure pressure × functional length or, alternatively, a measurement of the area beneath the urethral pressure profile curve.

The shape of the urethral profile is of diagnostic importance. In the normal male the most important part of the profile, from a functional point of view, is that between the bladder neck and the membranous urethra. The distal bulbar and penile urethra are very variable in length and are not usually described. Certain constant features are seen in male profiles. The presphincteric part of the trace shows, even in boys, a pressure increase due to prostatic tissue (Fig. 3.80). The presphincteric pressure area blends with the pressure zone attributed to the distal urethral sphincter mechanism, which in itself should be more or less symmetrical. As the male patient gets older the length of the presphincteric profile (prostatic length) increases and the pressure within this area may become higher. This is not necessarily abnormal within certain limits.

The normal female urethral pressure profile is symmetrical in shape (Fig. 3.81) and asymmetry is generally due to a faulty measurement technique, e.g. the saw-tooth profile.

Classification of Urethral Pressure Profile Abnormalities

Abnormalities may be classified according to the part of the urethra affected and the sex of the patient.

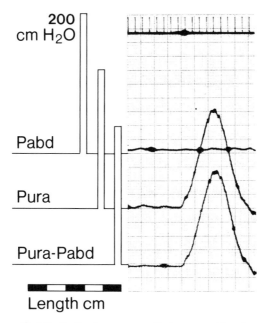

Fig. 3.81 Urethral pressure profile in a normal female.

Presphincteric abnormalities are usually seen in male patients with bladder neck or prostatic problems. Commonly, the prostatic plateau may be elevated or elongated. This plateau may be flat or there may be a prostatic peak between the bladder neck and the distal urethral sphincter mechanism (Fig. 3.82). The significance of this peak is uncertain. If it is at the region of the bladder neck then

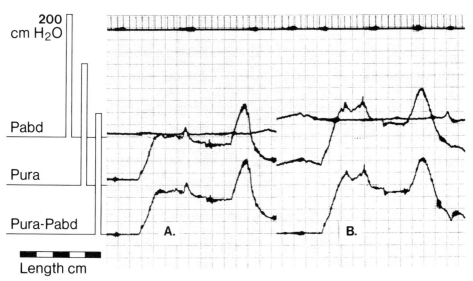

Fig. 3.82 Urethral pressure profile showing a bladder neck and prostatic peak in a man of 60. These peaks are not so prominent in the supine position (A) as they are in the erect position (B).

it is sometimes due to bladder neck hypertrophy. A bladder neck peak may also occur on penile erection. A peak in the mid-prostatic region may be related to the meeting of the lateral lobes of a hyperplastic gland. Presphincteric abnormalities in the female are usually produced by surgery where an elongation is related to operations which suspend the bladder neck.

Sphincteric abnormalities are confined to the area of the main urethral pressure peak: mid-urethra in the female and just near the prostatic apex in the male. The pressure here is either too low or too high and may be assessed either at rest or during voluntary contractions, as well as in relation to postural and bladder volume changes. Low pressure is related to damage, atrophy or denervation (Fig. 3.83).

An abnormally high pressure is usually related to involuntary sphincter overactivity or sphincter hypertrophy. In the latter case the high pressure is seen only on voluntary contraction when the pressure may reach about 300 cmH$_2$O and this is most commonly encountered while investigating adult enuretics of both sexes with unstable bladders. Recently described by Fowler has been a group of women with difficulty in voiding due to sphincter overactivity. Many of these patients have abnormally high urethral pressures due to overactivity of the intraurethral strited muscle.

Postsphincteric abnormalities are less common. Rigid urethral strictures are not well demonstrated by the profile techniques. Adequate demonstration of a stricture depends on the recording catheter being of exactly the same gauge as the stricture, or slightly larger. A small peak, because of mental stenosis, may be seen in females. Occasionally the urethral pressure from the bulbocavernosus muscle in the male will be greater than that at the region of the distal urethral sphincter

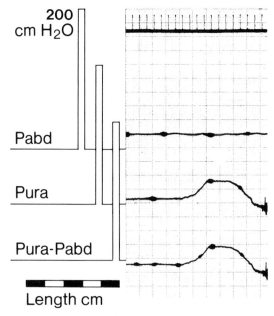

Fig. 3.83 Abnormally low urethral pressure profile in a woman of 84.

mechanism. The significance of this findings and other changes, with age and sexual activity, have not been investigated.

The "Stress" Urethral Profile

This concept of the "stress" profile was introduced by Asmussen and Ulmsten in 1976. Bladder pressure measurement can be made simultaneous with urethral pressure if a suitable dual-lumen catheter is used. For accurate measurement the catheter tip transducer system is recommended. The measuring catheter is withdrawn very slowly through the urethra (1 to 2 mm/s), as described above, with the patient coughing at regular intervals. An alternative method is to hold the measuring catheter stationary at 0.5 cm intervals down the urethra while the patient performs a Valsalva manoeuvre to a predetermined pressure. This method measures the efficiency of pressure transmission into the proximal

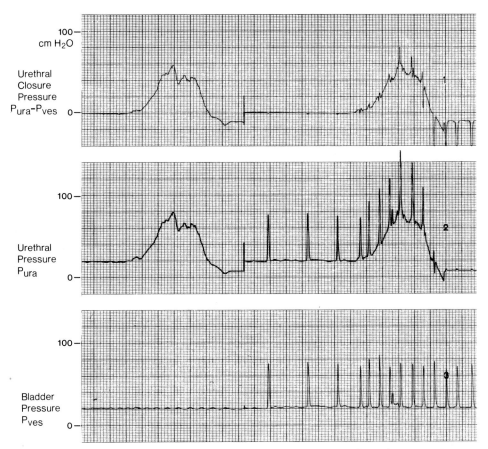

Fig. 3.84 Urethral closure pressure profile (*left*) and "stress" urethral profile (*right*) in a continent female patient. The urethral closure pressure (*upper trace*) does not become negative until the point of maximum urethral pressure has been passed.

urethra from the abdominal cavity. It is now well known that decreased conduction of increased intra-abdominal pressure is associated with genuine stress incontinence. The transmission may be expressed as the closure pressure, which is the urethral pressure minus the intravesical pressure. If the closure pressure becomes negative on coughing then leakage is likely to occur. Closure pressure may be derived electronically by subtracting intravesical pressure from intraurethral pressure, and this may be displayed on the chart recorder (Fig. 3.84, *previous page*) The best correlation between genuine stress incontinence and the findings on stress UPP is found if the test is done with a full bladder and the patient in the exact position. In GSI the classical stress UPP shows dips in close pressure below the 0 cmH$_2$O baseline (Fig. 3.85). Equivocal stress UPPs show dips in the closure pressure trace without reaching the zero line (Fig. 3.86). As with

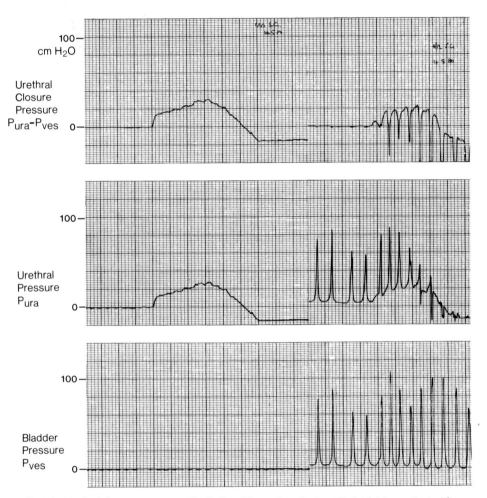

Fig. 3.85 Urethral closure pressure profile (*left*) and "stress" urethral profile (*right*) in a patient with a low urethral closure pressure, and poor transmission of cough pressure to the urethra. The urethral closure pressure becomes negative on coughing.

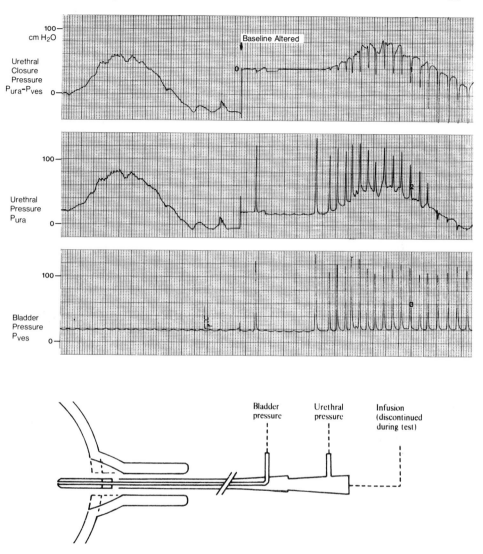

Fig. 3.86 "Equivocal stress UPP", where the negative dips on the upper trace reach but don't go below the 0 baseline. The patient has an acceptable static maximum urethral closure pressure of 60 cmH$_2$O.

static UPP, there is lack of specificity when normal stress UPPs are analysed against the presence or absence of GSI, there being many false negatives where the stress UPP is normal yet the patient on filling cystometry can be demonstrated to have GSI. The stress UPP has greater diagnostic specificity when it is abnormal or equivocal, when most patients will be found to have GSI.

There is probably little role for stress UPP unless it is carried out in the erect patient with a full bladder: the easiest position in which to demonstrate GSI.

However we have used the supine position with 200 ml in the bladder, because the erect position is more difficult from the technical point of view; for example, the withdrawal device must be held vertically and the catheter tends to fall out unless carefully supported.

Fluid Bridge Test

The fluid bridge test is designed to test bladder neck competence. As Fig. 3.87 shows, the principle of this technique is to position a catheter just distal to the bladder neck; when the patient coughs, if the bladder neck opens then there is a continuous water (urine) column and there will be leakage from the catheter. This test has never gained popularity, because movement artefacts have been suspected as a problem: it has been suggested that if the bladder neck is poorly supported by the pelvic floor and pubourethral ligaments then the bladder neck may move downwards, leading to the catheter tip entering the bladder lumen and therefore mimicking bladder neck incompetence. The same argument may be directed at the accurate measurement of stress UPP, particularly in the first centimetre of the urethra measured from the bladder neck. Also of importance is the videourodynamic finding that 50% of continent postmenopausal women have incompetent bladder necks at rest or on coughing.

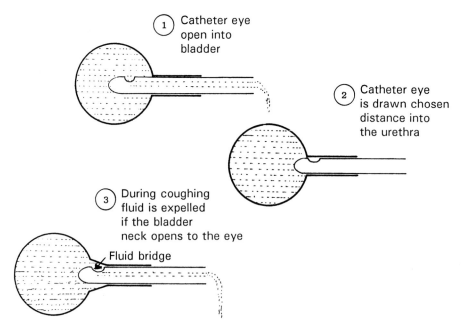

Fig. 3.87 Fluid bridge test.

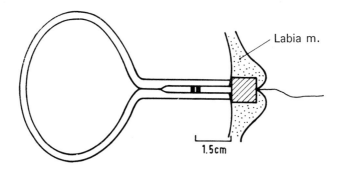

Fig. 3.88 Distal urethral electrical conductance test.

Urethral Electrical Conductance (UEC)

This is an electrical fluid bridge test and can be measured either at the bladder neck (BNEC) or in the distal female urethra (DUEC). The DUEC can distinguish between the shortlived increase in conductance seen in GSI and the more lengthy increase seen when incontinence is secondary to DI. The principle of both methods is that the resistance to the current flow between the two electrodes on the catheter will reduce, resulting in an increase in current, if there is urine in the area between the two electrodes (Fig. 3.88).

The UEC has little place in diagnostics but has been used in two particular circumstances:

- In needle suspension surgery for GSI the BNEC can be used to determine how tightly the sutures must be tied in order to achieve bladder neck closure.
- In patients with sensory urgency the BNEC has been used as part of a bio-feedback technique to teach patients how to voluntarily close the bladder neck and abolish the symptoms of urgency.

Urethral Leak point Pressure Measurement

This technique was described by McGuire and seeks to define overall urethral function in terms of the intravesical pressure at which urine starts to leak from the urethra. It is also known as Valsalva leak point pressure (VLPP) and the Valsalva manoeuvre (expiration against the closed glottis) is the easiest and most controlled way of achieving a graded increase in intravesical pressure. The technique is based on the assumption that the urethral catheter present during the test does not significantly alter the seal of the urethra. It also assumes that straining does not produce urethral distortion, which might falsely raise the VLPP. The third assumption is that there is no pelvic floor relaxation or con-traction during the test. While the technique has not been examined as closely from the technical point of view, as urethral pressure profilometry, it is clear that there is an association between poor urethral function and a low VLPP.

The VLPP has been used:

- To identify those women with GSI who have intrinsic urethral failure rather than hypermobility as the cause of their incontinence (abdominal LPP).
- To predict which meningomyelocele children will develop upper tract dilatation secondary to obstructed voiding due to well-preserved sphincter function (detrusor LPP; see Chapter 5).

Indicators for Urethral Function Testing

Specific indicators for testing have been discussed in the sections on urethral electrical conductance and leak point pressure measurement. In view of the poor specificity of stress UPP, its use has declined significantly. The measurement of static UPP has several uses:

- In postprostatectomy incontinence there is a close association between sphincter damage and reduction in maximum urethral closure pressure (MUCP).
- In women with GSI there is some evidence that a preoperative MUCP of less than 20 cmH$_2$O is associated with poor outcome. If further research bears this out then UPP measurement may define a group of women who require "obstructive" surgery in order to become continent.
- In women with unexplained incontinence measurement of MUCP for a period of minutes may show urethral instability (Fig. 3.89).
- In patents being considered for undiversion the MUCP gives a good indication as to whether implantation of an artificial sphincter or bladder neck suspension is necessary. If the MUCP is greater than 50 cmH$_2$O then the patient will be continent if a good-volume, low-pressure reservoir is created.

Neurophysiological Testing

There are no urodynamic centres using routine neurophysiological assessment in Great Britain. Some centres in North America, Continental Europe and Japan do use these techniques more frequently. There is no doubt that neurophysiological testing has been, is and will be most important in developing a better understanding of lower urinary tract function. The question is, "What additional information do these tests give that helps patient investigation and management?"

There are two situations where testing may influence diagnosis or help in management:

- In women who have voiding difficulty or who are in retention, by using bipolar urethral sphincter electromyography Fowler has shown a high percentage to have electrically bizarre sphincter activity as the likely cause.
- In children with dysfunctional voiding perineal, skin surface patch electrodes can be used, as part of biofeedback, to train the child to properly relax the pelvic floor muscles during voiding.

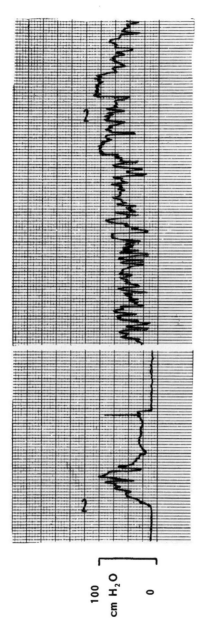

100
cm H₂O

0

M.U.C.P.

Fig. 3.89 Urethral instability. The left-hand trace shows static urethral pressure profilometry with normal maximum urethral closure pressure (MUCP) but an irregular shape. The right-hand trace is recorded by positioning the catheter at the MUCP: marked dips in pressure were recorded giving the diagnosis.

One of the reasons why many urodynamicists believe there is little role for these tests in clinical practice is that, with the exceptions above, almost all tests are only found to be abnormal in the presence of a clinically detectable neurological deficit. Hence careful physical examination coupled with a detailed analysis of UDS can provide the same answers that neurophysiological tests can give.

In the 1988 ICS collated report (see Appendix 1, Part 2) there are definitions and descriptions of the neurophysiological tests that can be used. The ICS report gives some idea of the complexity of neurophysiological testing. These tests require specific skills and are best carried out separately from urodynamic studies in an appropriately staffed and equipped neurophysiological laboratory.

References

Videourodynamics

Enhorning G, Miller ER, Hinman F (1964). Urethral closure studied with cineroentgenography and simultaneous bladder-urethra pressure recording. Surg Gynaecol Obstet 118:507–516.

Norlen LJ, Blaivas JG (1986). Unsuspected proximal urethral obstruction in young and middle aged men. J Urol 135:972.

Perkash I, Friendland GW (1985). Real-time gray-scale transrectal linear array ultrasonography in urodynamic evaluation. Semin Urol 3:49–59.

Versi E, Cardozo L, Studd JWW, Brincat M, O'Dowd TM, Cooper DJ (1986). Internal urinary sphincter in maintenance of female continence. Br Med J 292:166.

Webster GD, Older RA (1980). Video urodynamics. Urology 16:106.

Ambulatory Urodynamics

Griffiths CJ, Assi MS, Styles RA, Neal DE (1987). Ambulatory long-term monitoring of bladder and detrusor pressure. Neurourol Urodyn 6:161–162.

James D. Continuous monitoring. (1979) Urol clin N Am 6: 125–135.

Kulseng-Hanssen S, Klevmark B (1988). Ambulatory urethro-cysto-rectometry. A new technique. Neurourol Urodyn 7:119–130.

Kulseng-Hanssen S, Klevmark B (1996). Ambulatory urodynamic monitoring of women. Scand J Urol Nephrol 30 suppl 179 pp 27–37.

Paseini-Glazel G. Cisternino A, Artibani W, Pagano F (1992). Ambulatory urodynamics. Preliminary experience with vesico urethral holter in children. Scand J Urol Nephrol suppl 141:87–92.

Robertson AS, Griffiths C, Neal DE (1996). Conventional urodynamics and ambulatory monitoring in the definition and management of bladder outflow obstruction J Urol 155:506–511.

Van Waalwijk van Doorn ESC, Remmers A, Janknegt RA (1992). Conventional and extra-mural ambulatory urodyamic testing of the lower urinary tract in female volunteers. J Urol 147:1319–1326.

Webb RJ, Ramsden PD, Neal DE (1991). Ambulatory monitoring and electronic measurement of urinary leakage in the diagnosis of detrusor instability and incontinence. Br J Urol 146:336–337.

Pad Testing

Jørgensen L, Lose F, Andersen JT (1987). One hour pad-weighing test for objective assessment of female urinary incontinence. Obstet Gynaecol 69:39.

Gosling JA (1979) The structure of the bladder and the urethra in relation to function. Urol Clin N Am 6:31–38.

Lose G, Versi E (1992). Pad-weighing tests in the diagnosis and quantification of incontinence. Int Urogynecol J 3:324.

Versi E, Orrego G, Hardy E, Seddon G, Smith P, Anand D (1996). Evaluation of the home pad test in the investigation of female urinary incontinence. Br J Obstet Gynaecol 103:162–167.

Neurophysiological Testing

Fowler CJ, Christmas TJ, Chapple CR, Parkhouse HF, Kirby RS, Jacobs HS (1988). Abnormal electromyographic activity of the urethral sphincter, voiding dysfunction, and polycystic ovaries: A new syndrome? Br Med J 297:1436–1438.

Siroky MB (1996). Electromyography of the perineal floor. Urol Clin N Am I 23:299–307.

Vodusek DB (1996). Evoked potential testing. Urol Clin N Am II 23:427–447.

Chapter 4

Patient Assessment

Introduction

The vast majority of patients with lower urinary tract dysfunction present with symptoms. An occasional patient will present "silently", with a palpable mass in the lower abdomen, due to an enlarged bladder, or perhaps the symptoms of uraemia. Despite our extensive experience of assessing patients with voiding disorders we remain impressed by the unreliability of symptoms, even when taken by a urodynamically trained and experienced clinician. This is one of the reasons for the use of urodynamic testing. We commend any approach that lends objectivity to diagnosis, and in particular the use of frequency–volume charts (urinary diaries). The frequency–volume chart forms the basis for the interview during which the clinician attempts to reach a diagnosis, evaluate the patient's most troublesome symptoms, judge the severity of these symptoms, assess the impact of the symptoms on the patient's life and judge the patient's expectations in terms of treatment.

During discussion of the patient's presenting complaints, the clinician should seek information on both the storage and the voiding phases of the micturition cycle. In our unit, history-taking is based on the completion of a proforma (Appendix 3) which leads the interviewer through the phases of bladder function, the storage phase, premicturition symptoms, voiding symptoms and post-micturition symptoms. If the symptoms are interpreted in the context of the normal function of the lower urinary tract then it may be possible to produce a provisional symptomatic diagnosis. Urodynamics and other investigations then become tests of a clinical hypothesis. If these steps are taken consciously then there is feedback from functional urodynamic information which helps to improve symptomatic diagnosis. Although symptoms have been considered individually in this section, they may be grouped together in symptom complexes, which have more diagnostic significance.

Frequency–Volume Charts

The clinician has to deal with a range of urinary symptoms, many of which are variable in nature. It may be unnecessary to proceed with urodynamic investigation, because the basic abnormality in many patients may be related not to detrusor or urethral dysfunction, but rather to alterations in renal excretion, circadian rhythms or the psychological control of micturition. In addition, minor abnormalities of bladder dysfunction may be exacerbated by alterations in renal function, and it is important to identify such alterations before instituting major surgical treatment. Over a period of more than twenty years we have obtained considerable experience in the use of frequency–volume charts completed by the patient. We have found these an essential method of investigating the function of the male and female lower urinary tracts. The charts were developed originally as part of a research project evaluating the response to treatment (Torrens 1974). While Fig. 4.1 represents our normal chart, it is possible to use more complex charts if more information is required, for example when evaluating a new treatment (Fig. 4.2, *overleaf*).

Name _____   Date of appointment 14 : 1 : 92

DAY	time / volume (mls.)	DAY-TIME	NIGHT-TIME	Number of pads used in 24 hour period
1	times	↑a.n. 08.30 09.30 13.30 15.00 17.20 22.30	00.30 05.00	3
	volume	200 50 50 200 W 200 150	50 200	
2	times	08.00 08.30 10.00 11.30 13.20 17.30 18.10 22.30	01.00 05.30	2
	volume	150 50 100 100 W — 100 150	100 200	
3	times	08.00 09.00 10.30 12.00 14.30 18.00 21.00 22.30	00.15 03.30 05.15	4
	volume	100 W W 100 200 W 200 100	200 200 200	
4	times	07.45 09.00 10.15 11.30 12.00 17.45 22.00	04.00 07.10	2
	volume	100 100 100 100 250 250 250	150 100	
5	times	08.00 09.15 10.30 13.45 16.00 17.15 22.30	01.30 04.45	3
	volume	100 100 100 100 W 100 250	200 200	
6	times	07.30 08.15 09.30 10.45 12.00 14.30 16.00 18.15 22.30	01.45 04.30 07.00	4
	volume	100 50 50 W W 200 100 100 200	200 200 100	
7	times	08.00 09.15 10.00 13.00 13.45 16.00 17.45 19.45 23.00	02.15 06.30	4
	volume	100 100 100 200 W 100 150 W 100	250 200	

Fig. 4.1 Standard frequency–volume chart. The time of voiding and the volume voided are recorded for each micturition. Incontinence episodes are recorded as "W", pad usage is recorded in the right-hand column and the fluid intake is estimated.

RECORD DATE, TIME, VOLUME, URGENCY, LEAKAGE AND NUMBER OF PADS USED AS SHOWN IN THE EXAMPLE BELOW

DATE	DAY-TIME (from time out of bed to time to bed)							NIGHT-TIME (in bed)			NO OF PADS
Example 15 Febr	9.00 175 1, +	11.30 150 1, ++	1.00 150 2, +	3.30 175 1, +	5.00 200 2,	7.15 175 2, ++	9.30 125 1, ++	12.30 175 1, +	3.00 150 2, +	5.50 125 1, ++	1 + 1 + 1 or = 3
MARCH 27	7.30 250 1	8.30 50 1	11.00 — 1	2.00p — 1	400 — 2+	6.30 150 1	7.45 945 10.15 100 300 100 2 1	3.00a.m. 500 2			1
28	6.30 100 1	8.30 100 1	11.30 100 1	1.00p 150 2	3.15 5.15 300 400 1 2+	8.00 1000 200 200 1 2+	10.30 100 1	3.30 450 2+			1
29	8.45 150 1	1.45p 100 1	4 150 2+	5.45 150 1	700 200 +1	8.15 100 1	10.30 350 2++	—			2
30	7.30 900 2+	9.30 — —	11.00 — —	12.45 — —	2.15 4.30 — —	8.00 1000 — —	11p —	3.15 500 2			1
31	9.00 300 1	10.45 100 1	12.30 150 1	1.30 150 2	500 650 300 150 2+ 1	8.00 900 300 100 2+ 1	11.45 200 2++	—			2
APRIL 1	8.30 400 1	10.00 50 1	1.00p 150 1	1.45 100 1	400 4.30 300 300 2+ 1	6.15 8.45 100 150 1 1	10.00 11.00 250 200 2 1	—			2
2	8.00 500 2	11.00 —	1.00 100 2+	400 150 1	5.45 200 2	7.00 8.00 250 350 2 2++	9.30 11.00 250 1.30 2 1	—			2

1 = No urgency   2 = Urgency   + = a little/wet pants   ++ = a lot/wet clothes or pads

Fig. 4.2 Frequency–volume chart also recording urgency (1 or 2) and degree of leakage (+ or ++)

For a period of seven days prior to an outpatient appointment the patient is requested to record, as accurately as possible, the time and volume of each micturition. In addition, the chart is used to record episodes of urinary incontinence, and can be used to record the degree of urgency at each micturition, and the use of incontinence aids, such as pads. The patient is not instructed to "hold on" until the bladder is very full, as suggested by some authorities (Turner Warwick et al. 1979), but told to void as normal. No effort is made to make a precise assessment of the patient's fluid intake, because this makes the chart too complex: however, the patient is asked to estimate how much they drink per day, in cups. More accurate estimates of intake are difficult, not only because socially it would appear strange to be measuring the volumes of fluids imbibed but also because food is a significant source of fluid. Patients on diets eating large amounts of fruit and vegetables are often mystified by their high urine output when they appear to be drinking relatively little.

We have found that these charts are well accepted, even by elderly patients and, in the majority of cases, are completed with accuracy and enthusiasm; and even when enthusiasm outstrips ability the patient is still able to provide useful information. The chart facilitates history-taking and avoids exaggeration of the patient's symptoms. By examination of the chart the clinician is able to obtain accurate information as to the exact frequency and nocturia, together with the maximum and average volumes of urine passed at each episode of voiding. This method is the only way of obtaining a value for the average functional bladder capacity, a parameter which is important when deciding what volume a patient's bladder should be filled to during cystometry.

From the frequency–volume charts, abnormalities in the circadian rhythm of urine production may be detected, and psychogenic voiding patterns are often identified. In addition, it has been shown that certain patterns suggest particular types of bladder or urethral pathology. Klevmark (1989) has classified frequency–volume charts into four basic types:

1. Normal volumes, normal frequency: as seen in normal patients with a normal twenty-four-hour urine volume.
2. Normal volumes, increased frequency: such patients have an increased twenty-four-hour urine production (polyuria), indicative of increased fluid intake. Most frequently this is high fluid intake by choice, but occasionally will indicate a significant pathology such as diabetes insipidus or uncontrolled diabetes mellitus.
3. Reduced volumes, day and night: indicative of abnormalities such as detrusor instability or sensory urgency due to conditions such as interstitial cystitis or carcinoma *in situ*.
4. Normal early morning void, reduced variable day volumes. This pattern usually indicates a psychosomatic cause for frequency. The patient sleeps well and voids a normal or even increased volume on rising but passes small, variable amounts during the day.

We would subdivide Klevmark's type 3 into:

3a. Reduced *fixed* volumes, day and night; this pattern is suggestive of an intravesical pathology, such as interstitial cystitis or carcinoma *in situ*.
3b. Reduced *variable* volumes, day and night. This pattern is often indicative of detrusor instability.

We would also add a further type.

5. Nocturnal polyuria: these patients void with normal frequency and normal volumes by day, but with increased frequency at night, with more than 30% of the twenty-four-hour urine production being passed during the eight hours of rest. This pattern is the classical one of nocturnal polyuria which may be due to congestive cardiac failure or abnormalities of antidiuretic hormone or atrial natriuretic hormone secretion, but is often idiopathic.

Alterations in Fluid Excretion

The normal daily fluid output from the kidneys varies between one and three litres every twenty-four hours. It is worth remembering in the context of deciding what filling rate to use during urodynamics that a urine output of 1.4 litres in twenty-four hours represents a renal excretion of 1 ml of urine per minute. Approximately 80% of this volume is excreted during the waking hours, and therefore in the normal condition it is not necessary to empty the bladder at night. Abnormalities of renal excretion may be induced by sudden increase in the volume of fluid ingested, or by an alteration in the normal circadian rhythm.

Alterations in the quantity of fluid imbibed may occur at times of stress and during periods of social change, for example at times of redundancy or retirement. An example is shown in Fig. 4.3 (*overleaf*), where a sudden change in lifestyle has resulted in a dramatic increase in the patient's fluid intake, leading to

Name _____								Date of appointment _____	

DAY	time / volume (mls)			DAY-TIME					NIGHT-TIME		
1	10·30 / 500	11·09 / 400	2·17 / 375	4·37 / 600	8·15 / 450	9·43 / 300			12·40 / 400	5·00 / 450 ·	
2	6·00 / 200	9·17 / 350	11·05 / 450	1·57 / 350	4·24 / 350	6·31 / 400	8·14 / 200	9·41 / 350	12·00 / 300	5·11 / 450	
3	9·00 / 250	11·34 / 325	2·26 / 400	4·02 / 300	6·08 / 350	7·59 / 450	9·36 / 300	11·00 / 500	6·50 / 200	6·15 / 150	
4	9·34 / 325	11·00 / 400	2·15 / 300	4·00 / 350	6·51 / 400	9·23 / 400	10·11 / 300		1·00 / 400	4·23 / 200	5·45 / 150
5	10·45 / 300	12·25 / 250	1·40 / 250	2·21 / 350	4·34 / 400	16·40 / 350	9·25 / 300 ·		1·15 / 200	4·05 / 300	5·45 / 250
6	10·30 / 350	11·26 / 375	12·33 / 300	1·22 / 400	3·13 / 700	4·56 / 350	9·04 / 400		1·12 / 300	4·00 / 200	
7	6·00 / 200	10·37 / 400	12·27 / 350	4·22 / 400	6·09 / 350	8·23 / 350	9·32 / 350	10·30 / 250	3·04 / 400	5·25 / 300	

AVERAGE DAILY FLUID INTAKE (in cups) = ___12___

Fig. 4.3 The recording chart for frequency–volume assessment showing an alteration in frequency due to excessive intake.

frequency and nocturia, with large volumes voided on each occasion: the subject had become the teaboy in a prison! Abnormalities of the normal circadian rhythm may be induced primarily by disease itself, such as renal failure or heart failure, or be secondary to drugs used in the treatment of such conditions, for example, diuretic therapy. It is important to identify such abnormalities as a renal cause at an early stage, as they may exacerbate minor abnormalities of bladder function. Nocturnal polyuria in elderly men appears to be secondary to subclinical cardiac failure which results in increased production by the right atrium of the heart of atrial natriuretic peptide (ANP), the powerful natural diuretic, enabling urine production to be increased. ANP provides the essential mechanism by which excess fluid is excreted at night. Lastly, alterations in circadian rhythms may be due to a primary defect in posterior pituitary function. Although such abnormalities are easily identified by examination of the frequency–volume charts, they may be resistant to treatment. Antidiuretic hormone (DDAVP) administration may be helpful but must be used with care.

Psychogenic Voiding Patterns

The bladder has often been referred to as "the mirror of the mind", and it is common for psychological problems to manifest themselves initially as urological symptoms. Such psychogenic voiding patterns are often "diagnoses of exclusion" following persistently negative urological studies. However, the frequency-volume chart may identify such abnormalities at an early stage. Such alterations in voiding patterns are those of frequency and sometimes nocturia, occurring at times of social and mental stress. In Fig. 4.4 it is shown that frequency is occurring during periods at work, but disappears at the weekend. We have also found that patients may be able to interpret these findings themselves and make a self-assessment of their condition if they are given the opportunity to complete a

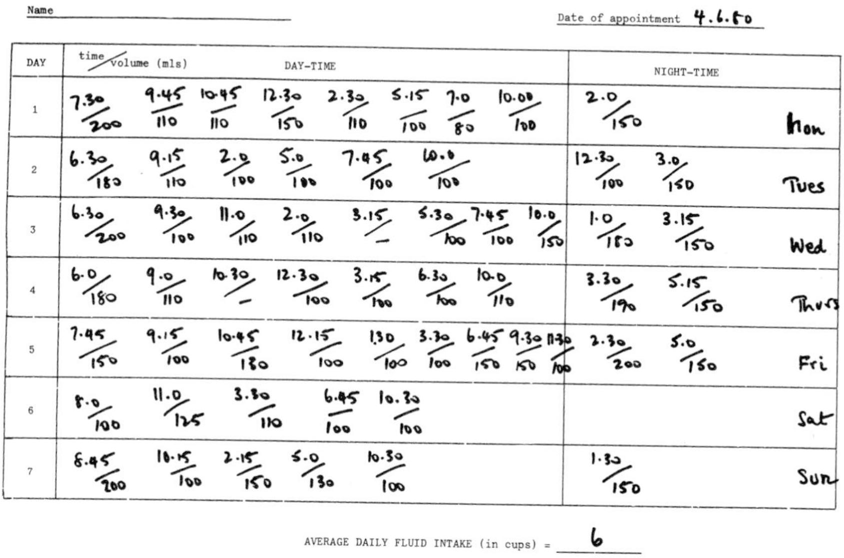

Name _____   Date of appointment **4.6.60**

DAY	time/Volume (mls)				DAY-TIME				NIGHT-TIME		
1	7.30/200	9.45/110	10.45/110	12.30/150	2.30/110	5.15/100	7.0/80	10.00/100	2.0/150		Mon
2	6.30/180	9.15/110	2.0/100	5.0/100	7.45/100	10.0/100			12.30/100	3.0/150	Tues
3	6.30/200	9.30/100	11.0/110	2.0/110	3.15/—	5.30/100	7.45/100	10.0/150	1.0/150	3.15/150	Wed
4	6.0/180	9.0/110	10.30/—	12.30/100	3.15/100	6.30/100	10.0/110		3.30/190	5.15/150	Thurs
5	7.45/150	9.15/100	10.45/180	12.15/100	1.30/100	3.30/100	6.45/150 9.30/50 11.30/100		2.30/200	5.0/150	Fri
6	8.0/100	11.0/125	3.30/110	6.45/100	10.30/100						Sat
7	8.45/200	10.15/100	2.15/150	5.0/130	10.30/100				1.30/150		Sun

AVERAGE DAILY FLUID INTAKE (in cups) = **6**

Fig. 4.4 Frequency–volume chart showing excessive frequency during periods at work. At the weekend daytime frequency becomes normal and nocturia reduces markedly.

frequency–volume chart. Another characteristic of the psychogenic voiding pattern is the absence of nocturia despite quite marked frequency during the day (Klevmark's type 4; see above).

Intravesical Pathology

Although serious bladder pathology (e.g. infiltrating carcinoma or carcinoma *in situ*) is usually associated with other symptoms including haematuria, such individuals may present with the symptoms of frequency and nocturia. These patients' frequency–volume charts frequently demonstrate a fixed functional bladder capacity with relentless frequency and nocturia. For example, Fig. 4.5 (*overleaf*) is from a patient who exhibited such characteristics and was subsequently shown to have bladder carcinoma. The finding of such a pattern on a frequency–volume chart should indicate the need for further investigations, including urgent cystoscopy.

Frequency/Urgency Syndrome

Following the exclusion of the abnormalities described above, there remain a group of patients in whom the basic pathology remains unclear. From the clinician's point of view the most important factor is to consider whether the patient's symptoms are related to bladder outlet obstruction or to an abnormality of detrusor function such as detrusor instability.

Name _____   Date of appointment **20·8·80**

DAY	time / Volume (mls) DAY-TIME	NIGHT-TIME
1	11·30AM 12·00 12·30 12·55 1·20 2·00 2·55 3·50 4·45 100 100 100 100 100 100 100 50 50	
↑	6·45 7·45 8·45 9·45 10·15 50 75 25 25 25	12·30 2·55 2·10 2·40 3·45 4·40 50 25 25 25 25 25
2↑	6·30 7·20 8·00 8·50 9·25 10·10 11·10 11·45 12·30 50 50 25 100 50 50 50 50 50	
↑	3·15 4·20 6·00 6·50 7·30 8·20 9·10 50 25 25 25 25 50 25	9·50 12·20 1·00 3·50 4·10 5·40 25 25 25 25 25 25
3↑	5·50 6·30 7·50 25 25 25	
↑		
↑		

AVERAGE DAILY FLUID INTAKE (in cups) = **4**

Fig. 4.5 Frequency–volume chart, showing frequency due to fixed bladder capacity in a patient with bladder carcinoma.

Patients with detrusor instability often show reduced but variable volumes of urine during the day. Their night-time volumes and the first void on waking in the morning are often of larger quantity.

Bladder Outlet Obstruction

We are not aware of any clear pattern on a frequency–volume chart that will allow the diagnosis of bladder outlet obstruction to be made.

Analysis of Symptoms

In this section each symptom is defined and explained in functional terms. The object, as ever, is to provide a pathophysiological understanding of the patient's complaints. Such an approach requires some conceptual thinking, but allows the clinician to develop a hypothesis as to the patient's underlying condition as the history is taken.

The interpretation of a patient's symptoms is modified by many factors, not least by the time the clinician is able to spend with the patient. The limits of normality are not adequately defined, and in an individual case may be what the patient, rather than the doctor, considers to be normal. The adequacy of communication is important, as are many preconceived ideas held by the medical staff. For this reason, for each symptom, a specific wording of the question to the patient about that symptom is suggested.

In the analysis of each individual symptom it is important not only to assess the presence or absence of any symptom, but also to define its frequency and

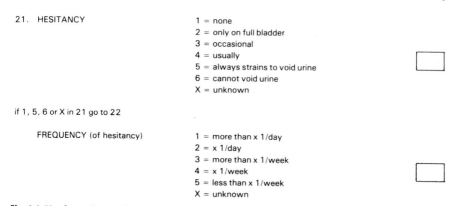

21. HESITANCY

1 = none
2 = only on full bladder
3 = occasional
4 = usually
5 = always strains to void urine
6 = cannot void urine
X = unknown

if 1, 5, 6 or X in 21 go to 22

FREQUENCY (of hesitancy)

1 = more than x 1/day
2 = x 1/day
3 = more than x 1/week
4 = x 1/week
5 = less than x 1/week
X = unknown

Fig. 4.6 Urodynamic questionnaire: an example of the question format with the presence/absence of the symptom followed by a supplementary question as to its frequency.

severity; as Fig. 4.6 shows, we now attempt to grade each of the symptoms in terms of frequency and/or severity.

Lower urinary tract symptoms (LUTS) should be divided into the phases of micturition: storage, voiding, post-micturition and others.

Storage Symptoms

Frequency of Micturition

Question: "*How often do you pass urine (your water) from the time you wake in the morning until the time you go to sleep at night?*"
Abnormality of urinary frequency is a change from that to which any particular patient is accustomed. There is surprisingly little objective data on frequency in the normal population, however two excellent papers by Larsson and Victor (1988) and Carter et al. (1992) give us information on women and men respectively. We would consider normal diurnal frequency to be between 3 and 7 voids per day.

Increased urinary frequency is seldom the patient's only complaint: it is usually associated with other symptoms – most frequently, urgency of micturition. Frequency of up to 10 to 12 times per day may be tolerated by many patients: above this it is usually socially embarrassing. However this statement must be modified according to the patient's occupation, and if the patient works on a factory production line, or is a long-distance lorry driver, then it becomes essential that they can hold urine for at least two hours. Patients are notoriously inaccurate in their assessment of urinary frequency, and for this reason an objective means of assessing frequency, such as the frequency–volume chart, is essential.

Mechanisms of Increased Urinary Frequency. It is useful in understanding the mechanisms of frequency if the causes are categorised according to the functional bladder capacity or voided volume.

1. Normal functional bladder capacity. We consider the normal maximum capacity to be 300 to 600 ml in the adult. Children's bladder capacity can be calculated on the basis of 30 ml plus 30 ml for each year of life, so that a child of three can be expected to void 120 ml at a time. In this group, with normal voiding volumes increased frequency must be due to an increased intake, resulting in increased output. This may be secondary to:

- Polydypsia, which may occasionally be psychotic, but is more usually because the patient enjoys a favourite beverage, be it tea, water or beer.
- An osmotic diuresis, e.g. diabetes mellitus.
- An abnormality of anti-diuretic hormone production, e.g. in diabetes insipidus.

2. Reduced functional bladder capacity. This term implies that the bladder capacity under general or regional anaesthetic would be normal, but the voided volumes are consistently small – less than 300 ml. The causes of reduced functional capacity include the following:

- Detrusor overactivity as in detrusor instability.
- A significant residual urine resulting either from bladder outlet obstruction, detrusor underactivity or a combination of the two.
- Non-inflammatory causes of increased bladder sensation, for example, anxiety or the idiopathic hypersensitive bladder.
- Inflammatory bladder conditions, e.g. acute cystitis, carcinoma *in situ* or bladder stone.
- A fear of urinary retention, especially in older male patients who experience increasing hesitancy as the bladder becomes full, and who compensate by voiding frequently.
- Fear of incontinence. Some patients, both with genuine stress incontinence and/or with detrusor instability, have increased frequency in order to keep their bladder volumes low, and minimise the risk of leakage.

3. Reduced structural bladder capacity. In this case the bladder capacity is smaller than normal under regional or deep general anaesthesia, resulting in consistently small voided volumes. The reduction in capacity may be due to:

- Post-infective fibrosis, e.g. tuberculosis.
- Non-infective cystitis, e.g. interstitial cystitis (Hunner's ulceration).
- Post-pelvic irradiation fibrosis, e.g. after radiotherapy for bladder or cervical cancer.
- After surgery, e.g. partial cystectomy.

Mechanism of Decreased Urinary Frequency. Infrequent voids of large volumes of urine usually provoke admiration rather than complaints. Decreased frequency may be due to the profession of the patient, for example, "check-out girls" working in supermarkets may develop the ability to hold their urine for long periods of time. Similarly lorry drivers working on the motorways may void infrequently. Reduced detrusor contractility and impaired bladder sensation may be factors that can lead to decreased frequency, or indeed result from the habit of holding large volumes.

When faced with patients, usually women, with recurrent urinary infections, it is important to ask the patient's voiding habits between infections, because quite frequently they can be discovered to be "infrequent voiders". Part of their management then consists of advising them to void at least four-hourly.

Nocturia

Question: *"How many times, on average, are you woken from your sleep because you need to pass urine?"*

Unless the clinician's definition of nocturia is made clear, the patient may include a void before going to sleep, or the first void in the morning. Furthermore the frequency of nocturnal voiding, in relation to age, needs to be considered when judging the significance of the symptom.

This complaint is dependent on age in both sexes. We have defined nocturia as being woken from sleep each night by the need to urinate. It is usual for men over 65 and women over 75 to be woken once at night in this way.

Other patients will attempt to include all voids during the hours of darkness, giving the paradox of increased nocturia during the winter, compared with during the summer. It is also important to ask whether the patient sleeps well, and whether he or she drinks during the night. Some patients sleep poorly for no apparent reason, and some because of a restless partner or chronic painful conditions such as arthritis. These patients, once awake, are often unable to settle until they have emptied their bladders, thus producing apparent nocturia. However most such patients have no increase in daytime frequency.

Mechanisms of Nocturia. Most causes of nocturia are the same as those described above for increased diurnal frequency. However, in addition, there may be increased nocturnal production of urine. Often this is due to the reabsorption of oedema fluid in patients with mild congestive cardiac failure: it is therefore important to examine the ankles and sacrum of all elderly patients for oedema fluid. However increased nocturnal urine production is often seen in the absence of demonstrable oedema, although oedema does not become clinically detectable until there is at least 1 litre of fluid lying in the interstitium. When the patient goes to bed, oedema fluid is reabsorbed into the circulation and the venous pressure increases. In the right atrium an increase in venous pressure results in the secretion of ANP (p. 122). Nocturia may also be due to loss or reduction of antidiuretic hormone production at night: a reversal of the diurnal pituitary rhythm. If there is diurnal frequency and urgency then nocturia is most likely to be due to detrusor instability.

Urgency

Question: *"When you get the feeling of wanting to pass your water, can you hold on or do you have to go immediately?"*

If the patient appears to have urgency then the following two supplementary questions may be useful:

"If you are watching your favourite TV programme, and get the feeling of wanting to pass urine, can you delay it until the programme has finished, or do you have to leave the room more or less immediately?"

"How much time does your bladder give you from the time you first feel you want to go until you think you are desperate and likely to leak – five minutes, ten minutes, half an hour?"

Mechanisms of Urgency. Urgency may be associated with two types of dysfunction:

- Detrusor instability, when urgency is often known as motor urgency. Motor urgency results frequently in urge incontinence.
- Bladder hypersensitivity, when it is known as sensory urgency. In this situation urgency is usually due to fear of increased pain or discomfort, and leakage is relatively uncommon. Common causes of sensory urgency would be acute cystitis or the idiopathic hypersensitive bladder.

Bladder Pain

Question: *"When your bladder fills do you have any pain in your bladder?"*
Although this symptom may share the same causes as urgency it is experienced differently. Bladder pain is felt suprapubically and increases slowly and gradually with bladder filling. The pain leads to frequency, not because of fear of incontinence, but due to increasing discomfort and fear of pain. Bladder pain, although often relieved by micturition, may persist after voiding, most classically in interstitial cystitis.

Mechanisms of Bladder Pain. Bladder pain may be due to:

- Inflammatory conditions of the bladder, e.g. acute cystitis or interstitial cystitis.
- Increased bladder sensation without inflammation but due to irritation by intravesical pathology such as bladder carcinoma ("malignant cystitis") or bladder stone.

Urinary Incontinence

Question: *"Do you ever leak urine or wet yourself?"*
The ICS defines incontinence as: "a condition in which involuntary loss of urine is a social or hygienic problem, and is objectively demonstrated" (Appendix 1, Part 2). Loss of urine through channels other than the urethra is defined as extraurethral incontinence, for example when due to a vesico-vaginal fistula. Strenuous effort should be made on history-taking to decide which type of incontinence is suffered by the patient.

It is unwise to ask patients if they are incontinent, because they will often answer "no", either through embarrassment or because they imagine that incontinence means being wet all the time.

Stress Incontinence

Question: *"Do you ever leak urine when you cough, sneeze, exercise, lift heavy objects or walk on rough ground or down hill?"*

Stress incontinence denotes a symptom, a sign or a condition. The symptom of stress incontinence indicates the patient's statement of involuntary urine loss during physical exertion. The sign of stress incontinence denotes the observation of urine loss from the urethra, synchronous with a physical exertion such as coughing. The condition "genuine stress incontinence" has been defined by the ICS as " the involuntary loss of urine occurring when, in the absence of a detrusor contraction, the intravesical pressure exceeds the maximum urethral pressure". Clearly, it is important that intra-abdominal pressure is measured during urodynamic studies in order to satisfy the needs of this definition.

Mechanisms of Stress Incontinence. The first line of continence is normal closure of the bladder neck throughout filling. The second line is a competent distal urethral sphincter mechanism. It follows that stress incontinence must involve a degree of inadequacy of both these mechanisms. The physiology of urethral incompetence has been discussed in Chapter 2.

The clinical situations in which bladder neck and urethral incompetence occur include:

- A weakened pelvic floor, especially in the obese and multiparous.
- A paralysed pelvic floor in lower motor-neurone lesions.
- Abnormally high pressures in a distended bladder where distension tends to open the bladder neck.
- Iatrogenic damage to the sphincter mechanisms, for example, following transurethral resection of the prostate.
- Congenital short urethra.

One important differential diagnosis is between genuine stress incontinence and stress-induced detrusor instability (see Chapter 3). It is important to ask the patient whether they have any sensation of urgency prior to leakage which occurs when detrusor instability follows coughing or change of posture.

Urge Incontinence

Question: *"When you want to pass urine, do you ever leak before you can get to the toilet because you can't hang on long enough?"*

This symptom is defined as the involuntary loss of urine associated with a strong desire to void (urgency). Most frequently there is no specific trigger for urge incontinence, but some patients do report certain provoking factors such as hand washing, answering the telephone or putting the key in the front door when returning home.

Mechanisms of Urge Incontinence. Urge incontinence may, as in the case of urgency, be associated with

- Detrusor instability, when it is known as motor urge incontinence.
- Increased bladder sensation (sensory urge incontinence).

- Urethral instability, which is defined as the inappropriate relaxation of bladder neck and urethra resulting in leakage; it is an unusual cause of urge incontinence.

Giggle Incontinence

This type of incontinence is usually a complaint of younger women. The history is clear and usually not associated with other urinary disturbance. Because of the problems of reproducing this symptom in the urodynamic laboratory the mechanism is not clearly understood. The definition is implicit in the name. Suggested mechanisms for giggle incontinence include urethral relaxation, detrusor instability and congenital urethral weakness.

Nocturnal Enuresis

Question: *"Do you ever wet the bed or your pyjamas (nightgown) when you are asleep, either at night or during the day?"*
Strictly speaking, enuresis can refer to any incontinence, day or night. However the term is most often used to mean a normal act of micturition occurring during sleep, that is nocturnal enuresis. Enuresis may be divided into primary, when the patient has never been dry at night, and secondary, when enuresis follows a period of nighttime continence. Nocturnal enuresis is often a significant factor in the past history of young adults with nocturia. A family history should be sought and the presence or absence of concurrent diurnal symptoms noted. When talking to children it is useful to assess diurnal symptoms by asking the questions, *"Do you have to leave the classroom in the middle of a lesson in order to pass urine?"* and *"Do you have to get up to pass urine when you are watching your favourite TV programme?"*

Mechanisms of Enuresis. Enuresis is fundamentally a disturbance of brain function whereby bladder distension, for one reason or another, cannot elicit normal cortical arousal. Various other factors may contribute to the situation, including:

- Increased nocturnal secretion of urine due to an inappropriately low level of ADH secretion at night.
- Reduced bladder or urethral sensation, such as in neuropathic patients.
- Detrusor overactivity.
- Inappropriate cerebral sedation, for example, by drugs or alcohol.
- Reduced bladder capacity.

It is very common to hear from parents that the enuretic child sleeps much more deeply than all the other children.

Reflex Incontinence

Reflex incontinence is defined as the loss of urine due to detrusor hyperreflexia and/or involuntary urethral relaxation in the absence of sensation, usually not

27. DEGREE OF INCONTINENCE

    1 = drops, wets underclothes
    2 = 'floods', wets outer clothes
    3 = 'floods', on floor
    X = not known

28. MANAGEMENT OF INCONTINENCE

    1 = no protective measures, no clothes change
    2 = changes underwear/clothes
    3 = pads for safety
    4 = pads for necessity
    5 = appliance
    6 = catheter
    7 = urinary diversion
    8 = other
    X = unknown

complete ONLY if 3 or 4 in 28

PADS PER DAY

PADS PER NIGHT

Fig. 4.7 Urodynamic questionnaire: the section enquiring as to the degree of incontinence and the measures taken to control leakage.

associated with the desire to micturate. This type of incontinence is seen only in patients with neuropathic bladder and/or urethral dysfunction.

Continuous Incontinence

Patients frequently complain of being "continuously incontinent". However, true continuous incontinence can only be due either to a fistula between the ureter, bladder or urethra above the distal sphincter mechanism, and the vagina, or to an ectopic ureter entering into the urethra below the distal mechanism or into the vagina in the female. Patients with severe sphincter weakness may be more or less continuously incontinent during the day, but when they lie down in bed they are usually dry for considerable periods of time.

When assessing incontinence it is essential to document the frequency and severity of incontinence. Figure 4.7 shows how we ask about severity and the measures the patient takes. In addition, if the patient uses pads then the type of pad, the proportion which are wet and the degree of wetness all need to be ascertained.

Incontinence During Sexual Intercourse

Incontinence may be related specifically to sexual activity. The commonest problem is leakage from the woman during intercourse. Penetration may precipitate involuntary contractions, and detrusor instability is a frequent finding in such cases. Leakage during intercourse may also occur in women with genuine stress incontinence. Leakage at orgasm in the woman may be secondary either to urethral sphincter weakness, or perhaps to urethral instability (relaxation). In the man, occasional ejaculation of urine with semen may occur, and this is most frequently seen in patients with neurological disease such as spina bifida.

It must also be recognised that incontinence can have a profound effect on the sexual activity of patients, and is frequently a cause of marital disharmony.

Because of the considerable psychological repercussions this can have, it is particularly important that the sexual history is taken in detail so that proper practical advice can be given.

Voiding Symptoms

Hesitancy

Question: *"After you have had the feeling that you want to pass water, and you are in the toilet and ready to urinate, does your urine come immediately or do you have to wait?"*

If the patient has hesitancy ask a supplementary question:

"How long do you have to wait, 10 seconds, 30 seconds, 1 minute or more than 1 minute?"

This symptom is defined as a delay in the onset of micturition when the patient wants to void and is ready to do so. The complaint of hesitancy should be assessed in terms of the volume voided. It may be normal for any individual to have hesitancy when trying to void with less than 100 ml in the bladder. Conversely, a patient may complain of hesitancy only with a full bladder; this is often taken as a sign of impending urinary retention. However, even a normal person may have problems initiating voiding if the bladder gets exceptionally full.

Mechanisms of Hesitancy. Hesitancy may be due to:

- Bladder outlet obstruction. Here the patient has to wait for the detrusor contraction to generate sufficient pressure to overcome increased outlet pressure
- Detrusor factors. These include detrusor underactivity, and either over- or underdistension of the bladder
- Urethral factors. For neurological reasons, or in some instances without obvious cause, the urethra may fail to relax, as in detrusor–sphincter dyssynergia (see p. 82). In neurologically normal patients it is difficult to know whether failure of urethral relaxation is the primary problem rather than an inability to initiate a detrusor contraction.
- "Psychological" factors. Many normal male patients are unable to void except when alone. Two patients spring to mind. The first was a man who could only void when locked in his toilet at home, having made sure that there was nobody else in the house. This man was impossible to investigate! The second man had sea fishing, as his hobby, which involved many hours at sea in an open boat. All his colleagues were able to micturate over the side of the boat, but he went into urinary retention, as he was too inhibited to "perform".
- Penile erection is an unusual but frustrating problem for some elderly men who, woken from their sleep, find that they have an erection due to a full bladder, and are then unable to void until the erection dies away.

Decreased Urinary Stream

Question: "*When you pass urine, does the flow come out in front of you in a good flow, or does it drop to your feet?*" (Brian Peeling's diagram is a useful way for the patient to visualise this question (Fig. 4.8).)

Urine flow rate depends on the volume voided, and therefore the patient should be asked about the quantities he voids, although this information should have been available from the frequency–volume chart. In addition to the question already mentioned, the patient should be asked about the characteristics of the stream. For example, is it thin and forceful, as would be seen in a patient who had a meatal stenosis? A patient with meatal stenosis might also notice that during micturition the penis enlarges because the penile urethra becomes distended by urine.

Mechanisms of Decreased Urinary Stream. A reduced urine flow may be due to:

- Any cause that reduces the voided volume and therefore any cause for frequency.
- Bladder outlet obstruction at any level from the bladder neck to the external meatus. Bladder outlet obstruction may be mechanical or functional. The commonest mechanical obstruction is prostatic hyperplasia, and the functional obstructions that may be noted are dysfunctional voiding, detrusor sphincter dyssynergia and isolated distal sphincter obstruction.
- Decreased detrusor contractility, which may be either neuropathic or myopathic. Myopathic abnormalities may be any primary disturbance of bladder muscle, any toxic influence upon bladder muscle, or secondary to over-stretching. There are a variety of neuropathic causes affecting both the upper and the lower motor neurones. Most classically underactivity would be associated with lower motor neurone damage, as for example after abdominal perineal resection of the rectum.

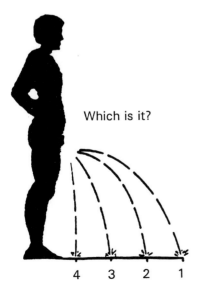

Which is it?

4   3   2   1

Fig. 4.8 Brian Peeling's figure to allow the patient to indicate his stream.

Intermittency

Question: "*Is your urine flow continuous or does it stop and start?*"
Figure 3.20 (p. 35) shows intermittency, which has in common many of the same causes as a variable stream when the stream is of varying strength without actual interruption.

Mechanisms of Intermittency. An interrupted or variable flow may be due to:

- *Urethral overactivity.* Actual closure or narrowing during voiding usually occurs at the level of the pelvic floor and is termed *dysfunctional voiding* in the neurologically intact and *detrusor sphincter dyssynergia* in those with neurological disease such as multiple sclerosis.
- *Detrusor underactivity.* A poorly sustained, wave-like detrusor contraction produces a variable or interrupted trace. Similar patterns are produced if the patient has an acontractile detrusor and has to strain to pass urine.
- *Straining during voiding* (see below).

Straining

Question: "*Do you strain either to start your stream or to keep it going?*"
Patients may strain through habit or necessity. If the bladder contains little urine it often helps to strain a little to initiate a detrusor contraction. Patients without outlet obstruction can increase their flow by straining, although men with BPO cannot. Patients with detrusor underactivity and/or urethral obstruction may rely on straining to achieve adequate bladder emptying.

Dysuria

Question: "*Does it hurt when you pass urine?*"
This term tends to be used in different ways. Some clinicians, particularly in Europe, mean difficulty in voiding. We reserve the term "dysuria" for the urethral pain typically felt in acute cystourethritis. Dysuria may be secondary to infection at any level in the urinary tract, but is usually indicative of urethritis, prostatitis or cystitis. Some patients with increased bladder sensation, without infection, for example, hypersensitive cases and those with the urethral syndrome, may also report dysuria.

Terminal Dribble

Question: "*Does your urine flow end quickly or do you have a dribble before you finish?*"
If the patient says there is a dribble they are asked how long it lasts. The patient should also be asked if he has terminal dribble, which can be defined as a prolongation of the urinary flow, and this may last 30 to 60 seconds or more. Terminal dribble is due to a failing detrusor contraction associated with bladder

outlet obstruction and must be distinguished from post-micturition dribble (see below).

Post-micturition Symptoms

Post-micturition Dribble

Question: *"After you have passed urine, dressed and left the toilet, do you leak in the next few minutes?"*

It is important to distinguish between terminal dribble and post-micturition dribble. Terminal dribble is continuous with the main flow of urine, whereas post-micturition dribble is defined as leakage coming after voiding has been completed. It usually occurs as the patient dresses, or soon after, and is seldom associated with any demonstrable abnormality. This type of leakage is most commonly seen in men.

Mechanisms of Post-micturition Dribble. This symptom may be due to:

- Failure of the bulbo-cavernosus and bulbo-spongiosus muscles to empty the penile urethra after micturition has ended.
- Failure of the normal "milk-back" mechanism whereby the urine lying between the distal urethral sphincter mechanism and the bladder neck, at the end of micturition, is returned to the bladder: leakage may occur later if the distal sphincter relaxes and the urine passes distally.
- In women, post-micturition dribble is due to urine being deflected by the external genitalia into the vagina, so that when the woman stands the urine drips from the vaginal lumen.

Feeling of Incomplete Emptying

Question: *"After you have passed your water, does the feeling of wanting to urinate go away, or are you left with any sensation?"*

The normal patient, after micturition, completely loses any awareness of the bladder. Persistence of symptoms is usually felt as incomplete emptying or sometimes as a continued desire to void. These symptoms may often be misleading, as the patient may be shown to have emptied the bladder completely.

Mechanisms of Sensation of Incomplete Emptying. The reasons include:

- Increased sensation, e.g. acute cystitis, interstitial cystitis, urethritis and prostatitis.
- Persistent detrusor contraction (after-contraction), in which the bladder contracts after it is empty, producing high post-micturition pressure. This phenomenon is not related to detrusor instability, and is not always felt, so that its significance is unknown. However on occasions it does give rise to a desire to void and to a feeling of incomplete emptying after micturition.

- Residual urine; many patients are unaware of the fact that they fail to empty their bladder, but others do have a feeling of incomplete emptying in this situation.

Post-micturition Bladder or Urethral Pain

Pain may also be felt after micturition, and this is often indicative of intra-vesical or intraurethral pathology and is frequently an indication for further investigation.

Strangury. Strangury describes a very unpleasant powerful feeling low in the pelvis, penis or urethra after voiding. It is usually indicative of an intravesical pathology such as a bladder stone or acute cystitis.

Other Symptoms

Haematuria

In almost every instance this symptom is an indication for further urological investigation and should never be ignored. Investigation of haematuria will usually take precedence over the investigation of other lower urinary tract dysfunction.

Loin Pain

It is unusual for the complaint of loin pain to be directly related to lower urinary dysfunction, although it can be secondary to vesico-ureteric reflux, or have an infective origin (pyelonephritis), and these conditions may occur in association with lower urinary tract dysfunction. Similarly calculus obstruction of the lower end of the ureter may present with a combination of upper and lower urinary tract symptoms. In a patient with lower urinary tract symptoms, loin pain is an indication for further investigation, most frequently an intravenous pyelogram.

Urinary Infections

It is appropriate to note here that there is a need for accuracy in the diagnosis of urinary infection. The condition is often diagnosed from symptoms or an inadequately taken "midstream specimen of urine" (MSU). If there is need for a midstream specimen then it should be properly supervised. If there is any doubt about the validity of an MSU, then either a suprapubic aspiration or a catheter specimen of urine may be taken. A catheter specimen should be sent to the laboratory at the commencement of urodynamic investigations. Alternatively a "Stix" test for nitrite has been shown to be an excellent and cost-effective alternative to the MSU.

Retention of Urine

The patient should be asked whether they have had any retention episodes. The most common causes of urinary retention are benign prostatic obstruction, pelvic surgery, childbirth, the commencement of drug therapy with agents having effects on the bladder or urethra (see p. Appendix 4), and acute neurological conditions such as prolapsed intervertebral disc. Hence a history of previous urinary retention should alert the clinician to the possibility of detrusor underactivity, asymptomatic bladder outlet obstruction or an underlying neurological cause.

Sexual History

Sexual function and lower urinary tract function are subserved by similar innervation and therefore sexual function should be discussed with most patients. Men should be asked whether erection is present or absent, whether ejaculation if present is forceful and clonic, or if emission is weak. In addition patients should be asked whether or not they have orgasm and questioned as to its character and acuity.

In the absence of previous surgical intervention, for example, surgery of the rectum, psychogenic factors are the most common cause of impotence. However these symptoms in the male patient may be due to demonstrable neurological disease, for example, after spinal cord injury or in multiple sclerosis. They may also be the first indication of a peripheral neuropathy, as in diabetes mellitus or alcoholism. Each of these pathological processes may also lead to lower urinary tract dysfunction.

Erection may occur as a reflex and is mediated by the sacral roots via the pelvic nerves, whereas a psychogenic erection requires intact cholinergic and sympathetic nerve fibres in the pelvic and hypogastric nerves. Ejaculation depends on the co-ordinated action of the striated musculature of the pelvic floor which is innervated by the pudendal nerves. Orgasmic sensation is a combined afferent bombardment through the sympathetic hypogastric and somatic pudendal nerves.

A sexual history should also be taken from female patients asking about orgasm and any associated urine symptoms such as incontinence (see p. 131).

Bowel Function

Bowel function is similarly closely related to lower urinary tract function, and patients should be asked about their frequency of bowel action as well as the mechanics of defecation, that is, do they relax or do they need to strain, or is it essential that they use some artificial means such as manual evacuation, suppositories or enemas to empty their bowel. They should also be asked about their control of bowel function, that is whether or not they ever soil or have an accident. In patients both with and without neurological disease, correction of bowel problems may produce a significant improvement in lower urinary tract symptoms.

Past Medical History

Obstetric History

The incidence of stress incontinence increases with the number of pregnancies and the difficulties of parturition. Electromyography has shown evidence of pelvic floor denervation that is associated with stress incontinence. This denervation is worsened by factors which affect the pelvic floor: the number of pregnancies, the length of labour, the size of the baby, any episiotomies or tears and the use of forceps during delivery. The use of post-partum exercises designed to improve pelvic floor tone may help to prevent stress incontinence.

Gynaecological History

The relationship between the lower urinary tract and the hormonal status of the woman is often significant; for example, patients with genuine stress incontinence frequently report that their symptoms are worse in the week before their period begins: this is probably due to increased progesterone levels and relative tissue laxity. Therefore it is important to inquire about not only the patient's menstrual cycle but also her menopausal status. Operations on the uterus may interfere with the innervation of the bladder or may lead to distortion of the lower urinary tract. Denervation, more properly termed decentralisation, is most likely after radical hysterectomy for neoplasia, and may act at both the bladder and urethral levels. Any history of vaginal or suprapubic procedures for prolapse or incontinence may be relevant, because such procedures can produce urethral or bladder neck distortion, scarring or narrowing.

Urological History

The significance of urological symptoms has already been discussed. The patient should be asked about his or her previous urological operations, as such operations have their complications, of which recurrent or persistent obstruction and sphincter damage after prostatectomy are the most common.

Surgical History

The operations most relevant to lower urinary tract function are those on the lower large bowel, where dissection at the side wall of the pelvis may result in nerve damage, especially during abdominal–perineal resection of the rectum.

Trauma History

Trauma to the urethra resulting in stricture formation and obstruction, or trauma to the spinal cord leading to an upper or lower motor neurone lesion, are the accidents most relevant to the lower urinary tract. Trauma to the urethra may be severe and obvious, as in a fractured pelvis with disruption of the pubic symphysis, but problems may follow an apparently trivial perineal injury from which the patient appears to recover in minutes or hours, only to develop a urethral stricture years later.

Other Significant Conditions

Systemic disease processes which influence the lower urinary tract may do so by affecting the innervation. Diabetes mellitus and multiple sclerosis are two such common conditions. Infections such as tuberculosis and schistosomiasis must be remembered. Degenerative disease of the cervical and lumbar spine, spinal tumours and many cerebral conditions may also present as incontinence. Pelvic radiotherapy may produce a post-irradiation cystitis with limitation of the bladder capacity frequency, together with increased frequency and sometimes bladder pain. Mucosal telangectasia following radiotherapy may occasionally cause haematuria.

Drug Therapy

Enquiries should be made as to any drugs the patient is or has been taking, and whether these drugs have any effect on bladder function or produce side-effects. Drugs may be taken intentionally to modify urinary function, or urinary symptoms may be a side-effect of a drug taken for another purpose. All drugs with enhancement or blocking effects on cholinergic, alpha-adrenergic or beta-adrenergic receptors and all drugs with calcium channel effects have a potential effect on lower urinary tract function. Most of these drugs are listed in Appendix 4.

Drugs Enhancing Bladder Emptying

Bladder emptying may be improved by giving drugs either to increase bladder contractility or to decrease bladder outlet resistance. In theory, cholinergic drugs increase bladder contractility and may produce frequency, whilst alpha-adrenergic blockers decrease outflow resistance, and may precipitate or exaggerate stress incontinence. Whilst alpha-blockers are thought to be effective, most clinicians have little faith in cholinergic medication designed to improve detrusor contractility.

Drugs Enhancing Bladder Storage

Bladder storage may be improved by increasing functional bladder capacity or by increasing bladder outlet resistance.

Anticholinergic drugs, which in patients with detrusor instability help to achieve continence and increase bladder capacity, may provoke retention of urine in normal or borderline obstructive patients. Whilst anticholinergic drugs are felt to be helpful in patients with detrusor overactivity during storage, their effectiveness is limited by side-effects: it is ironic that the most troublesome of these is dry mouth, which encourages the patient to drink more! Alpha-adrenergic stimulating drugs are used to increase bladder outlet resistance, although they have only a marginal effect.

Other Drugs

Other drugs of significance include the *diuretics*, which increase urinary frequency in a variable way. The action of diuretics varies in accordance with the patient's age in particular, and the onset of the resulting increased urine output may also vary according to the gastrointestinal absorptive function. *Antidepressants*, such as the tricyclic drugs, of which Chlorpromazine is an example, often have effects on lower urinary tract function: these drugs have anticholinergic actions which tend to increase storage and decrease voiding efficiency. *Oestrogen* therapy may improve lower urinary tract symptoms, decreasing urinary frequency and improving the symptom of dysuria.

Full discussion of the actions of drugs on the lower urinary tract is beyond the scope of this book. Some further information is provided in the chapter on anatomy and physiology, or the reader is referred to the excellent book edited by Marco Caine, *The Pharmacology of the Urinary Tract*, and the writings of Alan Wein. It is suggested that if the patient is on a drug prescribed to them to influence lower urinary tract function, or on a drug with urinary side-effects, then the investigator should interpret the urodynamic findings in the light of the known drug effects. In certain circumstances the clinician may prefer to withdraw the relevant drug two weeks before urodynamic testing, or before completion of a frequency–volume chart.

General Patient Assessment

Whilst discussing the presenting symptoms with the patient, the clinician will have made a subjective assessment of the patient. It is clear that there is a considerable interaction between the patient's personality and mood on the one hand, and the urinary symptoms on the other. It is a common experience that anxiety leads to urinary frequency and even urgency. Such factors as age, degree of stoicism, degree of neuroticism and mood should be assessed. Some patients are extremely tolerant of symptoms that other patients would refuse to accept, and the presence of nocturia is a good example. Whilst the factors mentioned above cannot be quantified easily, they remain important when the clinician comes to interpret the patient's symptoms and urodynamic findings, particularly with respect to proposals for treatment. It will be necessary occasionally to seek a psychiatric or psychological opinion where the clinician is uneasy about the patient's mental state, but cannot define the abnormality in its relation to urinary symptoms.

In addition to the mental state, the mobility and dexterity of patients can have a profound influence on management. Are they well motivated? Could they manage a urinary appliance? Would they be continent if more mobile and able to reach a toilet? Will they co-operate with follow-up or take drugs reliably? Often the fact that these aspects of assessment are overlooked prevents the subsequent urodynamic diagnosis and efforts at management from achieving the optimal result.

Physical Examination

It is assumed that a general examination of the patient has been undertaken already. This section will discuss only aspects of examination that are of special relevance to the lower urinary tract.

Abdominal Examination

It is appropriate that the lower abdomen should be palpated and percussed in an attempt to demonstrate the bladder. In an adult, only a bladder containing in excess of 300 ml is likely to be palpable or can be percussed above the pubic symphysis. Even though a patient is in urinary retention the bladder may be difficult to palpate, although it should be demonstrated readily by percussion. Other enlarged bladders reveal a clearly palpable outline. The poorly defined ("floppy") bladder is associated with lower intravesical pressures and normal upper tracts, whilst the firm and tense bladder is often associated with high intravesical pressures and upper tract dilatation. In most cases seen in the urodynamic laboratory the patient is unaware of their bladder distension. However, pressing on the suprapubic region, and asking if the patient feels a need to void, if positive, is a good indication of a full or enlarged bladder. Suprapubic examination also reveals the degree of sensitivity of the bladder in some cases where bladder pain is a symptom. The degree of obesity of the patient should be noted.

Examination of the External Genitalia

In the female, abnormalities such as meatal stenosis or fusion of the labia are found occasionally. In male patients, phimosis should be excluded, and the foreskin retracted to reveal the external meatus which should be examined carefully for stenosis. The urethra should be felt for fibrous thickening, which may indicate inflammation or stricture in either sex.

Vaginal Examination

Initially the introitus should be viewed with the patient lying on her back with the legs flexed and abducted.

- Part the labia and inspect the introitus: the position and appearance of the meatus should be noted. The clinician should look to see whether there is evidence of wetness at the introitus, whether the introital mucosa is well oestrogenised, showing a pink, moist and healthy appearance or whether there are signs of oestrogen deficiency when the mucosa appears thin, red and atrophic. If the mucosa is red and there is an offensive discharge it is likely that the patient is suffering an infective vaginitis.

- Test for urine leaking by firstly asking the patient to cough repeatedly and secondly by asking the patient to bear down (strain), observing the meatus for urine leakage.
- Assess prolapse: prolapse can be divided into three categories: I, where the prolapse does not reach the introitus; II, where the prolapse reaches the introitus; III, where the prolapse is through the introitus. The presence and degree of anterior vaginal wall descent and posterior vaginal wall descent should be assessed. Uterine descent and/or enterocele will often be missed in this position.
- Assess vaginal capacity and mobility. This has particular significance in choosing the type of surgery in patients with genuine stress incontinence. In order to perform a repositioning procedure, e.g. a colposuspension, it is necessary to evaluate the vagina on both sides of the urethra, and place it in contact with the back of the symphysis pubis. The Bonney test, whereby a finger is put either side of the bladder neck, will successfully assess vaginal mobility, but should not be relied on as a test of continence as the elevating fingers may well compress the bladder neck andurethra.

The woman should now be asked to turn on to the left lateral position and examined using the Sim's speculum to systematically assess the four possible elements of prolapse:

- Use a Sim's speculum to retract the posterior vaginal wall, and assess the resting position of the bladder neck/bladder base and the degree of descent of the anterior vaginal wall on straining. It may be easier to demonstrate incontinence on coughing in this position. Any vaginal scarring should be noted.
- Assess posterior vaginal wall by using the Sim's speculum to retract the anterior vaginal wall (the second blade of the speculum passes over the anterior abdominal wall).
- Assessment of vault prolapse (interior descent or enterocoele) can be achieved by retracting both anterior and posterior vaginal wall either using the Sim's speculum plus a long forceps or by using Cuscow's speculum. Cuscow's speculum cannot be used to assess anterior or posterior vaginal wall prolapse.
- The vaginal examination is an excellent opportunity to assess the voluntary contractile ability of the patient's perivaginal muscles. These muscles are part of the pelvic floor and the ability to contract them forms the basis of the pelvic floor exercises. An alternative method of assessing pelvic floor function is to use a perineometer (Fig. 4.9).

Rectal Examination

Rectal examination should also be systematic.

- *Inspection.* Does the anus appear normal? If a hand is placed on the perineal skin either side of the anus and lateral traction exerted then in patients with poor anal function the anus will begin to open.

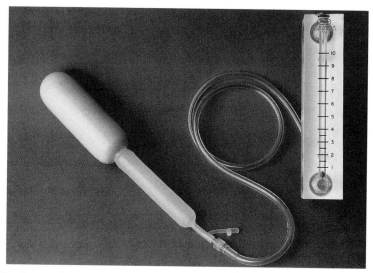

Fig. 4.9 Simple perineometer: the vaginal probe measures pelvic floor contraction and can be used to train and improve pelvic floor function.

- *Perineal sensation.* Because the dermatones S_2, S_3 and S_4 serve the perineal region, intact sensation is likely to mean that the innervation of the bladder and urethra, and indeed the rectum and anal canal is intact.
- *Anal reflex.* If the perineal skin is scratched the anus should "wink" at the investigator. This is best seen in patients with upper motor neurone lesions, for example, high spinal cord injury.
- *Anal tone.* As the examining finger passes into the anal canal the tone of the anal sphincter can be assessed. In lesions such as meningomyelocele anal tone may initially appear good, but after removal of the examining finger the anus may remain open.
- *Voluntary squeeze.* Patients should be able to increase anal sphincter pressure by voluntarily contracting the levator ani. If a woman has been unable to contract the perivaginal muscles during vaginal examination then the rectal examination may provide more stimulation, allowing her to appreciate which muscles need exercise as part of pelvic floor rehabilitation.
- *Faecal impaction.* If the rectum is impacted the subsequent urodynamics will be affected both because of the difficulty of inserting and monitoring the position of a rectal catheter but also because rectal distension inhibits bladder contraction.
- *Prostate evaluation.* In men the prostate gland should be assessed for size, shape, consistency and abnormal tenderness.

Neurological Examination

All patients must have a simple neurological examination, including a gross assessment of sensation, reflexes and muscle function in the legs. In particular, special attention should be paid to the sensory sacral dermatomes, the motor divisions of which supply the bladder (S_2 S_3 S_4). In patients found to have, or known to have, neurological abnormalities, a full neurological examination should be performed. In injuries to the spinal cord, the level of the lesion and whether or not the lesion is complete should be documented.

Certain reflex responses are described in the assessment of sacral function. The anal reflexes are listed by pricking the perianal skin and watching to see if the anal sphincter contracts reflexly. This is quite easy to do at the time of rectal examination. The second reflex is the bulbo-cavernosus reflex, and this involves digital squeezing of the glans penis (or clitoris) and the observation of contraction in the anal sphincter or bulbo-cavernosus muscle. In the neurologically intact patient this procedure may provoke a certain amount of discontent and perhaps encourage them to be less co-operative. In any case a positive response is present only in 70% of normal people. If the reflex is considered to be important then it should be demonstrated electrophysiologically.

As a result of neurological examination the patients can be crudely grouped into four:

- Normal.
- Lower motor neurone: with decreased muscle tone, decreased power, decreased reflexes and absent sensation. This picture occurs in low spinal cord injury patients, affecting the conus medullaris.
- Upper motor neurone: upgoing Babinsky responses, increased muscle tone, increased reflexes, muscle spasms and absent sensation. This is typically seen in a high spinal cord injury patient
- Mixed: lower motor neurone and upper motor neurone such as in spina bifida.

Investigations

Urinalysis

A catheter specimen of urine should be obtained at each urodynamic investigation. If the urine is obviously infected then urodynamics should not be performed because of the risk of provoking bacteria or septicaemia. It is sensible, in patients who have a past history of infection, to cover the urodynamic investigations by antibiotics. If investigation is essential in a patient who has an infection and has not been treated, then an adequate dose of the correct antibiotic should be given intravenously in order to ensure an adequate blood level at the time of investigation. The urine specimen should be routinely tested and may be sent for microscopy and culture. Alternatively, the urine can be tested for the presence of nitrite, an excellent indicator of infection: only those testing positive for nitrite are sent to the laboratory.

Cytology

Cytological studies of urine, vagina or cervix may be indicated. Patients with widespread *in situ* bladder carcinoma, which carries a poor prognosis, may present with the symptoms of cystitis or bladder hypersensitivity. In these patients the urine specimen often shows white cells or red cells, and urine for cytology is likely to show malignant cells. In female patients with lower urinary tract symptoms the hormonal status of the patient may be assessed by lateral vaginal wall cytological smear. It has been shown that the urinary symptoms of patients whose vaginal cells show oestrogen deficiency often improve with oestrogen therapy.

Radiology

Non-contrast Radiology

A plain X-ray of the abdomen and pelvis should be performed in every patient. The X-ray should be critically examined to look at soft tissue abnormalities such as an enlarged bladder, bony abnormalities such as spondylosis, spina bifida or metastasis, and for opacities such as bladder or ureteric stones.

Intravenous Urography

Traditionally many patients with lower urinary tract symptoms had an intravenous urogram (IVU) performed, but there is no evidence to show that in patients with lower urinary tract symptoms the IVU gave any useful information. This is because static films give very little idea of function: bladder shape may alter during contraction and diverticula may appear; the evaluation of residual urine is also notoriously inaccurate. Equally the absence of residual urine or of a basal prostatic filling defect does not exclude significant bladder outlet obstruction.

An IVU is indicated however, if the patient has blood in the urine or an abnormal plain x-ray. Similarly if the patient reports haematuria or has localised upper tract symptoms an IVU is essential. It should also be carried out in patients who have undiagnosed continuous incontinence, as it may reveal a duplex kidney, suggesting an ectopic ureter. In patients with a proteus urinary tract infection, an IVU may show an infected "matrix" renal calculus which can be difficult to see on a plain film.

Micturating Cystourethrography

The conventional micturating cystourethrogram (MCUG) consists of visualisation by a radiologist of abnormally fast filling, followed by emptying of the bladder: a number of spot films are taken at appropriate (or inappropriate) occasions. However, this can be a valuable assessment of lower urinary tract structure, because changes may be seen during the micturition cycle. It is appropriate to make the most of the investigation and to provide the maximum amount of clinical information to the radiologist. In order to do this the whole investigation should be recorded on videotape. The MCUG is a "second best" investigation to videourodynamics. However if videourodynamics is not available then MCUG should be performed (see "Videourodynamics" in Chapter 3).

Endoscopy

Endoscopy is not indicated in the assessment of lower urinary tract functions unless there are specific symptoms or signs. Endoscopy is indicated if the patient complains of bladder pain or haematuria or if there is an abnormal MSU or abnormal radiology. Occasionally clinical "desperation" may be an indication for endoscopy.

Endoscopy should always consist of urethroscopy followed by cystoscopy. It is particularly important that urethral inspection is not omitted, as it may give information as to the site of obstruction in patients with obstructed voiding. However, if the obstruction is functional rather than structural, for example, detrusor–bladder-neck dyssynergia or detrusor–sphincter dyssynergia, then the site of obstruction will not be demonstrated by endoscopy. Bladder neck and/or bladder wall hypertrophy does not indicate obstruction, nor does trabeculation of the bladder. If urethroscopy is normal and the urodynamic assessment has shown obstructed voiding then videourodynamics is the investigation of choice. The correlation between endoscopy and urodynamic findings is discussed further in the next chapter under "Urodynamics in Men".

Ultrasound

Considerable progress has been made in the level of sophistication in ultrasound technology. In assessing patients with lower urinary tract problems, ultrasound can be used in several ways:

- As basic screening test in place of the plain abdominal X-ray.
- To assess bladder emptying. Simple hand-held machines are now available which can be used during urodynamics, in the outpatient clinic, on the ward and even in the patient's home (Fig. 3.24).
- To exclude upper tract problems. It is useful to be able to scan the kidneys as in some situations vesico-urethral dysfunction can result in upper tract dilatation (see "Neuropathic Bladders" in Chapter 5). However renal ultrasound is probably best left to the radiologists.
- Vaginal ultrasound. Ultrasound can be used as an alternative to X-rays in videourodynamics (see Chapter 3).
- Rectal ultrasound: this can be used to visualise the prostate in men, and the lower urinary tract in both men and women.

References

Abrams P, Klevmark B (1996). Frequency volume charts: An indispensable part of lower urinary tract assessment. Scand J Urol Nephrol 30 suppl 179.

Bailey R, Shepherd A, Tribe B (1990). How much information can be obtained from frequency/volume charts? Neurourol Urodyn 9:382–385 (abst).

Caine M (1984). The pharmacoloogy of the urinary tract. London: Springer-Verlag.

Carter P (1992). The role of nocturnal polyuria in nocturnal urinary symptoms in the healthy elderly male. MD Thesis University of Bristol.

Donovan JL, Abrams P, Peters TJ, Kay HE, Reynard J, Chapple C, de la Rosette JJMCH, Kondon A (1996). The ICS-'BPH' study: the psychometric validity and reliability of the ICS male questionnaire. Br J Urol 77:554–562.

Jackson S, Donovan J, Brookes S, Eckford S, Swithinbank L, Abrams P (1996). The Bristol female lower urinary tract symptoms questionnaire: development and psychometric testing. Br J Urol 77:805–812.

Klevmark B (1989). Objective assessment of urinary incontinence. The use of pad-weighing and frequency-volume charts. Dan Med Bull Special Supplement Series 8:28–30.

Larsson G, Victor A (1988). Micturition patterns in a healthy female population, studied with a frequency–volume chart. Scand J Urol Nephrol supp. 4:53–57.

Larsson G, Abrams P, Victor A (1991). The frequency/volume chart in detrusor instability. Neurourol Urodyn 10:533–543.

Larsson G, Victor A (1992). The frequency/volume chart in genuine stress incontinent women. Neurourol Urodyn 11:23–31.

Nørgaard JP (1991). Pathophysiology of nocturnal enuresis. Scand J Urol Nephrol suppl. 140.

Robinson D, McClish DK, Wyman JF, Bump RC, Fantl JA (1996). Comparison between urinary diaries completed with and without intensive patient instructions. Neurourol Urodyn 15:143–148.

Reynard JM, Lamond E, Abrams P (1993). The significance of abdominal straining and intermittency in men with prostatism. Proc ICS 23rd Annual meeting Rome.

Torrens MJ (1974). The effect of selective sacral nerve blocks on vesical and urethral function. J Urol112:204–205.

Turner Warwick R, Milroy E (1979). A reappraisal of the value of routine urological procedures in the assessment of urodynamic function. Urol Clin N Am 6:63–70.

Chapter 5
Urodynamics in Clinical Practice

Introduction

The principles of urodynamics having been discussed and the reader provided with a proper understanding of urodynamic techniques, it is important to place urodynamic studies in a proper clinical context. The purpose of this chapter is to show how urodynamic tests can help the clinician to improve diagnosis and treatment. There are four main ways in which this is possible:

- The investigations may assist in the evaluation of an individual case, providing objective evidence on which to base decisions.
- The analysis of groups of patients may, over a time, improve both the understanding of pathophysiology and the selection of patients for treatment.
- Urodynamics may provide objective information before and after therapeutic intervention, allowing the clinician to monitor the results of treatment more accurately.
- The tests assist the continuing education of clinicians themselves.

As the clinician becomes more experienced in the urodynamic investigation of patients their confidence in their diagnostic ability as to the significance of symptomatic complaints increases. This increase in confidence is only partially justified. We shall refer to the study in which the diagnostic ability of the urodynamic investigations was tested. The computer proforma (Appendix 3 Part 1) contains a question that is asked of the investigator at the end of the symptomatic enquiry, i.e. they are asked to predict the urodynamic findings from the symptomatic complaints. Even for the experienced investigator the results are salutary!

The urodynamic diagnosis is used by us as the "arbiter of truth". This statement assumes that the explanation for the patient's symptomatic complaints will unfold as the urodynamic investigations proceed. If the symptomatic history and

Table 5.1. 1995 urodynamic workload (children are defined as ≤ 16 years old)

	Children	Female	Male	Total
Ambulatory UDS	1	79	3	83
Pad test	0	61	0	61
Routine UDS	5	809	418	1232
Uroflowmetry	27	133	1589	1749
Video UDS	48	190	175	413
Total	81	1312	2185	3578

the urodynamic investigations are at variance then the studies should be repeated or extended.

In 1995 we investigated 3578 patients in our unit. By far the most common investigation was urine flow studies with the ultrasound estimation of residual urine. Table 5.1 shows the proportions of children, men and women investigated and the investigations these patients had. The median age of women investigated was 52 years and that of men 66 years.

Urodynamics in Children

Three main groups of children are considered for urodynamic studies (UDS):

- Children with neurological disease and possible vesicourethral dysfunction.
- Children with lower urinary tract symptoms and/or dysfunction.
- Children with non-neurological congenital abnormalities and possible vesico-urethral dysfunction.

Children with Neurological Disorders

These are most commonly related to dysgenesis of the spine and the associated nervous system. The neurological deficit is frequently more complicated than that in acquired neurological problems, and this makes the interpretation of bladder dysfunction more difficult.

The largest group of children with neuropathic bladders are those with myelodysplasia. It is important to recognise that the level of the neurological lesion does not correlate with the functional classification of the bladder. This is true in many types of neurological disease, but is particularly evident in these children, most of whom have spina bifida in addition to their neurological lesion. The role of urodynamics is to make the crucial functional distinctions between a high-pressure bladder (unsafe) and a low-pressure one (safe), the former being associated with the worse prognosis. Blaivas et al. (1977) emphasised that there was no statistical correlation between the pressure generated in the bladder and the level of the neurological lesion. They noted that detrusor–urethral dys-synergia can occur in both "high-" and "low-pressure" bladders. The timing of UDS in these children is much debated. McGuire has been the protagonist for early UDS, within the first few months of life. Using leak point pressure measurements he advocates the early use of clean intermittent catheterisation to

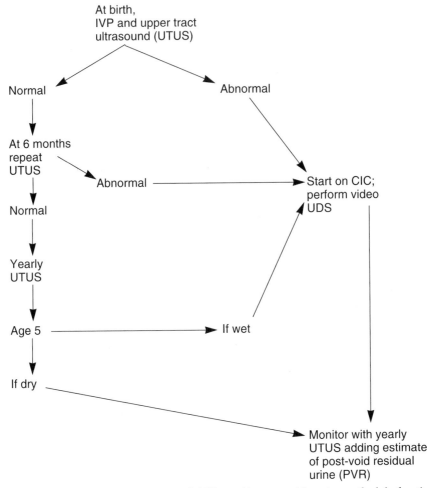

Fig. 5.1 Algorhythm for the investigation of children with neuropathic vesico-urethral dysfunction based on upper tract ultrasound (UTUS) and the use of clean intermittent catheterisation (CIC).

prevent upper tract drainage being compromised. It has been our habit to invest-igate these children later when continence would normally be expected to develop, at around 5 years of age. Figure 5.1 describes our protocol.

VUDS will have to be repeated if an interventional therapy such as ileo-cystoplasty or artificial sphincter implantation is planned. VUDS are used in these children in view of the relatively high incidence of abnormalities such as vesicoureteric reflux and sphincteric obstruction during voiding.

The keenly felt differences in views represent differences in experience, which are probably related to patient populations that differ significantly. With the reducing incidence of meningomyelocele births many born now have minimal defects and develop normal bladder and bowel function. The principles of management of these children are similar to that of the adult neuropathic patient and are discussed later.

Children Born with Non-neurological Defects

There are two main groups in this category:

- *Urethral valves.* Boys born with urethral valves have often been diagnosed prenatally and are treated very early in life. However there are often long-term sequelae to valves, with poor bladder compliance and upper tract dilatation. These boys need to be followed in a similar fashion to the meningomyelocele children with early urodynamics if there is upper tract dilatation.

- *Ano-rectal abnormalities.* The frequency of voiding dysfunction in these children depends on the extent of the abnormality and the presence of associated sacral bony defects: the higher the lesion the more likely the child is to have disturbed voiding. Urodynamic studies before and after pelvic surgery, aimed at restoring bowel continuity to the anus, give useful information, although it is unclear whether or not UDS are essential in management or whether the "watch and wait" policy outlined above is adequate.

Normal Children with Vesico-urethral Dysfunction

These children have no physical abnormality and fall into several main groups, but present chiefly with enuresis and daytime incontinence or recurrent urinary infections. On urodynamic investigation the main abnormalities found in children are detrusor instability, dysfunctional voiding and vesico-ureteric reflux, and these may occur alone or in combination.

- *Detrusor instability.* The toddler's bladder goes from the reflex organ of the infant to the adult bladder by the age of five in most individuals. Between, there is a stage at which children have partial control over bladder activity. All those who have brought up children are familiar with the techniques children use to control their overactive bladder: boys pinch the end of their penis and girls squat pushing the heel into the perineum. In performing these manoeuvres both boys and girls are probably using the bulbo-cavernosus reflex to inhibit an unstable contraction. In this period toddlers often make mistakes whilst playing a favourite game, delaying too long and wetting themselves. However by the age of 5, 90% of children are reliably dry, day and night, although the remaining 10% continue to have problems. Parents and some children understandably become distressed by continued poor bladder control with the wet beds and embarrassing daytime incidents that result. There is considerable pressure on the health care professionals to "do something". However we know that 90% of those wet at 5 will become dry by adulthood and therefore resist the pressure for any interventional treatments.

    Enuresis may or may not be associated with detrusor instability and it has to be remembered that enuresis is a phenomenon with a number of possible causes in addition to detrusor instability: low bladder capacity, reduced bladder sensation, failure of arousal from sleep and overproduction of urine at night are the most important. For those readers interested in this topic, the work of the Aarhus group in Denmark has been most important. They have shown that a proportion of children have deficient production of antidiuretic hormone at night and therefore fail to concentrate their night-time urine and produce higher volumes. Such children are better treated by synthetic antidiuretic hormone (DDAVP) than by an anticholinergic drug.

Management involves a presumptive diagnosis followed by empiric treatment, although in our view children should be screened by urine flow studies (UFS) and ultrasound estimates of residual urine, as UFS show that a small proportion of enuretic children exhibit disordered voiding, that is, dysfunctional voiding.

- *Dysfunctional voiding.* This term is reserved for those children unable to micturate with a continuous flow because of pelvic floor overactivity during voiding. The cause of the overactivity is not understood, although such children may also have bowel problems (chronic constipation) and often exhibit behavioural difficulties. The pelvic floor overactivity produces an interrupted flow pattern that looks very similar to detrusor–sphincter dyssynergia. As far as we know dysfunctional voiding is not seen commonly in asymptomatic children. An effect of stream interruption is to lead to detrusor inhibition before the bladder is emptied, resulting in an increasing residual urine. Voiding occurs against a partially closed sphincter, and that may be the reason that most children have detrusor instability during filling. This combination may produce detrusor hypertrophy, resulting in reduced bladder compliance with upper tract dilatation as well as incontinence, enuresis, infections and vesico-ureteric reflux.

  This condition was first described by Himan in 1956 and later by Allen in 1977. They used the term "non-neurogenic neurogenic bladder", which is confusing in many senses – the term "dysfunctional voiding" is to be preferred.

- *Children with vesico-ureteric reflux (VUR).* VUR is likely to be discovered after a child has presented with urinary tract infection often complicated by secondary enuresis. If screening studies, flow rates and ultrasound estimates of residual urine, together with upper tract ultrasound, are normal then urodynamics is not indicated. If reflux and upper tract dilatation coexists then urodynamics is indicated. However the interpretation of bladder compliance in the presence of gross reflux, or indeed a diverticulum, is very difficult because the refluxing ureter and kidney increase bladder compliance. In such children any change in compliance should be regarded as dangerous to the upper tract and renal function.

Modifications of Urodynamic Technique in Children

In children there may be specific problems in using conventional techniques for two main reasons, namely the small size of the child or lack of co-operation from the child.

The small size of children requires obvious alteration in techniques such as reducing the speed of bladder filling: Nijman recommends that the bladder should be filled at 10% of the expected bladder volume per minute. Expected bladder volume can be calculated by the formula 30 ml + (30 ml times age), giving a 3-year-old a capacity of 120 ml, i.e. 30 + (3 × 30). In children with compromised neurology resulting in reduced urethral sensation, or who have been taught to do clean intermittent catheterisation, a urethral catheter can be used for pressure measurement and the 6 Fr dual-channel catheter works well. The combination of an epidural catheter for pressure recording and a 6 Fr catheter for filling can be used. It is wise to record two fill and void sequences in children, as recommended by Griffiths and Scholtmeyer, because this allows the child to become used to the strange environment of the urodynamic room: a more relaxed micturition is often seen on the second void.

If the child is likely to be upset by urethral catheterisation, and this will apply to most neurologically normal small children not doing intermittent self-catheterisation (ISC), there are two choices: perform urodynamics under sedation, or prior to urodynamics put in suprapubic catheters under anaesthetic. Urodynamics under sedation works well for infants and toddlers under one year. They are admitted to the paediatric ward, where they receive an appropriate dose of a sedative such as Vallergan. The baby comes with its mother to the laboratory and can be breast-fed, given a bottle or given a dummy or comforter if they cry. In older children sedation is not so satisfactory and the child becomes very difficult to pacify if roused; we would prefer to use suprapubic catheters (two epidural catheters, one for filling and one for the measurement of p_{ves}, or a single dual-channel 6 Fr catheter). The suprapubic route allows the fill-and-void cycle to be repeated.

Passage of the rectal catheter for p_{abd} measurement can be a problem in children who are fearful of rectal examination. Most children over 5 can be calmed, provided the atmosphere is relaxed and the child is not pressurised. We once advocated the exclusion of parents from the urodynamic room, but this is now socially unacceptable and even the parent who adds to the child's anxiety has to be accepted. Our urodynamic laboratory has a plentiful supply of children's books and videos which have proved an excellent distraction: the child is invited to bring their favourite video.

Who Should Do Paediatric Urodynamics?

Paediatric UDS should only be performed in centres with an active urodynamic unit with staff expert in dealing with children and where there is active collaboration with the paediatricians and paediatric urologist (see Chapter 7).

Indications for Urodynamic Investigation in Children

Because these studies are often upsetting for children we only use UDS if:

- The results will affect management.
- Empirical treatment has failed and invasive therapy is contemplated requiring confirmation of the presumptive diagnosis.
- Screening tests have been shown to be abnormal.

We are still asked to do urodynamics in children with enuresis who have failed to respond to bladder training, enuretic alarm and anticholinergics. We refuse, but ask to do screening flow studies and offer to become involved in their management as their medical therapy may not have been aggressive enough. Only if invasive therapy such as ileocystoplasty is being contemplated would we agree to do full urodynamics.

Urodynamics in Women

UDS in women should be set in a therapeutic context. Incontinence in women forms a large part of the workload of any urodynamics unit; two-thirds of the women referred to the Bristol unit fall into this category. Stress incontinence is almost entirely a female problem which may occur alone or be associated, to a variable extent, with urgency. Leakage associated only with urgency (urge incontinence) is also a common problem. The symptom complex allows an index of suspicion about the nature of the functional disorder, but it is not entirely reliable. One of the principal roles for urodynamics is the identification of the main cause of incontinence, detrusor or urethral, in any particular case.

Table 5.2 shows the distribution of the different types of incontinence among patients referred to our unit; 64 % complain of either stress or urge incontinence. The reason why female incontinence is more frequent, and more troublesome, than in males is that the predisposing factors work together to compound the problem. While there is a natural tendency for the bladder to become overactive with advancing age, there is also a tendency for the urethra to become less competent. The pattern of presentation therefore varies with age (Table 5.3) and the overall prevalence increases with age.

As incontinence occurs with a high prevalence in the community, it is unrealistic and indeed unnecessary for all women to have urodynamic studies to confirm a diagnosis. Treatment should begin in the community and only if this is unsatisfactory or fails should urodynamic referral be made (see Chapter 6).

Table 5.2. Different types of female incontinence categorised by symptoms

Incontinence (types)	%
None	22.3
Stress	19.0
Stress/urge	25.1
Urge	14.4
Urge/enuresis	5.1
Enuresis	2.9
Post-micturition dribble	0.8
Continuous	6.4
Other	4.0

Table 5.3. Percentage of female patients presenting with incontinence according to age

Age	Stress	Stress/urge	Urge
20 to 30	14%	15%	15%
40 to 50	30%	34%	16%
60 to 70	12%	32%	20%

Symptom Presentation in Women

There are several common types of presentation:

- Stress incontinence
- Frequency–urgency syndrome
- Urge incontinence
- Mixed urge and stress incontinence
- Urinary infections

Urodynamics has a role in further defining the underlying vesico-urethral disorders when empirical treatment has failed.

Stress Incontinence

In the first edition of this book we stated that if the patient had pure stress incontinence then UDS were not indicated. Our attitudes have changed somewhat and there are several advantages to performing UDS on all women before invasive surgery:

- Confirmation of incontinence and its cause.
- Definition of detrusor activity during filling.
- Assessment of detrusor voiding function.
- Assessment of degree of sphincter weakness.
- Assessment of pelvic floor function.

Both the confirmation of incontinence and the definition of its cause is highly desirable. 12% of women with apparently pure stress incontinence can be shown to have detrusor instability rather than GSI as the cause of their symptoms. Very careful physical examination is a reputable way of making a clear diagnosis of GSI if leakage is synchronous with the first cough, but only in a minority of women with GSI can this be shown. The reason for this is clear on video, when many women will leak after the third or fourth cough as the bladder neck is progressively opened by successive coughs (Fig. 5.2). Even if the woman leaks on the

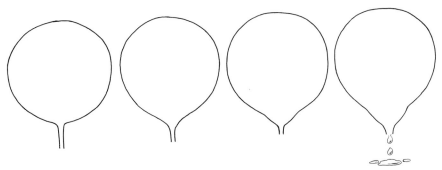

Fig. 5.2 Diagram of the video appearance of the bladder neck changing with successive coughs: leakage occurs after four coughs.

first cough and a diagnosis of GSI is certain, UDS do give further information on other aspects of urethral and detrusor function. These other pieces of information allow the surgeon to counsel the woman on the likely outcome of surgery. If the detrusor is underactive or acontractile on voiding then it is reasonable to warn the patient that spontaneous voiding may be delayed and that it might be necessary for her to go home with a catheter for a period of time. In some patients with apparently pure stress incontinence, detrusor instability (DI) may be found. In recent reports on the findings of ambulatory urodynamics in GSI patients it has been suggested that asymptomatic DI preoperative becomes symptomatic after GSI surgery. Certainly if DI is found preoperatively then the patient should be told that GSI surgery is for stress incontinence and cannot be guaranteed to cure DI. UDS also allows the assessment of urethral and pelvic floor function. If despite GSI the patient has reasonable urethral function as judged by the maximum urethral closure pressure (MUCP) and can effectively interrupt voiding using her pelvic floor then the outcome of GSI surgery is likely to be excellent. If however the MUCP is low (below 20 cmH_2O) then there is evidence that the outcome for simple repositioning procedures such as Burch colposuspension or needle suspension is less successful.

The Diagnosis of GSI

Much nonsense has been talked about videourodynamics being the "gold standard" test for the diagnosis of GSI. In fact, the "gold standard" is seeing urine leak from the external meatus when the patient raises her intra-abdominal pressure in the absence of a detrusor contraction. Videourodynamics is *not* necessary for the routine diagnosis of GSI, and indeed it is easy to miss the loss of a few drops of urine if the urodynamicist watches the TV monitor rather than the patient. Urodynamics is always an embarrassing investigation for patients, and much effort must be made to put the woman at her ease, so that she will tolerate the investigator "staring" at her perineum. To demonstrate GSI the patient should be seated as in all female UDS. If GSI is not demonstrated then it is useful to ask the patient to flex and abduct one thigh to open the introitus: this reduces the support offered by the pelvic floor and may allow the demonstration of GSI (Fig. 3.56).

Other urodynamic tests such as urethral profilometry may provide interesting and useful information but cannot be used to diagnose GSI if it is not seen during filling cystometry. Figure 3.78 shows how the maximum urethral pressure, whilst significantly lower in GSI patients, has inadequate specificity to be used for diagnostic purposes. If despite carrying out UDS as described above GSI is not demonstrated in patients with the symptom of stress incontinence, and if surgery is being contemplated then ambulatory urodynamics (AUDS) is the test of choice. If after AUDS no incontinence can be demonstrated then the patient should be told that surgery would not be wise when the cause of incontinence remains to be defined.

The Frequency–Urgency Syndrome

This syndrome includes detrusor instability and bladder hypersensitivity. In *detrusor instability* (DI), frequency and urgency may precede the onset of urge incontinence. In the nulliparous woman the pelvic floor has significantly better function than after childbirth and the patient can often use her pelvic floor to retain continence until the unstable contraction fades. In DI, bladder sensation is usually normal with the exception that the desire to void becomes accentuated.

However in patients with *bladder hypersensitivity*, bladder sensation is often described differently, as an irritating sensation. In hypersensitivity the first desire to void occurs at low volumes and persists, distracting the patient from normal activities: sometimes the patient will describe the sensation as developing into pain. Interstitial cystitis (IC) produces an extreme form of bladder hypersensitivity in which there is a consistently low functional capacity due to increasing bladder discomfort or pain as filling continues. In IC the pain is relieved by micturition, but often only after some 5 or 10 minutes. Although conditions such as IC, bladder tumours, bladder stones and bacterial cystitis may produce a hypersensitivity picture they usually have pain as part of the symp-tom complex. Bladder pain is a symptom that warrants further urgent investigation including repeat urine microscopy, urine cytology and usually cystourethroscopy.

Symptoms are inadequate to distinguish the cause of the frequency urgency syndrome and if a definitive diagnosis is required then UDS are essential.

Urge Incontinence

Although most urge incontinence follows urgency through fear of leakage, in other words it is a normal although increased desire to void, some patients have urge incontinence owing to increasing discomfort or pain. Hence some women with bacterial cystitis will have urge incontinence because bladder wall inflammation makes it more desirable to be a little wet rather than suffer extreme pain as the bladder fills. Evidence from ambulatory urodynamics is increasingly showing that in women with urge incontinence without any stress incontinence symptoms the cause of incontinence is almost always detrusor instability, whereas conventional urodynamics show that only two-thirds have DI. Because the association of urge incontinence and DI in this group of women appears so strong, UDS are not needed except in the research setting, for example trials of new drugs, and if invasive therapy is being contemplated after conservative and drug therapy have failed.

If all investigations fail to show DI in patients with urge incontinence then an alternative mechanism needs to be proposed. In DI incontinence occurs either because the increased bladder pressure overcomes the combined resistance of the intrinsic urethral muscle plus help from the pelvic floor or because the urethra relaxes as part of a preactivated micturition reflex. Urge incontinence in the absence of a detrusor contraction is known as "sensory urge incontinence" and can only happen if urethral relaxation occurs. Here there exists an overlap and some confusion with the term "urethral instability". Urethral instability has been defined as a fall in urethral pressure of greater than 20 cm H_2O recorded when measuring the maximum urethral closure pressure, during bladder filling or at capacity. However it is very unusual to witness urethral instability leading to incontinence whilst doing UDS, and we believe it to be an unusual single cause of incontinence. Nevertheless we have seen the occasional woman who has flooding incontinence without any prior warning, such as the feeling of urgency. In such patients, if conventional UDS fail to show a cause for incontinence then it is helpful to record urethral pressures over a 5 to 10 minute period, at capacity, to see if the MUCP fluctuates (see Fig. 3.89, page 117). In other women, for example, those with genuine stress incontinence, urethral instability might make incontinence worse if the fall in urethral pressure corresponds to an increase in intra-abdominal pressure due to coughing or straining.

Mixed Urge and Stress Incontinence

This combination is experienced by the largest group of women referred for UDS. Initial treatment is conservative (see therapy for LUTD, p. 173) but if this fails then UDS are required to direct future management. The assessment of mixed incontinence should be both symptomatic and urodynamic, and the key questions are:

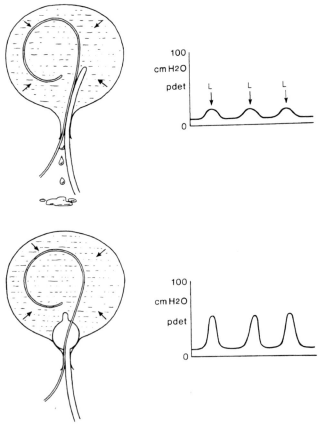

Fig. 5.3 Technique for assessing detrusor instability in women with poor urethral function (L signifies leakage).

- Is urge or stress incontinence most frequent?
- Is urge or stress incontinence most troublesome?
- Are both GSI and DI seen on UDS?
- Do the symptoms and the urodynamic findings correlate?

Because DI can be regarded as the premature activation of the micturition reflex, urge incontinence usually involves a larger loss which occurs more rapidly and which may be too much for any incontinence pad the woman is wearing. Hence even though incontinence secondary to DI may occur less frequently in a woman with mixed incontinence, it is often judged more troublesome.

When assessing DI during filling cystometry it should be remembered that the pattern of DI is dependant on urethral function. It is easy to underestimate the severity of DI in a woman with poor then urethral function: if the MUCP is 20 cmH$_2$O and the pelvic floor function poor, when the intravesical pressure rises to 20 or 30 cmH$_2$O due to an unstable wave, incontinence will occur and the pressure will fall. However after surgery which improves overall urethral function the DI often appears much more spectacular on UDS, with high pressures during filling: this is particularly true after implantation of an artificial sphincter. When judging the significance of DI in a woman with poor urethral function the degree of symptoms and frequency of unstable waves are good guides to the problems she may face after GSI surgery. DI can be more accurately assessed in women with poor urethral function if a Foley balloon catheter is used for filling and the balloon is pulled down to occlude the bladder neck (Fig. 5.3). This manoeuvre should only be used after conventional studies have demonstrated DI, because the presence of a balloon catheter has been shown to increase the incidence of DI in older men.

In our unit 45% of women with symptomatic mixed incontinence are found to have both GSI and DI. However a high proportion of those women with GSI who complain of urge incontinence do not have DI demonstrated on conventional UDS. There has been no large study to investigate such women by ambulatory UDS which might confirm the diagnosis of DI. It remains a clinical impression that women with symptoms suggestive of DI, but without DI on UDS, do better from GSI surgery. The symptoms of urgency and urge incontinence in these patients may reflect the fact that the woman is well aware that, as the bladder fills towards capacity, she is more likely to leak and it therefore becomes a matter of "urgency" to empty the bladder in these circumstances.

Urinary Infections

These are common in women and are not usually associated with voiding dysfunction except in the elderly. Poor bladder emptying due to bladder outlet obstruction (BOO) is rare in women. BOO has a variety of structural causes: meatal strictures, urethral distortion secondary to genito-urinary prolapse, urethral obstruction secondary to prolapsed ureterocoele, urethral cancer or stricture after surgery, but may also be functional (see "Dysfunctional voiding", p. 83). Detrusor underactivity (DUA) as a cause of poor bladder emptying is more common. Although DUA may be secondary to drugs (tricyclic antidepressants), surgery (for example after hysterectomy (Wertheims most classically), or rectal operations), injury (spinal cord trauma) or spinal disease, it is most commonly idiopathic and seen in elderly women.

Urinary infections are the most common presentation of voiding dysfunction, because few women complain of poor stream and hesitancy. UDS have little part to play, although we use urine flow studies and ultrasound estimates of residual urine to screen older women with recurrent infections. Flow patterns will usually give an indication if BOO is present, because the maximum flow rate will be consistently reduced. If poor emptying is due to DUA then the flow pattern will often show that reasonable flows can be achieved, often with the help of abdominal straining, but ultrasound shows that the bladder does not empty. We often catheterise the patient in outpatients to exclude any significant mechanical obstruction to flow, to obtain a urine specimen for microscopy and culture, and to accurately measure post-void residual.

Urodynamics in Men

In men, lower urinary tract symptoms (LUTS) are generally due to three main causes of lower urinary tract dysfunction (LUTD):

- Detrusor instability (DI)
- Bladder outlet obstruction (BOO)
- Detrusor underactivity (DUA)

Detrusor Instability

This may persist from childhood or develop in middle or old age, when it may or may not occur in the present of BOO. Because genuine stress incontinence does

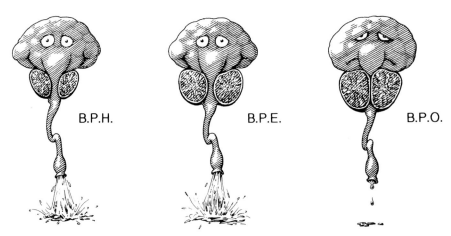

Fig. 5.4 Diagrammatic representation of benign prostatic hyperplasia (BPH), benign prostatic enlargement (BPE) and benign prostatic obstruction (BPO) when BPH leads to BPE, which in turn results in bladder outlet obstruction.

not occur in men, the confusion of symptoms that occur between stress and urge incontinence is not a problem. Hence a man with urgency and urge incontinence almost always has DI as the cause and UDS are only indicated if invasive therapy is being contemplated after conservative treatment has failed.

Bladder Outlet Obstruction

The suspicion of BOO is the usual reason for performing UDS in men. All men should be screened by urine flow studies (UFS) and the ultrasound estimate of post-void residual (PVR). In older men the prostate gland has been traditionally held responsible for many of the symptomatic complaints of male patients, and there has been a tendency to use prostatectomy as a panacea for lower urinary tract symptoms. The need for objective evaluation of these symptoms was answered by the introduction of pressure–flow analysis of micturition. Urodynamic studies have provided alternative explanations for certain symptoms and they have contributed to our understanding of some of the common disorders. However, they have not in any way superseded the importance of a careful and methodical clinical assessment. The history and clinical examination, followed by the routine urine and appropriate radiological investigations, remain the basis for urological management.

The correlations between symptoms and urodynamic diagnosis are poor, and the only symptom with a reasonable urodynamics correlation is urge incontinence with DI. Symptoms have been found to be neither sex- nor age-specific. For these reasons the term "prostatism" should be abandoned in favour of the term "LUTS", divided into "storage" and "voiding" symptoms, and not the old terms "irritative" and "obstructive" symptoms (Table 5.4). The terms referring to prostate histology (benign prostatic hyperplasia: BPH), prostatic size (benign prostatic enlargement: BPE) and the coexistence of BPE and BOO (benign prostatic obstruction: BPO) should be used appropriately and consistently so that clinicians and urodynamicists can communicate clearly about both individual patients and groups of patients. As Fig. 5.4 shows, the presence of BPH or BPE may have no impact on voiding but BPO does, producing the classic urodynamic finding of low flow rate and high voiding pressure. If the terms LUTS, BPH, BPE, BPO and BOO are used then misleading terms such as "clinical BPH", "symptoms of BPH", "symptomatic BPH" and "prostatism" can be abandoned.

Should all older men with LUTS have pressure–flow studies (pQS)? The answer depends on the treatment intentions of the patient and clinician. If conservative

Table 5.4. LUTS

Storage symptoms	Voiding symptoms
Frequency	Hesitancy
Nocturia	Straining to void
Urgency	Poor stream
Urge incontinence	Intermittent stream
Stress incontinence	*Dysuria*
Enuresis	Feeling of incomplete emptying
Bladder pain	Terminal dribble

Table 5.5. Predictive ability of first flow rate for a voided volume of 150 ml or more

Flow rate ml/s	Number	Pressure flows	
		Obstructed	Not obstructed
< 10	135 (38%)	119 (89%)	16 (12%)
10 to 15	130 (37%)	92 (71%)	38 (29%)
> 15	91 (26%)	44 (48%)	47 (52%)
Total	356 (100%)	255 (71%)	101 (28%)

AG number = $p_{\text{det}, Q_{\max}} - 2Q_{\max}$.

treatment is planned then basic urological tests should be performed after a routine physical examination and an analysis of symptoms, but unless there are definite indications for surgery then no urodynamic tests are needed at this stage (see treatment of LUTD). If conservative treatment has failed and the patient remains symptomatic to the extent that he wishes to consider surgery then urine flow studies (UFS) and the ultrasound estimate of PVR should be carried out. If the maximum flow rate ($Q_{\max}$) is below 10 ml/s then the chance of the patient having BOO is 90%; 38% of our patients would fit into this category. However if the $Q_{\max}$ is 10 to 15 ml/s then the incidence of BOO falls to 71% or less (Table.5.5).

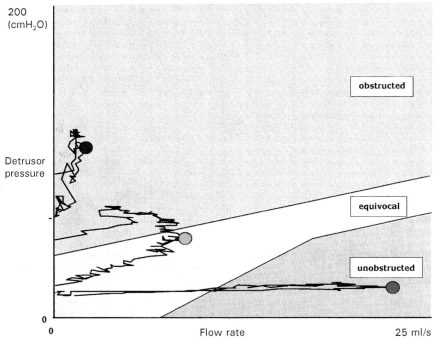

Fig. 5.5 Abrams–Griffiths nomogram divides three typical patients into obstructed, equivocal and unobstructed.

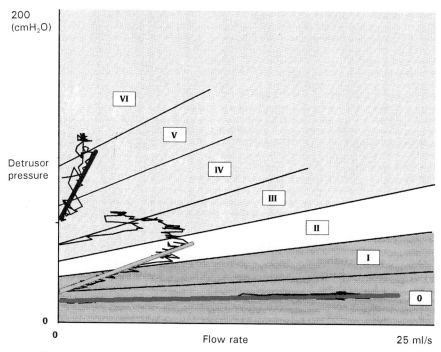

Fig. 5.6 Linear passive urethra resistance ratio (LPURR) classification divides patients into obstructed (III to VI), slightly obstructed (II) and unobstructed (0 and I); same three patients as Fig. 5.5.

Because 29% of these patients will not be shown to have BOO, we believe that *all patients with a Q_{max} of 10 ml/s or more should have pQS before invasive therapy.*

How is the diagnosis of BOO made? In some men either flow is very low (<10 ml/s) or voiding pressure is so high ($p_{det, Q_{max}}$ >100 cm H_2O) that BOO is highly likely. However for most patients the diagnosis of BOO is made by plotting the maximum flow rate (Q_{max}) against detrusor pressure at Q_{max} ($p_{det, Q_{max}}$) into one of the commonly used nomograms: Abrams–Griffiths (AG; Fig. 5.5), LPURR (Fig. 5.6) or URA (Fig. 5.7, *overleaf*). If the clinician wishes to describe the degree of obstruction then either the AG (by calculating the AG number) or the URA gives a precise figure, whereas the LPURR nomogram gives 7 grades from 0 to VI. The AG number can be calculated and BOO diagnosed without reference to the nomogram from the simple equation

$$\text{AG number} = p_{det, Q_{max}} - 2Q_{max}$$

If the AG number is greater than 40 then BOO exists; if it is below 40 then no definite BOO exists. By further analysing the urodynamic trace it is possible to categorise those patients with an AG number of less than 40. To do this the minimum detrusor pressure during voiding ($p_{det \, min, \, void}$) must be read from the trace: usually this is seen at the end of voiding. If both the $p_{det \, Q_{max}}/Q_{max}$ point and the point of $p_{det \, min, \, void}$ are plotted then the LPURR (linear passive urethral

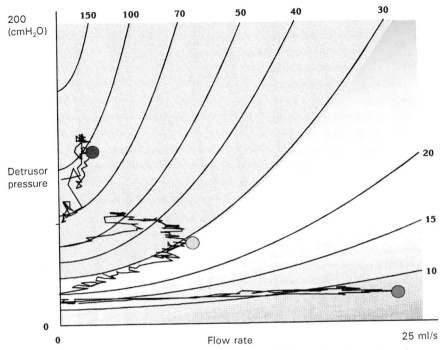

Fig. 5.7 URA nomogram divides patients into obstructed (URA > 28) and unobstructed.

resistance ratio) is obtained. The $p_{det, min\ void}$ point is where the flow–pressure curve reaches the pressure axis. For an AG number less than 40, BOO exists if:

- The $p_{det\ min,\ void}$ is 40 cmH$_2$O or more.
- The slope of the LPURR line is greater than 2 cmH$_2$O per ml per s. The slope of the LPURR line is calculated in cmH$_2$O/ml/s simply by the following equation:

$$slope = (p_{det,\ Q_{max}} - p_{det\ min,\ void})/Q_{max}$$

Many clinicians have been baffled by the various methods for diagnosis and grading BOO, but the degree of agreement in the diagnosis of obstruction is very high (95%), with the AG number and the LPURR being identical. It is probably advisable for clinicians to choose one of the three methods and become familiar with it. Research on more complex methods continues but in our view is unlikely to offer large patient benefits

Conventional, video or ambulatory UDS? The older the man the less likely that there will be a functional disorder producing BOO. However in younger men with poor flow there is a higher likelihood of either bladder neck obstruction (BNO) or detrusor underactivity (DUA) being the cause, and therefore video UDS are the investigation of choice. Whilst ambulatory UDS are more physiological and give interesting results they are unnecessarily complex for routine use in the male patient. In fact there are few instances when AUDS are indicated. Hence for the majority of male patients, that is the group of older men with LUTS suggestive of BOO, basic (conventional) UDS are the investigation of choice.

Detrusor Underactivity (DUA)

This is responsible for the symptoms of a significant minority of patients. As defined earlier, DUA either results in a significant post-void residual urine or results in the bladder being emptied more slowly than normal. DUA cannot be diagnosed with certainty from the flow trace, although an irregular flow curve with Q_{max} occurring in mid-trace is highly suggestive. DUA is a diagnosis made after pressure–flow studies (pQS): 10 to 20% of men with low flows have a degree of DUA. On the pQ trace DUA can appear as a low sustained contraction or as a wavelike contraction. If urethral relaxation is normal during voiding then the flow trace will reflect these pressure changes. However the patient with DUA will often uses training to assist micturition and the pQ curves can look confusing as a result.

What are the interrelationships between DI, BOO and DUA? These three common urodynamic diagnoses are not exclusive of each other, and commonly DI and BOO are found together (in up to 40% of patients). In fact the largest sub-group of older men, whose lower tract function has been defined by UDS, have both DI and BOO. DUA can exist with prostatic obstruction, but it is likely that most men with DUA and severe BOO will develop urinary retention early on. DUA and DI together are uncommon in the neurological intact male patient. Whilst DUA seems to occur with a similar prevalence in most age groups, the prevalence of DI rises with age, so that 50% of asymptomatic men of 70 can be shown to have DI on UDS, although DI may not give the patient troublesome symptoms and may be interpreted as a *normal* desire to void.

Urodynamics in the Younger Man

Video UDS are the investigation of choice after screening flow studies. Bladder neck obstruction and inadequate urethral relaxation are observed in younger men. Such abnormalities appear to be functional rather than structural abnormalities. Younger men are less phlegmatic than older men when investigated and require more careful handling. Fainting (syncope) is most common in this group and if the patient goes quiet, looks worried and pale and starts to sweat, lie him down! It is wise to stop the filling and allow the patient at least 20 minutes to recover. Usually the patient can then stand and the UDS can be continued. If the patient is very inhibited by the investigation then it may be necessary to leave him to void alone, in which case the video part of the study may have to be abandoned.

It should be reiterated that all patients should be screened by flow studies and the flow study results compared with the flow on the pQS: if they are not similar the pQS should be repeated. This rule should apply to all patients investigated by urodynamics.

Postprostatectomy Problems

Patients with postprostatectomy problems present as three main symptomatic groups:

- Persistent symptoms of bladder overactivity.
- Persistent symptoms suggestive of obstruction.
- Incontinence.

Therefore, several symptom complexes are seen which may suggest a single disorder or, as in the non-operated patient, a combination of symptoms suggesting, for example, overactivity and obstruction. The symptoms of frequency, nocturia, urgency, urge incontinence and bladder discomfort are suggestive of persistent DI: the symptom of slow stream, persistent BOO. The symptom of incontinence is likely to be regarded even more seriously by the patient after surgery than before operation. The patient should be asked the frequency and severity of his incontinence and whether or not he suffers social restriction or has to take protective measures to safeguard his clothes. It is also important to establish whether or not the incontinence was present before operation and then to determine what kind of leakage the patient suffers. The incidence of postprostatectomy incontinence has been estimated at 1 to 3%. Videourodynamic studies (VUDS) are the investigation of choice and urethral pressure profilometry can be very useful.

Persistent Symptoms of Bladder Overactivity

Those patients with persistent symptoms suggestive of bladder overactivity are shown by the cystometric findings to have a high incidence of DI and bladder hypersensitivity. The symptoms of DI are known to improve after prostatectomy and 62% of unstable bladders revert to normal on postoperative cystometry (Abrams 1978). However, 19% of patients continue to show bladder instability after an adequate prostatectomy. Price et al. (1980) have shown that those patients with the symptoms of urgency and urge incontinence and with demonstrable severe DI before operation are most likely to have persistent problems after operation. The reason for the conversion of bladder instability to normal detrusor behaviour on cystometry is unclear. It has been suggested that lower voiding pressures after prostatectomy, or the denervation of the bladder neck and posterior urethra resulting from surgery, may be important factors.

Persistent Symptoms Suggestive of Obstruction

The postoperative complaints of slow stream and hesitancy have in the past led to repeated transurethral resections with the increased likelihood of damage to the intrinsic urethral sphincter mechanism. The urodynamic results of this group of patients show clearly that the minority of such patients with reduced flow have persistent outlet obstruction. A higher proportion of patients have a slow stream due to an underactive or acontractile detrusor. If urethral pressure profilometry shows no residual prostatic tissue (Fig. 5.8) then a second prostatectomy will not help the patient. However, should profilometry show the presence of residual prostatic tissue (Fig. 5.9) then transurethral resection of the remaining prostatic tissue may be expected to improve voiding, even when the detrusor is underactive.

When assessing postprostatectomy problems a reasonable time interval following the operation should be allowed for the gradual improvement of symptoms,

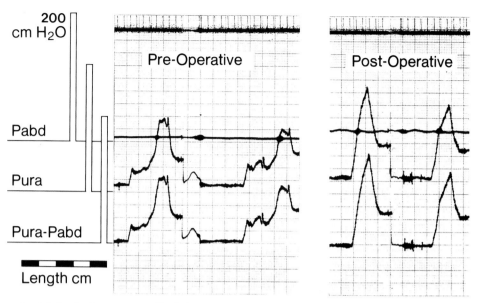

Fig. 5.8 Urethral pressure profiles before and after prostatectomy. There is no residual prostatic pressure area post-operatively.

which can be expected to occur for six months following surgery. The appearance of new complaints after surgery suggests that a change has occurred in the lower urinary tract. Symptoms of overactivity may be due to a urinary tract infection and those of obstruction to a developing stricture. If a patient complains of urge incontinence following prostatectomy then he will usually have had the symptoms of urgency and possible urge incontinence prior to operation. Because

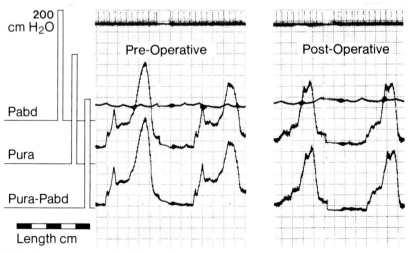

Fig. 5.9 Urethral pressure profiles before and after prostatectomy. In this case enough prostatic tissue remains to produce a presphincteric pressure rise.

these symptoms may fail to improve after operation, patients with urgency prior to operation should be counselled, explaining that although an improvement in urine flow rate is anticipated, one cannot be similarly confident about the symptoms of DI, which may persist.

Incontinence

Incontinence following prostatectomy is either urge incontinence, stress incontinence or very occasionally a mixture of the two types. The symptom of stress incontinence in neurologically normal male patients does not occur in the unoperated case. Therefore, the appearance of this symptom following surgery implies per-operative damage to the distal urethral sphincteric mechanism, or possibly the weakening of the pelvic floor support to the sphincter mechanism by removal of a large adenoma at open operation. In urological practice it is relatively common to see transient stress incontinence following open pro-statectomy. Persistence of stress incontinence, in our view, indicates per-operative sphincteric damage. In male patients stress incontinence is effectively treated by implantation of an artificial sphincter (see treatment of lower urinary tract dysfunction, in Chapter 6).

Urodynamics in the Elderly

Many patients we investigate are elderly and we like to distinguish only the *frail elderly* from other patients. If an old person is clearly in the last few years of their life then our approach to urodynamic investigations will be different because the therapeutic options will be limited. For example, if a frail old man has failed to respond to anticholinergic treatment for urge incontinence that persists after prostatectomy then there is little point in confirming that DI is the cause as he will never be considered for ileocystoplasty. However this will not be the case if the man is 70 and walks or exercises daily. Our use of urodynamics is governed by an assessment of the patient's *biological and not chronological age*.

The prevalence of DI increases with age and if there is mental impairment then DI is almost inevitable. Urodynamics on patients who are confused is often upset-ting for the patient and difficult for the urodynamic staff. Whilst we are always pre-pared to do studies if they will help the management of patients, UDS in general need to be limited in the frail elderly. However urine flow studies and the estima-tion of post-void residual (PVR) is often helpful in excluding significant BOO or DUA. If a significant PVR is seen then it may be beneficial to treat this by catheter-isation and thereby improve the quality of the patient's life. Many of the very elderly may be troubled by recurrent infections made worse by a failure to achieve proper bladder emptying: knowledge of the PVR in these patients will aid treatment.

Urodynamics in the Neurological Patient

There are a number of neurological conditions which commonly lead to lower urinary tract dysfunction and in these patients urodynamics are often a vital part of the investigation and management process. These conditions may be congenital, for example meningomyelocele or sacral agenesis, or else acquired, including multiple sclerosis, cerebrovascular accidents, spinal cord trauma and Parkinson's disease.

In the neurological patient symptoms may be altered or absent even though marked vesico-urethral dysfunction exists. For example in spinal cord trauma or meningomyelocele there can be changes in bladder behaviour that threaten kidney function even though the patient notices little change in symptoms. Therefore in the neuropathic patient urodynamics have a surveillance role in several conditions such as those mentioned above: spinal cord trauma and meningomyelocele. Neurological disease produces two important dysfunctions:

- *Detrusor hyperreflexia (DHR)* is the term often given to detrusor instability in the neuropathic patient. There are no real differences in urodynamic appearances between DHR and DI.
- *Functional bladder outlet obstruction* secondary to urethral overactivity occurs classically in spinal cord injury, meningomyelocele and multiple sclerosis (MS). The functional obstruction is due to either intermittent urethral overactivity, as in spinal cord injury or MS when it is known as *detrusor–sphincter dyssynergia*. Meningomyelocele patients may have a continuous obstruction to voiding known as *isolated distal sphincter obstruction* (IDSO). The effect of urethral overactivity is to produce a reduced interrupted flow rate and incomplete bladder emptying: in IDSO, the interrupted flow is due to the patient needing to strain to overcome the functional obstruction.

In the neurological patient, bladder behaviour is difficult to predict from the neurological signs, although broad principles apply in complete lesions. If there is damage to the lower motor neurones, for example after an injury to the lower part of the lumbar spine, then:

- Bladder sensation is lost.
- Detrusor contractility is absent.
- Bladder compliance may be reduced.
- Sphincter function is reduced.
- Voiding is by straining.

If the upper motor neurone is damaged within the central nervous system, for example by a high spinal cord injury:

- Bladder sensation is lost.
- Detrusor overactivity is likely.
- Bladder compliance may be reduced.
- Sphincter function is normal during filling but may be overactive during voiding.
- Voiding is reflex.

In conditions like MS and meningomyelocele the neurological lesions are more complex and the pattern is less constant because the lesions are incomplete.

Urodynamic Technique in the Neuropathic Patient

For reasons that are poorly understood the neuropathic bladder is particularly sensitive to the speed at which it is filled. Hence fast filling tends to produce artefactual low compliance. In neuropathic patients the bladder should *not* be emptied at the start off UDS unless the patient is on intermittent self-catheterisation and it is their normal time to catheterise. It is better to fill slowly on top of the residual.

Filling rate. A flexible approach needs to be taken. From the patient's frequency–volume chart and knowledge of the patient's residual urine (usually from ultrasound estimates) a policy for that patient can be defined. Generally filling should start at 10 ml/min. If there is no rise in the detrusor pressure this can be increased to 20 or 30 ml/min. However if pressure begins to rise then filling should be stopped for 5 to 10 minutes until the pressure has settled, and then restarted at 10 ml/min. In the neuropathic child the filling rate should be slower, 2 to 5 ml/min.

Patient position. Many male neuropathic patients will not be able to stand or even sit, either to be filled or to void. In neurological disease bladder behaviour is less dependent on patient position and if the patient has to lie down throughout filling and voiding this is likely to give appropriate information. Patients with paraplegia have to be investigated lying, because few can manage to sit for UDS. With the patient lying the voiding phase presents problems but in male patients urine can be voided so that it flows down a tube (a piece of builder's drainpipe) to the flowmeter; (after a considerable delay) the flow is eventually registered by the flowmeter.

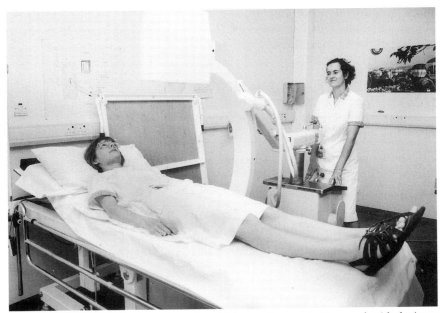

Fig. 5.10 Neuropathic patient being investigated lying on the examination couch with the image intensifier in position over the lower abdomen.

Which tests? In the neuropathic patient video UDS are the investigation of choice in view of the higher incidence of anatomical abnormalities, such as vesico-ureteric reflux and prostatic duct reflux. VUDS also make it easier to study any abnormalities of co-ordination between the detrusor and the urethra, for example, detrusor–sphincter dyssynergia. As VUDS are required, if the patient needs to be investigated lying, the couch has to be suitable for X-ray investigation (Fig. 5.10) Special problems exist in the neuropathic, such as muscle spasms and autonomic dysreflexia which produce particular difficulties during VUDS. Leg spasms in spinal injury patients may make it difficult to pass the catheters, but usually spasms settle during the investigations. *Autonomic dysreflexia* tends to occur in patients with high spinal cord injury. It is a dangerous syndrome where stimuli such as bladder filling or urinary infection lead to dramatic increase in blood pressure, increased pulse rate and sweating. If this occurs during VUDS the bladder should be emptied immediately and the situation will resolve.

Occult neuropathy. Neurological disease may present with lower urinary tract dysfunction (LUTD) before the onset of neurological signs: MS regularly presents to the urodynamicist, who is the first to suspect the diagnosis. The sudden onset of LUTD in a younger person, and the occurrence of voiding difficulties in patients with back or neck pain, are two relatively common indications that an underlying neurological disease may be present.

References

Abrams P (1978) Urodynamic changes following prostatectomy. Urol Int 33:181–186.

Abrams P (1994). New words for old. Lower urinary tract symptoms for 'prostatism'. Br Med J 308:929–930.

Allen T (1977). The non-neurogenic bladder. J Urol 177:232–238.

Andersen JT, Bradley WE (1976). Abnormalities of detrusor and sphincter function in multiple sclerosis. Br J Urol 48:193–198.

Andersen JT (1988). Urodynamics terminology and normal values in children, females and males. Scand J Urol Nephrol suppl 114.

Bhatia NN, Bergman A (1986). Urodynamic appraisal of vaginal pressure versus rectal pressure recording as indication of intraabdominal pressure changes. Urology 27:482.

Blaivas J, Labib KL, Bauer SB, Retik AB (1977). Changing concepts in urodynamic evaluation of children. J Urol 117:778–781.

Byrne DJ, Hamilton Stewart PA, Gray BK (1987). The role of urodynamics in female urinary stress incontinence. Br J Urol 59:228–229.

Chancellor MB (1993). Urodynamic evaluation after spinal cord injury. Physical medicine and rehabilitation clinics of North America 4:273–298.

Gierup J (1970). Micturition studies in infants and children. Scand J Nephrol 5:12 suppl.

Griffiths DJ, Scholtmeijer RJ (1982). Precise urodynamic assessment of meatal and distal urethral stenosis in girls. Neurourol Urodyn 1:89.

Houle A, Gilmour R, Churchill B et al. (1993). What volume can a child normally store in the bladder at a safe pressure. J Urol 149:561.

Koff S (1982). Estimating bladder capacity in children. Urology 21:248.

Lim CS, Abrams P (1995). The Abrams-Griffiths Nomogram. World J Urol 13:34–39.

Mayo ME, Chetner MP (1992). Lower urinary tract dysfunction in multiple sclerosis. Urology 39:67–70.

McGuire EJ (1994). Idiopathic detrusor instability. In Kursh ED, McGuire EJ (eds): female urology. Philadelphia: Lipincott p 95.

Nijman R (1994). Course on paediatric urodynamics. Utrecht.

Philp T, Read DJ, Higson RH (1981). The urodynamic characteristics of multiple sclerosis. Br J Urol 53:672–675.

Price DA, Ramsden PD, Stobbart D (1980) The unstable bladder and prostatectomy. Br J Urol 52:529–531.

Poulsen A, Schou J, Puggaard L, Torp-Pedersen S, Nordling J (1994). Prostatic enlargement symptomatology and pressure/flow evaluation: interrelations in patients with symptomatic BPH. Scand J Urol Nephrol suppl 157:67–73.

Shepherd AM, Powell PH, Ball AJ (1982). The place of urodynamic studies in the investigation and treatment of female urinary tract symptoms. J Obstet Gynaecol 3:123–125.

Chapter 6
Management of Lower Urinary Tract Dysfunction

Urodynamic data provides the basis for sound management of lower urinary tract dysfunction (LUTD). However as explained in Chapter 4, UDS follow a proper evaluation of the patient by symptom analysis, physical examination, urine microscopy and abdominal X-ray or ultrasound. This assessment may provide the basis for an initial period of empiric treatment, because precise diagnosis by UDS in every woman with incontinence and every older man with LUTS is not practical in most areas of the world. This chapter is intended to provide no more than the principles involved in treatment and their relationship with urodynamic investigation at different levels. The principles of treatment are common to all patient groups, although some treatments are not applicable initially; for example, bladder training for detrusor instability cannot be used, in the accepted sense, in patients without bladder sensation.

Storage Phase Problems

The principal patterns of the storage phase are bladder overactivity and urethral sphincter incompetence.

Detrusor Overactivity

Detrusor instability (DI), detrusor hyperreflexia (DHR) and reduced bladder compliance may lead to problems in three main ways:

- Frequency–urgency syndrome
- Incontinence (urge type)
- Upper tract dilatation leading to renal impairment

Treatments for detrusor overactivity can be divided into three main groups: conservative, medical, and surgical.

Conservative Treatments

These consist of:

- *Advice on fluid intake* including the twenty-four hour total and the timing and type of fluid intake, for example:
  - Don't drink before going out.
  - Don't drink before going to bed or during the night.
  - Maintain an adequate fluid output: one to two litres.
  - Avoid fluids that produce symptoms, for example containing caffeine or alcohol.
- *Bladder training.* The use of the voiding diary to encourage the voiding of increasing volumes at increasing intervals.
- *Pelvic floor exercises.* Increasing pelvic floor strength may work by reflex inhibition of the detrusor or by aiding urethral closure until the unstable wave has passed and the detrusor has relaxed.
- *Other treatments* such as biofeedback, in which the patient is given information on bladder activity so that when the detrusor pressure rises they can see an increasing number of lights illuminated, hear a louder sound or see the pressure tracing change.

Medical Management

For detrusor overactivity this is confined to drugs with an anticholinergic action such as oxybutynin, trospium, propantheline and the tricyclic antidepressants. It is ironic that their principal side-affect is dry mouth, which encourages the patient to drink more. These treatments are given using the principle of dose titration. The drug should be started at low dosage and increased slowly until the patient starts to experience side-effects. Oxybutynin is the most frequently used and should be started at 2.5 mg twice daily in children and the elderly and 2.5 mg three times per day in adults. The dose can be increased by one tablet per week until the optimum dose in reached, for example, in the second week 2.5 mg four times per day (or 5 mg twice a day) then 5 mg twice daily plus 2.5 mg once per day, to the maximum dose for most patients of 5 mg three times per day.

New possibilities exist for medical therapy of DI but at the time of writing none of these drugs has undergone a clinical trial beyond phase III.

Surgical Management

There are no effective managements between conservative and medical treatments on the one hand and major surgery on the other. Bladder augmentation or substitution is the most effective procedure for the symptomatic relief of bladder overactivity (DI, DHR or low bladder compliance). Augmentation cystoplasty can be achieved in a variety of ways by using ileum (ileocystoplasty), colon (colocystoplasty) or stomach (gastrocystoplasty); ureter (ureterocystoplasty) is used when the kidney is being removed for non-function and a widely dilated ureter is available).

In all these procedures the bladder is first split either side to side (coronally) or front to back (sagitally). The bowel segment (15 to 30 cm long) is also split along its length, on the antemesenteric border, and sewn into the bladder defect. The ureters are left undisturbed unless there is reflux, when the surgeon may wish to reimplant them. Bladder substitution is used if the bladder wall is excessively thick or diseased. For substitution cystoplasty similar techniques are used, although ileum and/or colon would be the tissues of choice and up to 45 cm may be needed: the ureters may require reimplantation although the trigone is usually preserved. Cystoplasty carries significant morbidity and the patient must be counselled in detail on the main complications, namely:

- *Intermittent self-catheterisation (ISC).* Owing to intentional weakening of the detrusor, Incomplete bladder emptying often occurs in up to 50% of patients. Because the resulting need for ISC is so frequent it is unwise for patients to undergo bladder augmentation until they have demonstrated their ability to perform ISC.

- *Mucus production from the bowel segment.* This can cause blockage, making ISC more difficult.

- *Urinary tract infections.* These are likely to occur with increased frequency after cystoplasty, probably due to mucus production and more difficult bladder emptying.

- *Tumour formation.* With time this may occur in the neobladder, but probably not for ten to twenty years. However the possibility will necessitate regular check cystoscopies.

Detrusor myectomy (autoaugmentation) is a newer procedure which is being assessed at present. It is inferior to bowel cystoplasty in producing symptom relief but is a more minor procedure without most of the longer-term risks of cystoplasty. If detrusor myectomy produces inadequate symptomatic effect then bowel cystoplasty can be performed.

Urethral Sphincter Incompetence

This can result in genuine stress incontinence and may be managed conservatively, medically, or surgically.

Conservative Therapy

This should be used in all patients who are suspected of having or who have been demonstrated to have genuine stress incontinence (GSI) by urodynamics. Such therapy includes:

- *General advice* on:
  - Fluid intake (see above)
  - Weight loss: losing weight reduces intra abdominal pressure and therefore increases the urethral closure pressure, resulting in reduced leakage.
- *Pelvic floor exercises (PFE).* In order to be effective, these should be performed repetitively, using the $10 \times 10 \times 10 \times 10$ rule. The woman is asked to increase

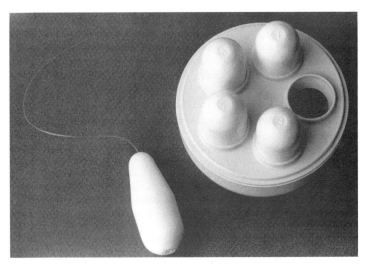

Fig. 6.1 Vaginal cones used for pelvic floor training. The cones contain graduated weights and are used for progressively longer periods at increased weight.

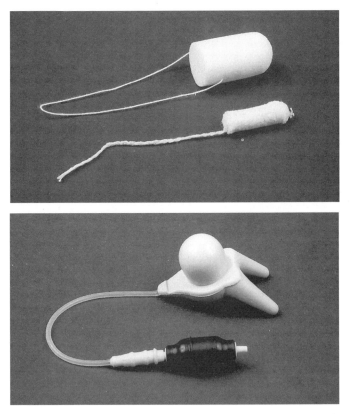

Fig. 6.2 Intravaginal devices designed to prevent stress incontinence: a large tampon for use during exercise compared with a standard tampon, and an inflatable prosthesis shown with the pump connected and the balloon inflated to press on the urethra.

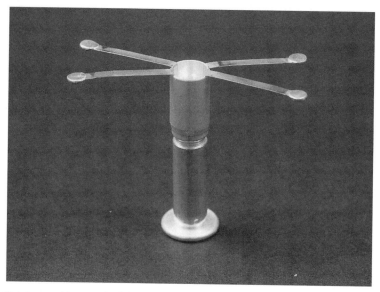

Fig. 6.3 Stainless steel intraurethral device inserted *per urethram*: the "wings" hold the device on the bladder base. The patient voids by straining and activating a sophisticated valve system.

her PFE until she does ten 10-second contractions, ten times a day (roughly hourly) for ten weeks. Most women cannot sustain a PF contraction for 10 seconds initially and a contraction held for 5 seconds with 5 to 10 seconds between contractions is more realistic at first.

If the patient is unable to contract her PF then it may be necessary to use "aids" such as perineometry, vaginal cones (Fig. 6.1) or electrical stimulation to help re-educate the muscles. Faradism is a technique which uses electrical stimulation as therapy rather than to re-educate the pelvic floor muscles.

- *Continence aids*. These have increased in number and variety. Originally only the vaginal ring pessary was available, but now there are both intravaginal and intraurethral devices. *Intravaginal devices* (Fig. 6.2) are designed to support the bladder neck and to prevent anterior vaginal wall descent. Intraurethral devices are relatively new (Fig. 6.3) and aim to prevent urine leakage by obstructing the urethra: voiding occurs either by a pressure-activated valve mechanism or by removing the device. A third type of device is stuck by adhesive hydrogel onto the external urethral meatus and removed for micturition (Fig. 6.4, *overleaf*). Most of these devices are not yet commercially available.

Medical Therapy

For GSI this is of disappointing efficiency. A few patients benefit from alpha-adrenergic agonists such as phenylpropanolamine (see Appendix 4). These drugs are not generally used except in patients with sphincter weakness associated with neuropathic vesico-urethral dysfunction.

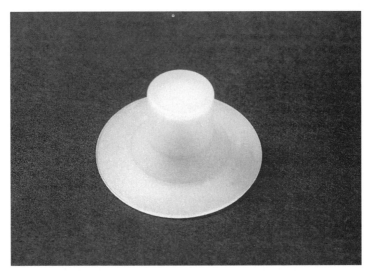

Fig. 6.4 Small "sucker" device applied directly over the external urinary meatus to be removed for voiding.

Surgical Treatment

For GSI this should be directed at one or other of the two basic causes of incontinence after proper assessment by vaginal examination and urodynamic testing.

Urethral hypermobility. This is best treated by repositioning procedures. There are three main classes of operation:

- *Retropubic techniques* including the Burch colposuspension, vagino-obturator shelf procedure and Marshall Marchetti Krantz operation have the best long-term results.
- *Needle suspension procedures* include the Pereyra, Stamey, Raz and Gittes operations. These have good initial results but on longer-term follow-up have shown an increasing failure rate from one to five years.
- *Vaginal procedures* such as the Kelly procedure are the least effective class of operation for the relief of GSI. Vaginal or anterior repair is the operation of choice for simple anterior vaginal wall descent.

The author's preference is for colposuspension for the young active and fit, and the Stamey procedure for the older, more sedentary or unfit. There must be adequate vaginal mobility for repositioning procedures to be used.

Intrinsic urethral sphincter weakness. This is usually not associated with anterior vaginal wall descent, being due to either neurogenic causes or trauma, for example after repeated procedures for GSI. Treatment may be by:

- *Periurethral injection.* Teflon (polytetrafluoroethylene) and Silastic (silicone rubber) are not now widely used because of fears over particle migration.

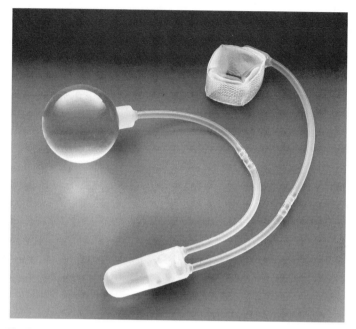

Fig. 6.5 Artificial urinary sphincter consisting of a pressure-regulating balloon, a periurethral cuff and an intrascrotal (or intralabial) control pump.

Collagen and fat are used and are safe but are probably quite easily absorbed, so that additional injections are required. More-stable, inert, yet naturally occurring compounds are currently being investigated.

- *Sling procedures.* These have an excellent reputation for cure of incontinence but may produce voiding dysfunction. Formerly these procedures had adverse publicity due to urethral erosion by the sling, but by using fascial material, either from the patient or from porcine sources, and by using low-tension techniques these problems have been largely overcome.

- *Artificial urinary sphincter (AUS).* Most of the treatments for GSI can only be used in women, although the sling procedure and injection have been used in men. The AUS can be used in men, women and children, and produces excellent results. Because the AUS (Fig. 6.5) is made from artificial material, infection can be a problem, in that an infected sphincter has to be removed.

Management of Intractable Incontinence

If age, physical status, mental state or disease prevents the use of the techniques described above then other methods of treatment may be needed. These methods can be divided into conservative and surgical.

Conservative Techniques

Included among these are:

- *Pads.* These vary in type from dribble pouches for the man with small-volume incontinence to a full-sized nappy for the incontinent adult. All patients should be properly assessed as to their pad needs, with the appropriate size of pad being given together with suitable incontinence pants to support the pad. All-in-one washable pants with fitted pads are preferred by many patients. Patients may require different protection at night from that used in the daytime. Better bed protection in the form of disposable or washable, reusable protective sheets should be provided.

- *Indwelling catheter.* There is a longstanding prejudice against permanent catheterisation, but it may be the only practical way of managing some patients. The situation has been improved by the use of long-term catheters and by proper systematic catheter care. Suprapubic catheterisation can be preferable to the urethral route, particularly if complications occur with urethral catheterisation: catheter blockage and leakage around the catheter are common problems.

Surgical techniques

If conservative methods fail then surgical techniques may be needed:

- *Urethral closure.* If despite an effective suprapubic catheter there is troublesome urethral leakage then the urethra may be closed surgically.

- *Urinary diversion.* Intractable incontinence in a patient with a normal life expectancy is a huge burden to both the patient and any carers. Formation of an ileal conduit can transform the life of a patient who has suffered urinary incontinence for years. It is easier for most carers to change or drain the urine drainage bag of a conduit than to change both the clothes and the bedclothes of an incontinent patient. The main indications for ileal diversion are in wheelchair-bound meningomyelocele patients with significant skeletal deformity and in multiple sclerosis patients.

The proper management of incontinence depends on a continence service which is properly integrated into not only the urodynamic but also the urological, gynaecological, neurological, paediatric and geriatric services.

Other Storage Phase Problems

Nocturia is a common and troublesome problem. Its causes are several (see Chapter 4). Treatment should be directed at the cause or causes. Where bladder outlet obstruction with associated residual urine has reduced functional capacity, then effective surgery will reduce nocturia. Similarly, effective treatment of detrusor instability will reduce nocturia if it is responsible for that symptom. Congestive cardiac failure (CCF) is a potent cause of nocturia and is often subclinical. If CCF is the cause of nocturia there will be nocturnal polyuria (more than one-third of urine produced during the eight night hours). If nocturnal polyuria exists then synthetic antidiuretic hormone (DDAVP) should not be used; treatment should aim to induce a relative diuresis in the second half of the day so that the patient goes to bed without oedema fluid. It should be remembered that at least a litre of oedema fluid must be present in the legs before it is clinically obvious. We use frusemide in a dose of at least 40 mg given at teatime (approximately 4 to 6 p.m.). DDAVP is useful in nocturia if there is no other obvious cause and may help in patients with detrusor overactivity: care should be taken in the elderly because of its potential for causing fluid retention, resulting in a low serum sodium.

Management of Voiding Problems

Voiding problems may be due to bladder outlet obstruction (BOO) or to detrusor underactivity (DUA). Most patients with BOO are male, although neurological conditions cause outlet obstruction in both males and females.

Bladder Outlet Obstruction

BOO either can be due to anatomical causes or may result from a functional obstruction to the bladder outlet. Treatment may be demanded by a variety of anatomical causes, for example in a child with congenital abnormality such as urethral valves, a young man with a stricture or an elderly man who has developed acute retention of urine. However most causes of BOO present with symptoms which can be managed conservatively, medically or by surgery.

Conservative Management

This may consist of:

- General advice such as regulation of the volume, type and timing of fluids.
- Bladder training: if BOO is associated with symptoms of detrusor instability, for example urge incontinence, then bladder training may be very helpful.
- Catheterisation: if the patient is unfit or unwilling to have definitive treatment then either intermittent self-catheterisation or an indwelling catheter can be used to allow proper bladder drainage.

Medical Therapy

If conservative treatment has failed after a reasonable trial period of three months then this can be considered. There are only two classes of drug that have been shown to be effective:

- *Alpha-adrenergic blocking agents.* These drugs act on alpha-receptors at the bladder neck, in the prostatic capsule and in the prostatic stoma.

- *5-alpha-reductase inhibitors.* The prostatic epithelial tissue shrinks when the conversion of testosterone to 5-dihydrotestosterone is blocked.

Drugs produce a moderate decrease in symptoms and some change in BOO with increased flow rates and some reduction in voiding pressure. Alpha-blockers are effective immediately, whereas 5-alpha reductase inhibitors take six months to have full effect. Although 5-alpha reductase inhibitors have little in the way of side-effects, alpha-blockers cause some problems by producing postural hypertension with dizziness and loss of energy. However, the newer alpha-blockers are more "prostate-specific" and have fewer side-effects. Neither class of drug has a dramatic effect and tends only to move patients from the obstructed group to the equivocal zone on the Abrams–Griffiths nomogram, whereas surgery in the form of transurethral resection of the prostate (TURP) moves most obstructed patients into the unobstructed zone. There is little evidence to support the use of other classes of drugs in BOO. Plant extracts, homoeopathic remedies and aromatase inhibitors have been investigated to a limited extent: none of these drug groups shows convincing evidence of efficiency.

It has been the view that in patients with BOO and detrusor instability (DI) the use of anticholinergic drugs is dangerous. There is little evidence for this view and a careful trial of an anticholinergic in the patient whose symptoms are predominantly storage in type is reasonable.

Surgical Treatment

For BOO this is the most effective treatment in reducing symptoms and obtaining relief. When there is a stricture then optical urethrotomy and occasionally urethroplasty in the male and urethral dilatation in the female are the treatments of choice. In the largest group of patients, the older males with BPO, there is currently great interest in alternative methods of treating BPO in particular. Whilst (TURP) (see above) remains "*le beau idéal*", a number of other options are being assessed:

- Visual laser ablation of the prostate (VLAP); techniques include non-contact and contact side-firing, as well as interstitial laser therapy.
- High-intensity focused ultrasound (HIFU).
- Transurethral needle ablation (TUNA) using high-frequency radio waves.
- Thermotherapy (TUMT), hypothermia and thermal ablation: these methods deliver microwave energy to the prostate from a urethral source.
- Pyrosurgery: the extracorporeal delivery of heat to the prostate is one of the latest techniques to be tried.

Transurethral incision of the prostate (TUIP) is rather better established and is useful in small glands (less than 30 ml). Bladder neck obstruction is quickly and easily dealt with by bladder neck incision (BNI) and it seems unlikely that laser incisions have more to offer.

Prostatic stenting and prostatic dilatation have been used but have few real indications. If patients are unfit then VLAP offers a "blood-free" and safe alternative to TURP. The ultimate places of therapies such as VLAP, HIFU, TUNA and TUMT remain to be defined and they should, at the time of writing, be used only in randomised controlled trials, in comparison with TURP and, perhaps, conservative treatment. It is safe to say that, at present, none of these techniques has the ability to reduce symptoms and relieve obstruction as effectively as TURP.

Treatment of Functional Obstruction

Functional causes of BOO are a good deal less common than anatomical causes, and functional BOO is generally associated with neurological disease (see Chapter 5), but there are two small but important groups of patients with no neurological signs who have voiding dysfunction:

- Dysfunctional voiding due to pelvic floor activity is normally seen in children (see Chapter 5). Its treatment is by biofeedback using either the flow traces or perineal surface electromyography. The patient by understanding the mechanism of their interrupted stream learns to relax the pelvic floor during voiding.
- Idiopathic sphincter overactivity: this syndrome is usually seen in women aged 20 to 40 and often results in the inability to void. At present there are no effective curative treatments and management is usually by intermittent self-catheterisation.

As discussed in Chapter 5, two relatively common conditions produce functional BOO in neurological patients:

- Detrusor–sphincter dyssynergia, classically seen in spinal cord injury patients and in multiple sclerosis.
- Isolated distal sphincter obstruction: this is found in meningomyelocele patients and in patients after radical pelvic surgery associated with denervation (for example, after Wertheim's hysterectomy or abdominoperineal resection of the rectum).

Treatments of functional BOO can be classed as conservative, medical or surgical.

Conservative Therapies

These include biofeedback as described above and catheterisation. ISC is used when possible, but in some patients an indwelling catheter will be necessary. ISC has revolutionised the management of functional BOO. It can be used by both sexes and all ages. If the patient is too young or too disabled then intermittent catheterisation can be performed by the parent or carer. The technique is remarkably free of complications, although urinary infections can be a problem in the first few weeks, and this has led clinicians to prescribe low-dose antibiotics for the first four to eight weeks of ISC.

Medical Therapy

This is rarely successful, although alpha-adrenergic blockers were formerly used in spinal cord injury patients. Occasionally women with idiopathic sphincter overactivity benefit from alpha-blocker therapy and a trial of treatment is worth while, particularly if it means avoiding the need for ISC.

Surgical Therapy

This was formerly the rule for these conditions: meningomyelocele girls were diverted and boys were subjected to urethral sphincterotomy. These procedures were usually performed for intractable incontinence or because of recurrent infections and or upper tract deterioration. With the advent of intermittent self-catheterisation (ISC) most surgical interventions can be avoided. Nevertheless, there is still a small place for surgery when patients are unable to perform ISC and have problems with indwelling catheters (either urethral or suprapubic). The ileal conduit is still appropriate in some patients, although an alternative is offered by the Mitrofanoff procedure, in which the bladder or augmented bladder is joined to the anterior abdominal wall by a conduit fashioned from appendix, small bowel, fallopian tube or ureter. Instead of performing ISC through the urethra the patient can catheterise using the Mitrofanoff stoma.

Some reputable centres perform VY plasty of the bladder neck if video studies show that the bladder neck fails to open and if the patient is unhappy to do ISC.

Treatment of Detrusor Underactivity

Detrusor underactivity (DUA) occurs in patients both with and without neuro-logical disease. In men the symptom complex in patients with DUA is indistinguishable from that suffered by patients with BOO. In the neurological patients it is common for DUA, and indeed BOO due to sphincter overactivity during voiding, to occur in combination with detrusor hyperreflexia during filling. DUA can be managed as follows:

- Conservative therapy is possible if there are no complications and the patient's symptoms are not troublesome. However if symptoms or complications occur and there is significant post-void residual urine (PVR) then ISC and the other measures discussed under the section on management of BOO may be required.
- Medical therapy aimed at increasing detrusor activity, for example by cholinergic drugs, is not effective. Some believe that DUA may be secondary to sphincter overactivity and would use alpha-adrenergic blockers to try to improve sphincter relaxation and indirectly enhance detrusor function.
- Surgical therapy can be considered if there is evidence of significant PVR and conservative therapy has failed. However there is little evidence that surgery will improve voiding function in men with DUA, although it is possible that bladder neck incision, prostatic incision or TURP may improve voiding by allowing more effective straining.

Management of Post-micturition Symptoms

Post-micturition dribble (PMD) is a common symptom in elderly men but is not due to BOO. PMD is due to urine left in the bulbous and penile urethra, at the end of micturition. This urine dribbles out and wets the underpants and occasionally the trousers after the man has dressed and left the toilet. Treatment is by explaining the cause and by suggesting that the man takes a little more care and time in voiding. If this fails to work, pelvic floor exercises help, as they lead to contraction of the periurethral musculature. Finally the patient should be taught how to manually express the subsphincteric urethra by exerting upward perineal pressure and slowly moving the pressure point down the urethra towards the tip of the penis.

This chapter has attempted to provide a frame work of management of LUTD, but readers are advised to consult other texts aiming more directly at treatment rather than investigation.

References

Abrams P (1994). Managing lower urinary tract symptoms in older men. Br Med J 310:1113–1118.

Anthuber C, Pigny A, Schussler B, Lacock J, Norton P, Stanton S. editors (1994). Pelvic floor re-education. Principles and practice, first edn 4.4.3. Clinical results neuromuscular electrical stimulation. London: Springer-Verlag pp 163–167.

Bakke A, Brun OH, Høisæter PA (1992). Clinical background of patients treated with clean inter-mittent catheterisation in Norway. Scand J Urol Nephrol 26:211–217.

Fall M, Lindstrøm S (1991). Electrical stimulation. A physiologic approach to the treatment of urinary incontinence. Urol Clin N Am 18:393–407.

Fantl JA, Wyman JF, McClish DK et al. (1991). Efficacy of bladder training in older women with urinary incontinence. JAMA 256:609.

Frewin WK (1979). Role of bladder training in the treatment of the unstable bladder in the female. Urol Clin N Am 6:273.

Kegel AH (1951). Physiologic therapy for urinary incontinence. JAMA 146:915–917.

Peattie AB, Plevnick S, Stanton SL (1988). Vaginal cones: a conservative method of treating genuine stress incontinence. Br J Obstet Gynaecol 95:1049.

Swami SK, Abrams P (1996). Urge incontinence. Urol Clin N Am II 23:417–426.

Wilson PD, Samarrai TA, Deakin M, Kolbe E, Brown ADG (1987). An objective assessment of physio-therapy for female genuine stress incontinence. Br J Obstet Gynaecol 94:575–582.

Chapter 7
Organisation of the Urodynamic Unit

The urodynamic unit must respond to the need for patient investigation from a variety of sources and must ensure that the studies are carried out to a consistently high standard. There is a need for three levels of urodynamic investigation:

- Basic urodynamics, including urine flow studies, filling cystometry, pressure–flow studies and pad testing.
- Advanced urodynamics, including urethral pressure profilometry and video-urodynamics.
- Complex urodynamics, including ambulatory urodynamics and neuro-physiological testing.

The requirements for each level is different, although all have common needs:

- Secretarial staff
- Technical/nursing support
- Medical physics backing
- Medical involvement
- Urodynamic records system

The basic organisation of our department can be illustrated by tracing a patient through the department.

Patient Referral

After reviewing the referral letter from the patient's general practitioner (family physician) or specialist, the patient is assigned to either the urgent category or the routine list. The patient details are entered into the patient administration system of the hospital if the patient has not yet received a hospital number. The recorded details are shown on the front sheet of the patient's urodynamic data proforma (Appendix 3, Part 1).

Making the Patient's Appointment

The individual patient's requirements are assessed so that an appointment of appropriate length and timing can be given. Appointment lengths are:

- 60 minutes: for routine appointments for either basic or advanced UDS in the neurologically normal patient.
- 90 minutes: for advanced UDS in neurological or disabled patients and children.
- 120 minutes: for complex UDS and for ambulatory UDS. The patient is warned they need to set aside 2 to 4 hours for the appointment.

For male patients who have not had screening uroflow in the referring centre, a morning appointment is made for the flow clinic and a 60 minute appointment for urodynamics in the afternoon. Female patients in whom there is a possibility that ambulatory studies (AUDS) may be needed are often investigated by video UDS in the morning with a provisional appointment for AUDS in the afternoon. If patients have to travel some distance to reach us then a late morning appointment is given.

All patients are sent a seven-day frequency–volume chart (Appendix 2, Part 1) for completion before attending their appointment. We offer appointments four weeks in advance and if the patient does not confirm the appointment, then it is offered by telephone to another patient. In the British system we have a problem with "no-shows" or "DNAs" (did-not-attends) as we call them: by insisting on confirmation of appointment we have significantly increased our efficiency.

For the urine flow clinic the patient is also sent a frequency–volume chart with their clinic appointment. Both urodynamic patients and flow clinic patients are sent information leaflets (Appendix 2, Part 2) which describe the investigations.

The Patient's Hospital Attendance

On arrival the patient presents at the clinic reception and the urodynamic technician or flow clinic nurse is informed.

Urodynamic Studies

The patient is shown to the urodynamic room where the technician describes the test procedure to the patient, emphasising the points raised in the information leaflet. The following sequence is then followed:

- *Urodynamic history.* We use a standard proforma which can be entered into our computer database either online or offline. We have computer terminals in each urodynamic room (Fig. 7.1, *overleaf*). The screens on the terminal follow the urodynamics answer sheet (Appendix 3, Part 2). If the clinician is unfamiliar with the computer system then he or she can complete an answer sheet and the technician will enter the data into the database later that day. A master questionnaire (Appendix 3, Part 1) is available in each room to aid the clinician if necessary.

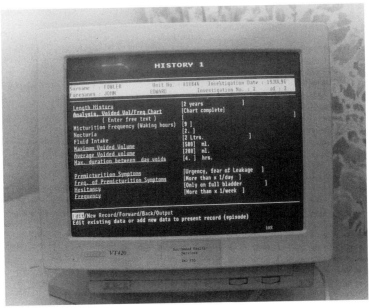

Fig. 7.1 Computer terminal within the urodynamic room.

- After the history has been taken, the patient undresses.
- *Urodynamic examination.* The examination as detailed in Chapter 3 is carried out and the findings entered into the computer or on the answer sheet.
- *Urodynamic investigations.* After the investigations the technician analyses the urodynamic traces and enters the urodynamic data into the computer.
- *Urodynamic report generation.* The doctor is given the skeleton urodynamic report (Fig. 7.2) by the technician so that the clinical information from the history and physical examination can be entered into the upper part of the report form while the urodynamic findings, management recommendations and arrangements for follow-up are detailed in the lower part of the report. The report is sent to the referring clinicians as well as other relevant doctors including the family physician (GP) and other appropriate persons such as the continence advisor.
- After completing the test the patient dresses and then the physician explains the finding of the tests to the patient, outlining the suggested management plan which will be communicated to the patient's doctor.

Urine Flow Clinic

We set up the flow clinic because of an awareness that we were often unable to get patients to do a flow study in the regular outpatients: usually the patient did not expect to be in the outpatients for more than half an hour and as we also wanted urine for microscopy and culture they were not prepared to stay for an additional test. As with UDS we follow a set protocol:

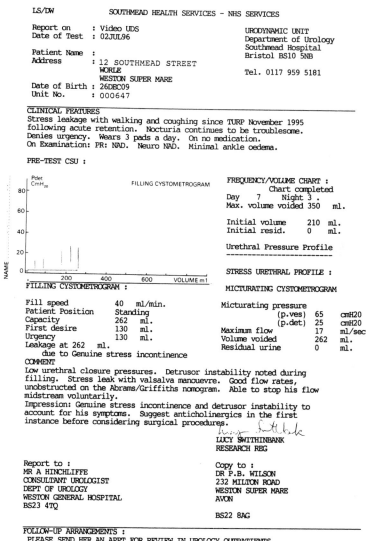

LS/DW   SOUTHMEAD HEALTH SERVICES - NHS SERVICES

Report on   : Video UDS
Date of Test   : 02JUL96   URODYNAMIC UNIT
                                                  Department of Urology
Patient Name   :   Southmead Hospital
Address   : 12 SOUTHMEAD STREET   Bristol BS10 5NB
                 WORLE
                 WESTON SUPER MARE   Tel. 0117 959 5181
Date of Birth : 26DEC09
Unit No.   : 000647

CLINICAL FEATURES
Stress leakage with walking and coughing since TURP November 1995
following acute retention. Nocturia continues to be troublesome.
Denies urgency. Wears 3 pads a day. On no medication.
On Examination: PR: NAD. Neuro NAD. Minimal ankle oedema.

PRE-TEST CSU :

FREQUENCY/VOLUME CHART :
                Chart completed
Day   7   Night 3 .
Max. volume voided 350   ml.

Initial volume   210   ml.
Initial resid.   0   ml.

Urethral Pressure Profile

STRESS URETHRAL PROFILE :

MICTURATING CYSTOMETROGRAM

FILLING CYSTOMETROGRAM :

Fill speed   40   ml/min.   Micturating pressure
Patient Position   Standing   (p.ves) 65   cmH20
Capacity   262   ml.   (p.det) 25   cmH20
First desire   130   ml.   Maximum flow   17   ml/sec
Urgency   130   ml.   Volume voided   262   ml.
Leakage at 262   ml.   Residual urine   0   ml.
     due to Genuine stress incontinence
COMMENT
Low urethral closure pressures. Detrusor instability noted during
filling. Stress leak with valsalva manoeuvre. Good flow rates,
unobstructed on the Abrams/Griffiths nomogram. Able to stop his flow
midstream voluntarily.
Impression: Genuine stress incontinence and detrusor instability to
account for his symptoms. Suggest anticholinergics in the first
instance before considering surgical procedures.
                                        LUCY SWITHINBANK
                                        RESEARCH REG

Report to :   Copy to :
MR A HINCHLIFFE   DR P.B. WILSON
CONSULTANT UROLOGIST   232 MILTON ROAD
DEPT OF UROLOGY   WESTON SUPER MARE
WESTON GENERAL HOSPITAL   AVON
BS23 4TQ
                                        BS22 8AG

FOLLOW-UP ARRANGEMENTS :
PLEASE SEND HER AN APPT FOR REVIEW IN UROLOGY OUTPATIENTS

Fig. 7.2 Completed urodynamic report form.

- Patients are sent their appointment 3 to 4 weeks in advance together with a frequency–volume chart.
- The patient is asked to drink a litre of fluid at home on the day of the appointment.
- On arrival at the hospital the patient is shown the flow room and the tests are explained.
- The first flow is taken when the patient has a comfortably full bladder – or in other words is getting slightly uncomfortable!

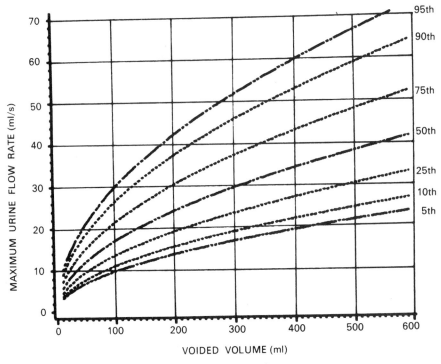

Fig. 7.3 Liverpool nomogram for women.

- Soft drinks or water are provided at the clinic and the patient is encouraged to drink.
- These three flow studies are recorded, with post-void residual urines measured by ultrasound.
- Report preparation: the flow results and PUR volumes are presented on one of three flow nomograms, for men under 50, men over 50, or women (Fig. 7.3) (see "Uroflowmetry" in Chapter 3).

If the patient has not been seen in the urology outpatients then the flow clinic appointment is arranged to coincide with the relevant urological clinic allowing the patient a single hospital visit. Flow clinic appointments for morning urology clinics are made for 9 a.m. and those for afternoon urology clinics at 11 a.m.

Planning a New Urodynamic Service

Since the first edition of this book urodynamics has become widely accepted and established in most centres in western countries. In some centres the organisation is suboptimal and below are suggestions for the basic structures that will determine the shape of a new unit.

What size of population will you serve? There is little point in establishing a unit if there are units in surrounding areas offering an efficient and comprehensive service. If your hospital serves a population of 250 000 then it is likely that you will need to perform basic urodynamics on 6 patients per week and flow studies on 12 to 15 patients per week.

What investigations do you plan to offer? Again the breadth of services will depend on existing services in surrounding areas and on the population you serve. It is probably unnecessary to offer advanced urodynamics (video-urodynamics etc.) unless the referrals for urodynamics amount to the equivalent of 15 patients per week. If there are 30 urodynamic referrals per week then complex urodynamics should be offered.

Where will you do the urodynamic studies? This will depend on the quantity and type of studies you offer. Our urodynamic unit is a separate part of a specialised urology outpatients. All patients – children, women and men – attend our unit with referrals from all specialities. If you do not have your own out-patient building then it may be more convenient to have the urodynamic unit close to the urology or gynaecology ward. Other suitable sites are in continence care areas or clinical investigation units which might also offer investigations, such as gastrointestinal studies and cardiac tests. Videourodynamics must be done either in the X-ray department or in a suitably screened room, in out-patients or on the ward, if an image intensifier is used. If imaging is by ultrasound then these limitations do not apply.

Above all, a friendly sympathetic atmosphere with proper privacy for the patient must be offered.

The unit must have:

- Changing facilities: these may be a curtained area in the investigation room (Fig. 7.4, *overleaf*).
- Sluicing facilities for disposal of urine and occasional faeces (Fig. 7.5, *overleaf*).
- Adequate storage space for catheters, catheter packs and other essential items.
- Adequate space for the urodynamic table, commode and equipment. The minimum size for basic urodynamics is 20 square metres and for video-urodynamics 30 square metres; Fig. 7.6 (page 194) shows why a relatively large room is needed.
- Waiting area for patients.

It is highly desirable to have the urodynamic area solely for urodynamic use. This enables the equipment to be left ready for use with tests being done at times con-venient for the patients and staff: this also allows a more relaxed approach to UDS. If the studies have to be done in shared space then there is pressure to com-plete the tests at a set time, resulting in an incomplete test if more time is needed than was appreciated. Similarly, if UDS are done in the X-ray department then it is necessary to fit into the timetable of the X-ray department where the expensive equipment and limited number of rooms demand highly efficient usage. UDS are an investigation that demands sensitivity and privacy and everything should be done to ensure that these quality issues are addressed.

Who will perform the urodynamic studies? We believe that a doctor must be involved in the urodynamic investigations and that technical assistance is also required. The doctor has to be suitably qualified and suitably trained. The best units have a variety of medical input:

- There should be a consultant (specialist) who leads, providing the link between investigation and therapy.

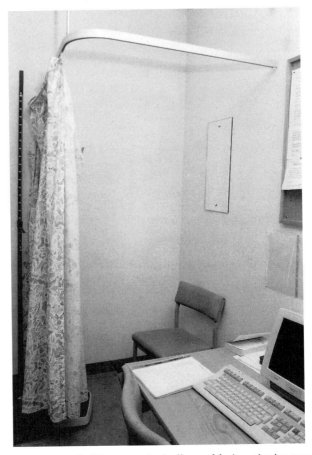

Fig. 7.4 Changing facilities: a curtained-off area of the investigation room.

- In large units there should be permanent medical staff to provide a continuity that ensures good quality control for the studies and enables doctors coming to the department to receive proper training in urodynamic theory and technique.
- Training-grade doctors may perform many of the tests in departments that are large or in small departments if the consultant is too busy to perform all UDS himself. Herein lies a danger, because relatively inexperienced doctors require supervision for several months before they are able to report reliably on the urodynamic findings.

In many departments the key personnel will be the technicians or nurses who assist with the tests and, like the consultant or other permanent staff, provide a continuity that allows the maintenance of an efficient and effective unit.

Who should assist at urodynamics? It is probably not important whether it is a nurse or a technician. The nurse brings the advantages of their training, whilst the technician brings their technical background into an investigation area where this is vital. Our unit started with technicians only but now has a mixture of

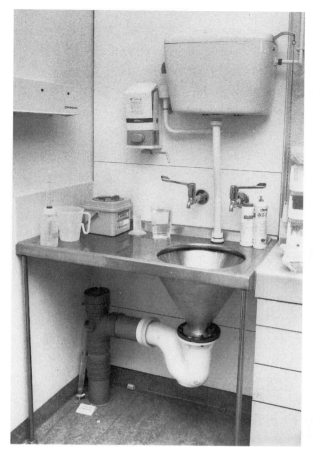

Fig. 7.5 Sluice for disposing of body fluids.

nurses and technicians. As medicine has become more complex most recently trained nurses are very comfortable with urodynamic apparatus. The principle responsibilities of the nurse/technician are to:

- Maintain and calibrate the urodynamic equipment.
- Ensure proper standards of cleanliness and sterility.
- Be responsible for the general care of patients.
- Work the urodynamic equipment during UDS.
- Analyse the urodynamic tracing and prepare the report.
- Be responsible for restocking the urodynamic room with disposables, catheters, infusion fluids and sterile gloves, etc.
- Liaise with the medical physics department.

In our department all the technicians and nurses have been women. This has arisen from the need to have a female to chaperone female patients when the investigating clinician is male.

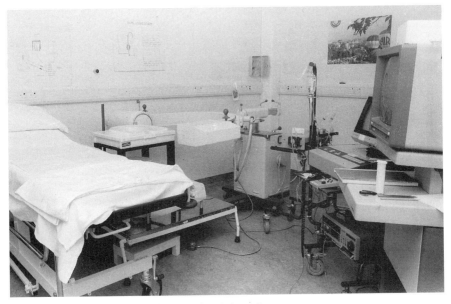

Fig. 7.6 Videourodynamics room.

What record system should be used? We have always kept our own records and now have 25 000 urodynamic patient files in our secretarial area. These files are separate from the general hospital patient record files. Hence we can obtain urodynamic records without delay. The urodynamic record files contain:

- The referral letter.
- The completed frequency–volume chart.
- The urodynamic tracing.
- The urodynamic report.

In addition the records may contain the urodynamic data sheet if the details of patient history, examination and urodynamic findings were put into the computer database offline.

Several of the new computer-based systems have a database and report generation capacity. It is useful if the system can link into the hospital patient administration system so that double data entry can be avoided. This should become possible with the increasing flexibility of computer systems and software and with the refocusing of these systems on the user rather than the organisation.

What equipment should you buy? The decision as to which system to buy depends on a number of factors:

- First decide what range of urodynamic tests will be offered.
- It is wise to involve the medical physics department of your hospital whose help can prove invaluable at times of crisis.
- It is sensible to talk to and visit colleagues who are using the equipment you wish to buy.

- Attend meetings which have trade exhibitions, because you will be able to have a demonstration and to handle the equipment on the commercial stand.
- Establish what service facility the company can offer. In a busy department losing a machine for a week, due to a breakdown, is a disaster!
- Ask for a demonstration in your own hospital so that you can invite colleagues including medical physics staff to see the equipment.
- Lastly make a cost-benefit assessment, going for reliability and service rather than equipment with a myriad of computer functions you are unlikely to use. The computerisation of urodynamics has brought problems as well as benefits. Computers allow the manipulation of data, but this facility can be a weakness as well as a strength. The raw data must be accurate and relevant to that patient: if it is not then any manipulation of data for the purpose of diagnosis, as in pressure–flow studies, will lead to the wrong diagnosis and possibly to inappropriate management. The key data points must be verified before computer programmes are used for diagnosis.

What relationships should exist with other departments? The urodynamic unit is a service department for other departments. However as discussed above, the lead specialist and permanent doctors will have or will develop the skills to advise on management. The important relationships will be with:

- Urology, which provides more than 50% of our referrals. In particular the flow clinic is largely used by male patients.
- Gynaecology, the next largest referral source. The director of our unit is a gynaecologist and she maintains the excellent relationships with the neighbouring departments of gynaecology.
- Paediatrics, since an increasing source of referrals come from paediatric urologist, paediatric surgeons (for example problems associated with ano-rectal anomalies), paediatricians, and paediatric nephrologists (with referrals of children who may have a lower urinary tract cause for renal impairment).
- Neurology/neurosurgery, which refers a significant number of patients with proven or suspected neurological abnormalities associated with vesico-urethral dysfunction.
- Geriatrics, a declining primary source of referral, and we have found it useful to screen the elderly in outpatients before requesting UDS.
- Gastro-enterology, and in particular surgeons with an interest in lower bowel dysfunction, who are moving into closer relationships with urodynamic units. They are forming collaborative links with gynaecologists and urologists interested in pelvic floor function. In our department ano-rectal measurements are carried out by our technicians with the colo-rectal surgeon.
- Nephrology, particularly where patients have renal failure which cannot clearly be attributed to intrinsic renal disease, and who often need to be assessed urodynamically prior to being transplanted.
- Radiology, an important link because it is often necessary to organise additional tests such as urethrography, micturating cystourethrography, pyelography and isotope scanning (DMSA and MAG 3 renography)
- Medical physics, who are useful friends and allies both for emergencies and for basic maintenance and problem-solving. They can also be useful in discussion with the equipment manufacturers.

The Investigating and Therapeutic Team

In terms of therapy the team approach should be continued and should consist of:

- Continence care staff under the direction of the continence adviser.
- A urologist and paediatric urologist.
- A gynaecologist.
- A colo-rectal surgeon.

The facilities should exist for joint outpatient sessions and joint operating lists where necessary.

Summary of Equipment Needs

Basic Urodynamics

Uroflow

- Uroflowmeter, commode, examination couch, ultrasound machine.
  - Private room with lockable door (Fig. 3.3).
  - Nurse/technician.

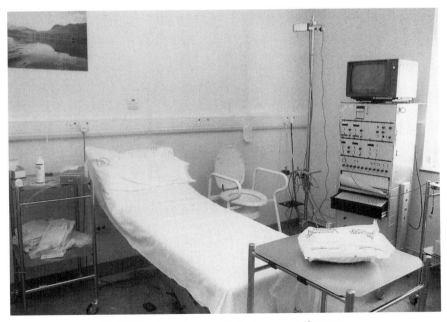

Fig. 7.7 Urodynamics room for basic pressure–flow tests.

Pressure–flow Studies

- Uroflowmeter, examination couch, commode, transducer stand, basic urodynamic equipment with transducers and infusion pump.
  - Room with 20 square metres of floor area (Fig. 7.7).
  - Doctor plus nurse/technician.

Advanced Urodynamics (Additional Requirements)

- Imaging apparatus (image intensifier, fixed X-ray unit or ultrasound machine). Motorised withdrawal pump for urethral pressure profilometry. Advanced urodynamic equipment.
  - Room with 30 square metres of floor area (Fig. 7.6).
  - Radiographer if studies performed in the X-ray department.

Complex Urodynamics (Additional Requirements)

- Electrophysiological equipment. Ambulatory urodynamic equipment.
  - Input from neurophysiologist/neurologist.

Appendix 1, Part 1
Urodynamic Equipment: Technical Aspects

J Med Engng Technol 11:57–64 (1987)

Produced by the International Continence Society[†] Working Party on Urodynamic Equipment

Chairman: David Rowan[†]
Members: E. Douglas James, August E. J. L. Kramer, Arthur M. Sterling and Peter F. Suhel

[†]*International Continence Society, Department of Clinical Physics & Bio-Engineering, 11 West Graham Street, Glasgow G4 9LF, UK*

Introduction

The two parameters that are most commonly measured in urodynamic studies are pressure and urinary flow rate. In each case a *transducer* is used to produce an electrical signal to represent these parameters in a form that can be readily recorded on chart paper or magnetic tape, displayed on an oscilloscope or stored digitally in a computer. Another useful parameter, the *electromyogram* (EMG), is already in an electrical form. Generally it is desirable to reproduce these parameters as "faithfully" as possible, without modifying the signal appearing at the source. This can usually be achieved by direct *amplification*. Often, however, more useful, and perhaps more readily interpretable, data can be acquired by modifying the original signal before it is eventually displayed. This, together with amplification, is referred to as *signal processing*. Interference from other physiological variables may be present in the recorded signal, appearing as if originating from the source. The recorded signals should therefore be interpreted with caution.

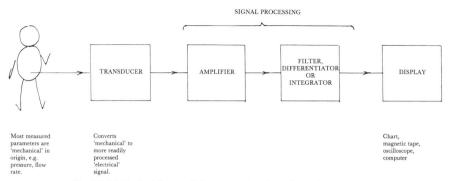

SIGNAL PROCESSING

| TRANSDUCER | AMPLIFIER | FILTER, DIFFERENTIATOR OR INTEGRATOR | DISPLAY |

Most measured parameters are 'mechanical' in origin, e.g. pressure, flow rate.

Converts 'mechanical' to more readily processed 'electrical' signal.

Chart, magnetic tape, oscilloscope, computer

Fig. A.1.1.1 Typical "system" for measuring physiological parameters.

Signal Processors

A typical electronic system used for measuring urodynamic parameters is shown in Fig. A.1.1.1, the design procedure taking into account the importance of maintaining compatibility between the various components in the overall system. Processors can be used to:

(1) Amplify the signal.
(2) Filter the signal.
(3) Differentiate the signal.
(4) Integrate the signal.
(5) Convert the analogue signal into digital form.

Amplification

The ideal amplifier changes the amplitude of an applied signal without distortion.

Signal Filtration

Signals which change their values with respect to time can be described as the sum of a number of components of different frequencies possessing different amplitudes. More rapidly changing signals contain higher frequencies. As examples, the changes that occur in bladder pressure on coughing are much more rapid compared to the slower changes that occur during detrusor activity. Other frequencies, perhaps even higher than those encountered physiologically, may also appear superimposed on the signal in the form of "noise". By limiting the frequency range of the measuring system, it is possible to reproduce signals which can adequately represent the parameter being measured, while at the same time filtering out the noise. To reproduce the rapidly changing signals quoted above, an amplifier with a frequency range of DC-15 Hz is required; however, for EMG measurements, this would have to be extended to several kilohertz (kHz).

The principle of filtering can be illustrated by reference to recordings obtained from urine flow rate meters which measure the rate at which urine is collected in

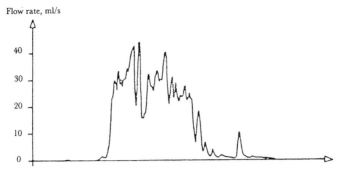

Fig. A.1.1.2a Flow rate recording, including mechanically-generated and "other" noise.

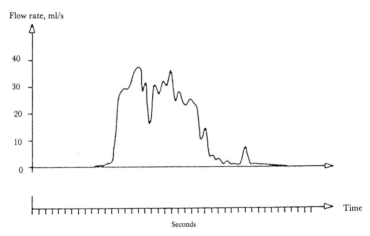

Fig. A.1.1.2b Following filtering the flow rate recording still contains adequate diagnostic data.

an external vessel. Inevitably *mechanical noise* is introduced during this measurement, which subsequently appears as electrical noise. Without adequate filtering the recorded signal could be difficult to interpret (Fig. A.1.1.2). Excessive filtering not only reduces the noise further but also prevents the important components of the signal from being recorded. The marked effects of different filters on pressure recordings are shown in Fig. A.1.1.3.

Differentiation

Often the rate of change of a signal with respect to time contains more useful information than the original signal. This information can be derived from the original signal by the process of *differentiation*. The most frequently encountered application of differentiation occurs in flow rate meters that measure the volume or mass of urine (Fig. A.1.1.4a). Following differentiation (Fig. A.1.1.4b), the signal represents the volumetric or mass flow rate (see section on "Flowmeters", p. 205).

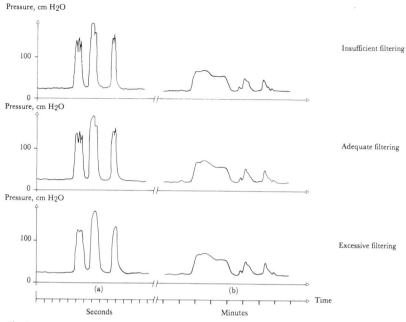

Fig. A.1.1.3 Coughs (rapid pressure changes) and detrusor spasms (slow pressure changes).

Integration

Integration, the reverse process of differentiation, is used to produce a signal to represent the area under a curve. For example, the area under the curve (Fig. A.1.1.4b) of a direct recording of urine flow rate (see section on "Flowmeters", p. 205) is equivalent to the total voided volume (Fig. A.1.1.4a).

Integrating techniques also find useful application in the processing of EMG signals. In common with differentiators, integrators have characteristics which define the range over which they can be operated.

Analogue-to-Digital Conversion

Signals representing urodynamic parameters normally appear in a continuous uninterrupted form (analogue). The signals can also be approximated by a series of discrete numbers (digital). It is often useful to convert analogue signals into digital form for direct presentation of numerical data such as "the volume of urine voided" or for feeding into a computer for further processing or analysis.

Pressure Transducers: Characteristics and Specifications

A *pressure transducer* is a device that converts an applied pressure into an electrical signal, the magnitude of which is proportional to the pressure. The pressure

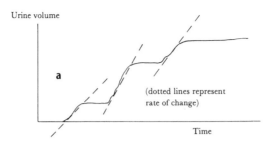

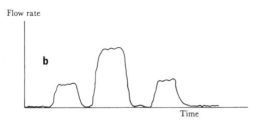

Fig. A.1.1.4 Differentiation: the original signal (**a**) representing the volume (or mass) of urine when differentiated appears as the flow rate signal (**b**).
Integration: the original signal, now (**b**), when integrated represents the volume (or mass) of urine voided (**a**).

to be measured, for example that within the bladder, may be transmitted to an external transducer using either an open-ended or sealed, liquid or gas-filled, catheter. Alternatively, the pressure may be measured by a small transducer mounted directly on the catheter. There are four principal types of transducer: resistive (strain gauge), capacitive, inductive and opto-electronic.

Units of Measurement

The SI unit of pressure is the pascal (Pa) although in urodynamics the unit cmH_2O (1 cmH_2O = 98.07 Pa) is still used. When parameters that are a function of pressure, for example compliance, are calculated, SI units must be used.[1]

Important Characteristics and Specifications of Pressure Transducers

Pressure Range

A pressure range of 0–300 cmH_2O (0–30 kPa) is adequate for pressure measurements in the urinary tract and in many cases a range of 0–200 cmH_2O (0–20 kPa) is acceptable (for example in the measurement of intravesical pressure).

Sensitivity

The sensitivity of a transducer is defined as the change in amplitude of its output signal per unit change in applied pressure. A change in sensitivity with temperature is called *sensitivity drift*. A drift of less than 0.1%/°C is desirable.

Linearity and Hysteresis

In an ideal transducer the electrical output is linearly related to the applied pressure. Non-linearity is specified as a percentage of the pressure range. In addition the output signal has a slightly different value for a given applied pressure depending on whether this is increasing or decreasing in amplitude. This effect is called *hysteresis*. It is common practice to give a combined Figure for linearity and hysteresis in terms of a specified percentage deviation over a stated pressure range. A value of not more than ± 1% over the range 0–100 cmH$_2$O (0–10 kPa) is acceptable.

Overload Pressure

Transducers can be permanently damaged by applying excess pressure. The maximum pressure that may be applied without affecting the transducer characteristics is called the *overload pressure*. Typical values are in the range 1500–5000 cmH$_2$O (150–500 kPa). The calibration over the working range should change by less than 1% after the overload pressure is removed.

A pressure above a certain level will destroy a transducer; this is defined as the *damage pressure level*.

Note: In practice it is very easy to exceed the maximum rated pressure if the transducer chamber is flushed out with a high resistance in the outlet (for example a fine bore catheter or a closed tap).

Zero Offset

All transducers have a small electrical signal output when the applied pressure is atmospheric (or zero in the present context); this is known as the *zero offset signal*. Provided this offset is constant, no errors in measurement will be introduced since the transducer signal conditioner can be adjusted to produce a zero output. The change in the offset signal with temperature, called *zero offset drift*, is more important than the absolute value. A zero offset drift of less than 0.1 cmH$_2$O/°C (10 Pa/°C) is desirable.

Zero Reference Level

A transducer is normally calibrated against atmospheric pressure. In urodynamics the zero reference level is taken as the superior edge of the symphysis pubis.[2] When a liquid-coupled system is used to measure pressure within the bladder, the transducer is subjected to two sources of hydrostatic pressure which tend to cancel:

(1) The pressure arising from the presence of liquid in the catheter.
(2) The pressure due to the depth of the catheter tip within the volume of urine.

With this type of system, therefore, the measurement of bladder pressure is substantially independent of the location of the tip of the catheter within the bladder. On the other hand, the pressure measured by micro-tip and sealed gas systems is dependent on the position of the membrane within the bladder.

Detrusor pressure is calculated by electronic subtraction of the abdominal pressure from the intravesical pressure.[2] To achieve a good approximation to detrusor pressure, both abdominal and intravesical pressure should be measured with reference to the standardized zero level (superior edge of the symphysis pubis) using liquid-coupled external transducers. However, for studies involving significant patient movement (for example, ambulatory monitoring) a liquid-filled system is unsuitable as the zero reference may vary and major artefacts are produced due to movement of the liquid in the catheter. In these cases a qualitative assessment of detrusor pressure can be made using a micro-tip or sealed gas system.

Volume Displacement

The pressure applied to a transducer produces a movement in its diaphragm. The volume change caused by a specified pressure is called the *volume displacement* of the transducer. Typical values are in the range $0.03\,mm^3/100\,cmH_2O$–$0.003\,mm^3/100\,cmH_2O$ ($0.03\,mm^3/10\,kPa$–$0.003\,mm^3/10\,kPa$). In general, for catheters and transducer chambers filled with similar fluids, the greater the volume displacement for a given applied pressure, the lower the frequency response.

Frequency Response

The response of most modern transducers used for physiological purposes is more than adequate when pressure measurements are made at source. However, if the pressure to be measured is transmitted to the transducer via a liquid-filled catheter, then the dynamic characteristics of the system are limited by the dimensions and compliance of the catheter and its connections. Thus the frequency response decreases as the internal diameter of the catheter decreases and as the length and the compliance of the coupling system increase. Since air is compressible, all air bubbles must be removed from the liquid coupling otherwise the response will be dampened. The response of a particular system can be measured by coupling it to:

(1) A hydraulic sinusoidal pressure generator of variable frequency; or
(2) A chamber in which the pressure can be very rapidly changed (step response).

The response required depends on the type of investigation. For example in filling cystometry, a frequency response of typically DC-4 Hz is adequate. On the other hand, when rapid changes of pressure, which occur on coughing or during patient movement, are to be studied, a frequency response of typically DC-15 Hz is desirable.

Complete Pressure Measuring System

When transducers are incorporated in complete pressure measuring and display systems, further detrimental effects may be introduced. The effect on the frequency response and any additional drifts introduced by the chart recorder must be specified by the manufacturer.

Flowmeters: Characteristics and Specifications

In urodynamic investigations a flowmeter is a device that measures and indicates the quantity of fluid (volume or mass) passed per unit time. Depending on the type of transducer used, either the *flow rate* or the *instantaneous accumulated amount* can be measured. Uroflowmeters normally indicate the *volumetric flow rate*.

Units of Measurement

The SI unit for volumetric flow rate is the cubic metre per second (m^3/s) and for mass flow rate is the kilogram per second (kg/s). However, the millilitre (ml) is also an acceptable unit,[1] and it is conventional in urodynamic work[2] to report volumetric flow rate in millilitres per second (ml/s). The unit cubic centimetre per second (cm^3/s) should not be used.

Conversion of Units

The volumetric flow rate and the accumulated volume are related as follows:
Volumetric flow rate
Q = rate of change of accumulated volume (V) with respect to time, i.e.
$$Q = dV/dt$$

Similarly, accumulated volume

V = integral of the volumetric flow rate (Q) with respect to time, i.e.
$$V = \int^t Q \, dt$$

Conversion between flow rate and accumulated volume is usually done electronically.

The mass and volume of fluid are related as follows:

$$m = \rho V$$

where m = mass of fluid
ρ = density of fluid
V = volume of fluid.

The conversion between mass and volume (or between mass flow rate and volumetric flow rate) can only be carried out provided the fluid density is known.

If a particular flowmeter measures the *accumulated mass of fluid*, the volumetric flow rate is obtained from:

Volumetric flow rate

Q = rate of change of accumulated mass (m) with respect to time divided by the density (ρ)

i.e.
$$Q = \frac{1}{\rho}\frac{dm}{dt}$$

The *mass flow rate* is obtained by electronic differentiation. The volumetric flow rate is obtained by dividing the mass flow rate by the fluid density.

Normally mass flowmeters are calibrated for water. When other liquids are used with densities significantly different from water, in particular a radio-opaque medium, the instrument must be recalibrated.

Types of Transducer

The most commonly used uroflowmeters employ one of the following methods.

Gravimetric method: these instruments operate by measuring the weight of the collected fluid or by measuring the hydrostatic pressure at the base of the collecting cylinder. In either case, the output signal is proportional to the mass of fluid collected. Gravimetric meters therefore measure accumulated mass and mass flow rate is obtained by differentiation.

Electronic dip stick method: in this method the electrical capacitance of a dip stick mounted in the collecting chamber changes as the urine accumulates. The output signal is proportional to the accumulated volume and the volumetric flow rate is obtained by differentiation.

Rotating disc method: the voided fluid is directed on to a rotating disc increasing the inertia of the disc. The power required to keep the disc rotating at a constant rate is measured and is proportional to the mass flow rate of the fluid. The accumulated mass is obtained by integration.

Many other metering techniques are known including electromagnetic, ultrasonic, radioisotope and drop spectrometry. However, these are not in general use.

Characteristics of Flowmeters

Static Characteristics

The most important static characteristic of a flowmeter is its accuracy over its usable range.

Zero offset: zero offset is the non-zero output signal of a flowmeter at zero input flow.

Linearity and hysteresis: the output signal of a flowmeter system should ideally be proportional to the input flow. In practice non-linearity and hysteresis errors are encountered similar to those described in the section on pressure transducers.

Accuracy: the offset should be set to zero and the sensitivity control adjusted during the calibration procedure. The accuracy will then be determined by the non-linearity and hysteresis.

It is common for manufacturers to state system accuracy only in terms of percentage full-scale error which can be readily misinterpreted (see section on accuracy).

Dynamic Characteristics

Time constant (τ) is a measure of the frequency response of a system. It is defined as the time required for a system to register 63% of its final reading when subjected to a step change in input (Fig. A.1.1.5). The larger the time constant, the lower the frequency response.

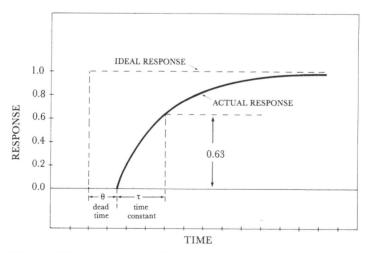

Fig. A.1.1.5 Typical dynamic response of a flowmeter system to a unit step change in input flow.

The time constant is increased by filtering, which can be introduced into the system mechanically or electronically. Mechanical filtering occurs primarily at the funnel. The degree of filtering is influenced by funnel design, by the location and angle at which the stream strikes the funnel and by the flow rate. The filtering effect of the funnel cannot be calculated *a priori*; it must be determined experimentally. Electronic filtering is designed into the system to reduce signal noise. The time constant of the electronics should be stated by the system manufacturer.

Use of Flowmeter in Pressure–Flow Studies

In many investigations urinary flow rate is measured in conjunction with bladder pressure. If the pressure events in the bladder are to be correlated with variations in the flow rate, the *dead time* between the pressure event and the flow event must be estimated.

Dead time (θ) is the delay between the exit of the urine from the bladder and its initial registration by the flowmeter (Fig. A.1.1.5).
Several factors contribute to the dead time:

(1) The time taken for urine to traverse the urethra.
(2) The time taken for urine to pass from the external meatus to the flowmeter funnel.
(3) The time taken for urine to pass via the funnel to the transducer.

System Specifications

Range

A meter with a flow rate range of 0–50 ml/s and a volume range of 0–1000 ml is adequate for clinical use. These ranges will be exceeded only in exceptional cases.

Time Constant

The time constant should be as short as possible. For most flowmeters on the market a time constant of 0.75 s is needed to achieve a reasonable compromise between noise reduction and loss of meaningful temporal information. This time constant should include the contribution of both the funnel and the electronics.

Accuracy

For clinical purposes the measured and indicated flow rate should be accurate to within ± 5% over the clinically significant flow rate range. It is therefore recommended that the calibration curve representing the percentage error over the entire range is made available.

The use of percentage full-scale error should be avoided as this can be mis-interpreted. For example, a flowmeter with a range of 50 ml/s and a quoted accuracy of ± 5% full-scale error could have a maximum absolute error of 2.5 ml/s. If this error occurred at a flow rate of 10 ml/s, the percentage error in the measured flow rate would be 25%.

EMG Measurements

Electromyography (EMG) is the recording of the electrical activity of contracting muscles and so no transducers are required. The electrical signals, however, are so minute that special amplifying techniques are needed. Consideration will be given only to the recording of EMG activity of striated muscles.

The functional contractile unit is the *motor unit*. Each motor unit while contracting has a *firing frequency* ranging from 10 to 100 discharges/s. Normal muscle activity results in the asynchronous contractions of many motor units, leading to an *interference pattern* in the EMG recording. This activity is detected by electrodes inserted into, or placed adjacent to, the muscle.

Electrodes

The electrical potential variations in muscle can be sensed either with respect to an unchanging reference value (*monopolar approach*) or as the potential difference between two points (*bipolar approach*) in or adjacent to the muscle.

Monopolar

The reference value, the potential level of the extra-cellular fluid, is sensed by an indifferent electrode. This electrode has a greater surface area than the active electrode and is placed remotely from it. The latter may be placed on the skin in the neighbourhood of the muscle (*surface electrode*) or in the bulk of the muscle (*tip electrode* or *coaxial needle electrode*). In the coaxial needle approach, the shaft of the needle acts as the indifferent electrode.

Bipolar

Bipolar surface electrodes are widely used in urodynamics; anal plug electrodes, urethral catheter electrodes and self-adhesive electrodes on the perineum are examples. The bipolar intramuscular approach (*bipolar wire electrodes*) is less popular than the use of the coaxial needle.

Types of Recording

Bipolar wire and coaxial needle electrodes have sensing ranges of about 1 mm around the tip of the electrode. They register the sum of the activities of all muscle fibres within this range (*motor unit potentials*). In the sphincteric muscles bi- or triphasic potentials lasting about 7 ms are mostly recorded. The amplitudes of these potentials are dependent on the arrangement of the intermingled fibres from the various motor units with respect to the electrode. With increasing contraction the discharge frequency of individual motor units and the number of asynchronously activated motor units increase leading to a complex record of potential variation known as *interference pattern*. Parameters of this pattern are only qualitatively related to the contraction strength.

Surface electrodes register potential variations from the bulk of the muscle. These electrodes are suitable for assessing the overall behaviour of large muscles. Reflex responses, sphincter activity in relation to bladder conditions and the patient's ability to voluntarily control muscle can be checked adequately by this technique.

EMG Amplification

Characteristics

To enable the EMG to be adequately displayed, an amplifier with a wide frequency range is required. The amplifier has also special characteristics to reduce signal distortion and electrical noise.

Specifications

A good-quality EMG amplifier should have the following specifications:

Input impedance:	Minimum of 100 megohms shunted by a maximum of 10 picofarads.
Common mode rejection ratio:	Greater than 1000 (80 dB)
Frequency range:	Flat characteristic from 10 Hz to 10 kHz
Voltage input range:	5 μV–50 mV
Overload recovery time:	Less than 100 ms
Output impedance:	50 ohms.

Artefacts

EMG recording is very sensitive to artefacts. These can be minimised by:

(1) Optimum positioning of electrodes and leads.
(2) Appropriate preparation of skin when surface electrodes are employed.
(3) Proper grounding of instrumentation and the use of an isolation amplifier for connection to the patient.

Processing of EMG Signals

A variety of processing techniques are available to assist in the interpretation of EMG signals. Rectification and smoothing are often used to produce a low frequency signal which provides information on the timing and relative strength of muscle contraction.

Recording and Display Systems

Electrical signals corresponding to physiological parameters can be displayed directly or stored for subsequent examination. This can be achieved in a number of ways:

(1) By displaying on a screen of a cathode ray oscilloscope.
(2) By recording directly on to a paper chart recorder.
(3) By storing on magnetic tape.
(4) By digital storage.

Cathode Ray Oscilloscope

Because this device can faithfully reproduce signals with a high frequency range, it is often used to display rapidly changing physiological parameters (for example EMG). The displayed data can be photographed for permanency or stored for short periods of time (say minutes) using special *storage oscilloscopes*.

The cathode ray tube is also incorporated in video display units (VDUs) of computers and in image intensifying systems. In the latter a video mixing unit is employed to enable the registration of physiological parameters simultaneously on the same screen (video-pressure-flow-cystourethrography). The combined information can be stored on a *video tape recorder*.

Paper Chart Recorders

These are employed in urodynamic investigations to produce continuous visual displays of one or more parameters, in most cases with respect to time. The basic components are:

(1) An electromechanical device to convert an electrical input signal to mechanical movement.
(2) A writing mechanism to produce on paper a visual record of the mechanical movement (pen, ink-jet or light beam). Recordings may be written in curvilinear or rectilinear form. Depending on the type of recorder, the paper is driven at appropriate selected speeds or held stationary as the writing mechanism operates. The parameters may be recorded with respect to time (X-t recorders) or with respect to one another (X-Y recorders/plotters).

The frequency response of a recorder is particularly important for accurate reproduction of the signal. The following features must be taken into account when selecting a recorder:

(*a*) Number of channels.
(*b*) Type of paper, writing principle and recording format.
(*c*) Input sensitivity and offset adjustment.
(*d*) Chart speed.
(*e*) Time and event markers.
(*f*) Writing span.
(*g*) Trace accuracy.
(*h*) Start-stop on front panel or by remote control.
(*i*) Power supply (a.c. or d.c.).

Most urodynamic signals are unlikely to contain frequency components greater than 15 Hz and can be recorded on almost any of the instruments described. For direct EMG recording, however, pen-type recorders are inadequate.

Magnetic Tape Recorders

Signals are stored on magnetic tape for subsequent display, processing and analysis. Only *instrumentation tape recorders* should be used.

Magnetic Tape Recording Techniques

Two recording techniques are employed for analogue recording, the most important being *frequency modulation* (FM) and the other the *direct mode*. The former is capable of recording signals with frequency components ranging from DC to several kilohertz. The direct mode covers the frequency range of, typically, 10 Hz–100 kHz.

In urodynamics the FM mode must be used for recording all parameters with the exception of raw EMG signals. These signals are best recorded using the direct mode.

To select a suitable instrumentation tape recorder the following features should be considered:

(1) Tape speed range.
(2) Flutter (tape speed stability) and flutter compensation.
(3) Maximum input signal.
(4) Signal-to-noise ratio.
(5) Number of signal and voice channels.

Digital Storage

The discrete data obtained when analogue signals are converted to digital form can be stored as follows:

(1) On magnetic tape using the technique of *Pulse Code Modulation* (PCM).
(2) Via a computer on to floppy disk, hard disk or non-volatile *Random Access Memory* (RAM). These techniques are known as data acquisition.

Electrical Safety Aspects

Any electrical equipment used in urodynamic investigations in common with all other medical instrumentation should comply with the recommendations of the International Electrotechnical Commission.[3] Prospective users of such equipment should seek advice from a suitably qualified engineer or physicist.

References

1. The International System of Units (1973). London: Her Majesty's Stationery Office.
2. Bates P, Bradley WE, Glen E, Griffiths D, Melchior H, Rowan D, Sterling A, Zinner N, Hald T (1979). The standardisation of terminology of lower urinary tract function. J Urol 121:551–554.
3. International Electrotechnical Commission (1977). Safety of Medical Electrical Equipment. Part 1. General Requirements (IEC 601–1, Geneva).

Appendix 1, Part 2
The Standardisation of Terminology of Lower Urinary Tract Function

Scand J Urol Nephrol, Supplementum 114, 1988

Produced by the International Continence Society Committee on Standardisation of Terminology; Members: Paul Abrams, Jerry G. Blaivas, Stuart L. Stanton and Jens T. Andersen (Chairman)

1. Introduction

The International Continence Society established a committee for the standard-isation of terminology of lower urinary tract function in 1973. Five of the six reports[1-5] from this committee, approved by the Society, have been published. The fifth report on "Quantification of urine loss" was an internal I.C.S. document but appears, in part, in this document.

These reports are revised, extended and collated in this monograph. The standards are recommended to facilitate comparison of results by investigators who use urodynamic methods. These standards are recommended not only for urodynamic investigations carried out on humans but also during animal studies. When using urodynamic studies in animals the type of any anaesthesia used should be stated. It is suggested that acknowledgement of these standards in written publications be indicated by a footnote to the section "Methods and Materials" or its equivalent, to read as follows:

"Methods, definitions and units conform to the standards recommended by the International Continence Society, except where specifically noted".

Urodynamic studies involve the assessment of the function and dysfunction of the urinary tract by any appropriate method. Aspects of urinary tract mor-phology, physiology, biochemistry and hydrodynamics affect urine transport and storage. Other methods of investigation such as the radiographic visualisation of the lower urinary tract is a useful adjunct to conventional urodynamics.

This monograph concerns the urodynamics of the lower urinary tract.

2. Clinical Assessment

The clinical assessment of patients with lower urinary tract dysfunction should consist of a detailed history, a frequency/volume chart and a physical exam-ination. In urinary incontinence, leakage should be demonstrated objectively.

2.1. History

The general history should include questions relevant to neurological and con-genital abnormalities as well as information on previous urinary infections and relevant surgery. Information must be obtained on medication with known or possible effects on the lower urinary tract. The general history should also include assessment of menstrual, sexual and bowel function, and obstetric history.

The urinary history must consist of symptoms related to both the storage and the evacuation functions of the lower urinary tract.

2.2. Frequency/Volume Chart

The frequency/volume chart is a specific urodynamic investigation recording fluid intake and urine output per 24 hour period. The chart gives objective information on the number of voidings, the distribution of voidings between daytime and night-time and each voided volume. The chart can also be used to record episodes of urgency and leakage and the number of incontinence pads used. The frequency/volume chart is very useful in the assessment of voiding disorders, and in the follow-up of treatment.

2.3. Physical Examination

Besides a general urological and, when appropriate, gynaecological examination, the physical examination should include the assessment of perineal sensation, the perineal reflexes supplied by the sacral segments S2-S4, and anal sphincter tone and control.

3. Procedures Related to the Evaluation of Urine Storage

3.1. Cystometry

Cystometry is the method by which the pressure/volume relationship of the bladder is measured. All systems are zeroed at atmospheric pressure. For external transducers the reference point is the level of the superior edge of the symphysis pubis. For catheter mounted transducers the reference point is the transducer itself.

Cystometry is used to assess detrusor activity, sensation, capacity and compliance.

Before starting to fill the bladder the residual urine may be measured. However, the removal of a large volume of residual urine may alter detrusor function especially in neuropathic disorders. Certain cystometric parameters may be significantly altered by the speed of bladder filling (see 6.1.1.4.).

During cystometry it is taken for granted that the patient is awake, unanaesthetised and neither sedated nor taking drugs that affect bladder function. Any variations should be specified.

Specify

(a) Access (transurethral or percutaneous)
(b) Fluid medium (liquid or gas)
(c) Temperature of fluid (state in degrees Celsius)
(d) Position of patient (e.g. supine, sitting or standing)
(e) Filling may be by diuresis or catheter. Filling by catheter may be continuous or incremental; the precise filling rate should be stated.
    When the incremental method is used the volume increment should be stated. For general discussion, the following terms for the range of filling rate may be used:
    (i)   up to 10 ml per minute is slow fill cystometry ("physiological" filling).
    (ii) 10–100 ml per minute is medium fill cystometry.
    (iii) over 100 ml per minute is rapid fill cystometry.

Technique

(a) Fluid-filled catheter – specify number of catheters, single or multiple lumens, type of catheter (manufacturer), size of catheter.
(b) Catheter tip transducer – list specifications.
(c) Other catheters – list specifications.
(d) Measuring equipment.

Definitions

Intravesical pressure is the pressure within the bladder.

Abdominal pressure is taken to be the pressure surrounding the bladder. In current practice it is estimated from rectal or, less commonly, extraperitoneal pressure.

Detrusor pressure is that component of intravesical pressure that is created by forces in the bladder wall (passive and active). It is estimated by subtracting abdominal pressure from intravesical pressure. The simultaneous measurement of abdominal pressure is essential for the interpretation of the intravesical pressure trace. However, artefacts on the detrusor pressure trace may be produced by intrinsic rectal contractions.

Bladder sensation. Sensation is difficult to evaluate because of its subjective nature. It is usually assessed by questioning the patient in relation to the fullness of the bladder during cystometry.
    Commonly used descriptive terms include:

First desire to void

Normal desire to void (this is defined as the feeling that leads the patient to pass urine at the next convenient moment, but voiding can be delayed if necessary).

Strong desire to void (this is defined as a persistent desire to void without the fear of leakage).

Urgency (this is defined as a strong desire to void accompanied by fear of leakage or fear of pain).

Pain (the site and character of which should be specified). Pain during bladder filling or micturition is abnormal.
    The use of objective or semi-objective tests for sensory function, such as electrical threshold studies (sensory testing), is discussed in detail in 5.5.
    The term "Capacity" must be qualified.

Maximum cystometric capacity, in patients with normal sensation, is the volume at which the patient feels he/she can no longer delay micturition. In the absence of sensation the maximum cystometric capacity cannot be defined in the same terms and is the volume at which the clinician decides to terminate filling. In the presence of sphincter incompetence the maximum cystometric capacity may be significantly increased by occlusion of the urethra e.g. by Foley catheter.

The *functional bladder capacity*, or voided volume is more relevant and is assessed from a frequency/volume chart (urinary diary).

The *maximum (anaesthetic) bladder capacity* is the volume measured after filling during a deep general or spinal/epidural anaesthetic, specifying fluid temperature, filling pressure and filling time.

Compliance indicates the change in volume for a change in pressure. Compliance is calculated by dividing the volume change (ΔV) by the change in detrusor pressure (ΔP_{det}) during that change in bladder volume ($C = \Delta V / \Delta P_{det}$). Compliance is expressed as ml per cmH_2O (see 6.1.1.4).

3.2. Urethral Pressure Measurement

It should be noted that the urethral pressure and the urethral closure pressure are idealised concepts which represent the ability of the urethra to prevent leakage (see 6.1.5). In current urodynamic practice the urethral pressure is measured by a number of different techniques which do not always yield consistent values. Not only do the values differ with the method of measurement but there is often lack of consistency for a single method. For example the effect of catheter rotation when urethral pressure is measured by a catheter mounted transducer.

Intraluminal urethral pressure may be measured:

(a) At rest, with the bladder at any given volume
(b) During coughing or straining
(c) During the process of voiding (see 4.4)

Measurements may be made at one point in the urethra over a period of time, or at several points along the urethra consecutively forming a *urethral pressure profile* (UPP).

Storage Phase

Two types of UPP may be measured:

(a) Resting urethral pressure profile – with the bladder and subject at rest.
(b) Stress urethral pressure profile – with a defined applied stress (e.g. cough, strain, Valsalva).

In the storage phase the *urethral pressure profile* denotes the intraluminal pressure along the length of the urethra. All systems are zeroed at atmospheric pressure. For external transducers the reference point is the superior edge of the symphysis pubis. For catheter mounted transducers the reference point is the transducer itself. Intravesical pressure should be measured to exclude a simultaneous detrusor contraction. The subtraction of intravesical pressure from urethral pressure produces the *urethral closure pressure profile*.

The simultaneous recording of both intravesical and intra-urethral pressures are essential during stress urethral profilometry.

Specify

(a) Infusion medium (liquid or gas)
(b) Rate of infusion.
(c) Stationary, continuous or intermittent withdrawal.
(d) Rate of withdrawal.
(e) Bladder volume.
(f) Position of patient (supine, sitting or standing).

Technique

(a) Open catheter – specify type (manufacturer), size, number, position and orientation of side or end hole.
(b) Catheter mounted transducers – specify manufacturer, number of transducers, spacing of transducers along the catheter, orientation with respect to one another; transducer design e.g. transducer face depressed or flush with catheter surface; catheter diameter and material. The orientation of the transducer(s) in the urethra should be stated.
(c) Other catheters, e.g. membrane, fibreoptic – specify type (manufacturer), size and number of channels as for microtransducer catheter.
(d) Measurement technique: For stress profiles the particular stress employed should be stated e.g. cough or Valsalva.
(e) Recording apparatus: Describe type of recording apparatus. The frequency response of the total system should be stated. The frequency response of the catheter in the perfusion method can be assessed by blocking the eyeholes and recording the consequent rate of change of pressure.

Definitions (Fig. A.1.2.1: Referring to profiles measured in storage phase).

Maximum urethral pressure is the maximum pressure of the measured profile.

Maximum urethral closure pressure is the maximum difference between the urethral pressure and the intravesical pressure.

Functional profile length is the length of the urethra along which the urethral pressure exceeds intravesical pressure.

Functional profile length (on stress) is the length over which the urethral pressure exceeds the intravesical pressure on stress.

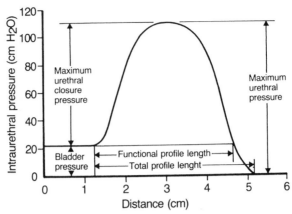

Fig. A.1.2.1 Diagram of a female urethral pressure profile (static) with I.C.S. recommended nomen-

Pressure "transmission" ratio is the increment in urethral pressure on stress as a percentage of the simultaneously recorded increment in intravesical pressure. For stress profiles obtained during coughing, pressure transmission ratios can be obtained at any point along the urethra. If single values are given the position in the urethra should be stated. If several pressure transmission ratios are defined at different points along the urethra a pressure "transmission" profile is obtained. During "cough profiles" the amplitude of the cough should be stated if possible.

Note: the term "transmission" is in common usage and cannot be changed. However transmission implies a completely passive process. Such an assumption is not yet justified by scientific evidence. A role for muscular activity cannot be excluded.

Total profile length is not generally regarded as a useful parameter.

The information gained from urethral pressure measurements in the storage phase is of limited value in the assessment of voiding disorders.

3.3. Quantification of Urine Loss

Subjective grading of incontinence may not indicate reliably the degree of abnormality. However it is important to relate the management of the individual patients to their complaints and personal circumstances, as well as to objective measurements.

In order to assess and compare the results of the treatment of different types of incontinence in different centres, a simple standard test can be used to measure urine loss objectively in any subject. In order to obtain a representative result, especially in subjects with variable or intermittent urinary incontinence, the test should occupy as long a period as possible; yet it must be practical. The circumstances should approximate to those of everyday life, yet be similar for all subjects to allow meaningful comparison. On the basis of pilot studies performed in various centres, an internal report of the ICS (5th) recommended a test occupying a one-hour period during which a series of standard activities was carried out. This test *can* be extended by further one hour periods if the result of the first one hour test was not considered representative by either the patient or the investigator. Alternatively the test can be repeated having filled the bladder to a defined volume.

The total amount of urine lost during the test period is determined by weighing a collecting device such as a nappy, absorbent pad or condom appliance. A nappy or pad should be worn inside waterproof underpants or should have a waterproof backing. Care should be taken to use a collecting device of adequate capacity.

Immediately before the test begins the collecting device is weighed to the nearest gram.

Typical Test Schedule

(a) Test is started without the patient voiding.

(b) Preweighed collecting device is put on and first one hour test period begins.

(c) Subject drinks 500 ml sodium free liquid within a short period (max. 15 min), then sits or rests.

(d) Half hour period: subject walks, including stair climbing equivalent to one flight up and down.

(e) During the remaining period the subject performs the following activities:
    (i)   standing up from sitting, 10 times
    (ii)   coughing vigorously, 10 times
    (iii) running on the spot for 1 minute
    (iv) bending to pick up small object from floor, 5 times
    (v)   wash hands in running water for 1 minute

(f) At the end of the one hour test the collecting device is removed and weighed.

(g) If the test is regarded as representative the subject voids and the volume is recorded.

(h) Otherwise the test is repeated preferably without voiding.

If the collecting device becomes saturated or filled during the test it should be removed and weighed, and replaced by a fresh device. The total weight of urine lost during the test period is taken to be equal to the gain in weight of the collecting device(s). In interpreting the results of the test it should be borne in mind that a weight gain of up to 1 gram may be due to weighing errors, sweating or vaginal discharge.

The activity programme may be modified according to the subject's physical ability. If substantial variations from the usual test schedule occur, this should be recorded so that the same schedule can be used on subsequent occasions.

In principle the subject should not void during the test period. If the patient experiences urgency, then he/she should be persuaded to postpone voiding and to perform as many of the activities in section (e) as possible in order to detect leakage. Before voiding the collection device is removed for weighing. If inevitable voiding cannot be postponed then the test is terminated. The voided volume and the duration of the test should be recorded. For subjects not completing the full test the results may require separate analysis, or the test may be repeated after rehydration.

The test result is given as grams urine lost in the one hour test period in which the greatest urine loss is recorded.

Additional Procedures

Additional procedures intended to give information of diagnostic value are permissible provided they do not interfere with the basic test. For example, additional changes and weighing of the collecting device can give information about the timing of urine loss. The absorbent nappy may be an electronic recording nappy so that the timing is recorded directly.

Presentation of Results

Specify

(a) collecting device
(b) physical condition of subject (ambulant, chairbound, bedridden)
(c) relevant medical condition of subject
(d) relevant drug treatments
(e) test schedule

In some situations the timing of the test (e.g. in relation to the menstrual cycle) may be relevant.

Findings

Record weight of urine lost during the test (in the case of repeated tests, greatest weight in any stated period). A loss of less than one gram is within experimental error and the patients should be regarded as essentially dry. Urine loss should be measured and recorded in grams.

Statistics

When performing statistical analysis of urine loss in a group of subjects, non-parametric statistics should be employed, since the values are not normally distributed.

4. Procedures Related to the Evaluation of Micturition

4.1. Measurement of Urinary Flow

Urinary flow may be described in terms of *rate* and *pattern* and may be *continuous* or *intermittent*. *Flow rate* is defined as the volume of fluid expelled via the urethra per unit time. It is expressed in ml/s.

Specify

(a) Voided volume.
(b) Patient environment and position (supine, sitting or standing).
(c) Filling:
    (i)   by diuresis (spontaneous or forced: specify regimen),
    (ii)   by catheter (transurethral or suprapubic).
(d) type of fluid.

Technique

(a) Measuring equipment.
(b) Solitary procedure or combined with other measurements.

Definitions

(a) *Continuous flow* (Fig. A.1.2.2)

Voided volume is the total volume expelled via the urethra.

Maximum flow rate is the maximum measured value of the flow rate

Average flow rate is voided volume divided by flow time. The calculation of average flow rate is only meaningful if flow is continuous and without terminal dribbling.

Flow time is the time over which measurable flow actually occurs.

Time to maximum flow is the elapsed time from onset of flow to maximum flow.

    The flow pattern must be described when flow time and average flow rate are measured.

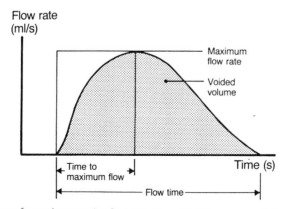

Fig. A.1.2.2 Diagram of a continuous urine flow recording with ICS recommended nomenclature.

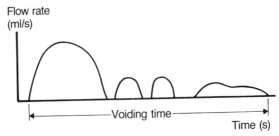

Fig. A.1.2.3 Diagram of an interrupted urine flow recording with ICS recommended nomenclature.

(b) *Intermittent flow* (Fig. A.1.2.3)

The same parameters used to characterise continuous flow may be applicable if care is exercised in patients with intermittent flow. In measuring flow time the time intervals between flow episodes are disregarded.

Voiding time is total duration of micturition, i.e. includes interruptions. When voiding is completed without interruption, voiding time is equal to flow time.

4.2. Bladder Pressure Measurements During Micturition

The specifications of patient position, access for pressure measurement, catheter type and measuring equipment are as for cystometry (see 3.1).

Definitions (Fig. A.1.2.4)

Opening Time is the elapsed time from initial rise in detrusor pressure to onset of flow. This is the initial isovolumetric contraction period of micturition. Time legs should be taken into account. In most urodynamic systems a time lag occurs equal to the time taken for the urine to pass from the point of pressure measurement to the uroflow transducer.

The following parameters are applicable to measurements of each of the pressure curves: intravesical, abdominal and detrusor pressure.

Premicturition pressure is the pressure recorded immediately before the initial isovolumetric contraction.

Opening pressure is the pressure recorded at the onset of measured flow.

Maximum pressure is the maximum value of the measured pressure.

Pressure at maximum flow is the pressure recorded at maximum measured flow rate.

Contraction pressure at maximum flow is the difference between pressure at maximum flow and premicturition pressure.

Postmicturition events (e.g. after contraction) are not well understood and so cannot be defined as yet.

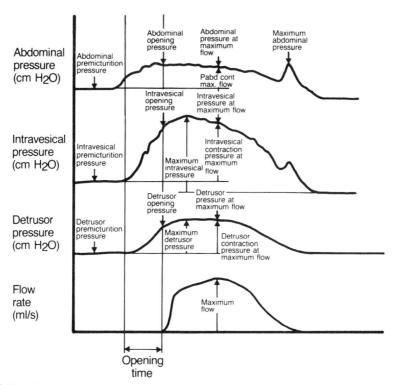

Fig. A.1.2.4. Diagram of a pressure–flow recording of micturition with I.C.S. recommended nomenclature.

4.3. Pressure–Flow Relationships

In the early days of urodynamics the flow rate and voiding pressure were related as a "urethral resistance factor". The concept of a resistance factor originates from rigid tube hydrodynamics. The urethra does not generally behave as a rigid tube as it is an irregular and distensible conduit whose walls and surroundings have active and passive elements and, hence, influence the flow through it. Therefore a resistance factor cannot provide a valid comparison between patients.

There are many ways of displaying the relationships between flow and pressure during micturition; an example is suggested in the ICS 3rd Report[4] (Fig. A.1.2.5). As yet available data do not permit a standard presentation of pressure/flow parameters.

When data from a group of patients are presented, pressure–flow relationships may be shown on a graph as illustrated in Fig. A.1.2.5. This form of presentation allows lines of demarcation to be drawn on the graph to separate the results according to the problem being studied. The points shown in Fig. A.1.2.5 are purely illustrative to indicate how the data might fall into groups. The group of equivocal results might include either an unrepresentative micturition in an obstructed or an unobstructed patient, or underactive detrusor function with or without obstruction. This is the group which invalidates the use of "urethral resistance factors".

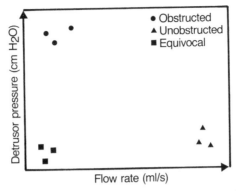

Fig. A.1.2.5 Diagram illustrating the presentation of pressure flow data on individual patients in three groups of 3 patients: obstructed, equivocal and unobstructed.

4.4. Urethral Pressure Measurements During Voiding (VUPP)

The VUPP is used to determine the pressure and site of urethral obstruction.

Pressure is recorded in the urethra during voiding. The technique is similar to that used in the UPP measured during storage (the resting and stress profiles 3.2).

Specify

As for UPP during storage (3.2).

Accurate interpretation of the VUPP depends on the simultaneous measurement of intravesical pressure and the measurement of pressure at a precisely localised point in the urethra. Localisation may be achieved by radio opaque marker on the catheter which allows the pressure measurements to be related to a visualised point in the urethra.

This technique is not fully developed and a number of technical as well as clinical problems need to be solved before the VUPP is widely used.

4.5. Residual Urine

Residual urine is defined as the volume of fluid remaining in the bladder immediately following the completion of micturition. The measurement of residual urine forms an integral part of the study of micturition. However voiding in unfamiliar surroundings may lead to unrepresentative results, as may voiding on command with a partially filled or overfilled bladder. Residual urine is commonly estimated by the following methods:

(a) Catheter or cystoscope (transurethral, suprapubic).
(b) Radiography (excretion urography, micturition cystography).
(c) Ultrasonics.
(d) Radioisotopes (clearance, gamma camera).

When estimating residual urine the measurement of voided volume and the time interval between voiding and residual urine estimation should be recorded: this is particularly important if the patient is in a diuretic phase. In the condition of vesicoureteric reflux, urine may re-enter the bladder after micturition and may falsely be interpreted as residual urine. The presence of urine in bladder divert-icula following micturition presents special problems of interpretation, since a diverticulum may be regarded either as part of the bladder cavity or as outside the functioning bladder.

The various methods of measurement each have limitations as to their applic-ability and accuracy in the various conditions associated with residual urine. Therefore it is necessary to choose a method appropriate to the clinical problems. The absence of residual urine is usually an observation of clinical value, but does not exclude infravesical obstruction or bladder dysfunction. An isolated finding of residual urine requires confirmation before being considered significant.

5. Procedures Related to Neurophysiological Evaluation of the Urinary Tract During Filling and Voiding

5.1. Electromyography

Electromyography (EMG) is the study of electrical potentials generated by the de-polarization of muscle. The following refers to striated muscle EMG The func-tional unit in EMG is the motor unit. This is comprised of a single motor neurone and the muscle fibres it innervates. A motor unit action potential is the recorded depolarisation of muscle fibres which results from activation of a single anterior horn cell. Muscle action potentials may be detected either by needle electrodes, or by surface electrodes.

Needle electrodes are placed directly into the muscle mass and permit visualisation of the individual motor unit action potentials.

Surface electrodes are applied to an epithelial surface as close to the muscle under study as possible. Surface electrodes detect the action potentials from groups of adjacent motor units underlying the recording surface.

EMG potentials may be displayed on an oscilloscope screen or played through audio amplifiers. A permanent record of EMG potentials can only be made using a chart recorder with a high frequency response (in the range of 10 kHz).

EMG should be interpreted in the light of the patients symptoms, physical findings and urological and urodynamic investigations.

General Information

Specify

(a) EMG (solitary procedure, part of urodynamic or other electrophysiological investigation).

(b) Patient position (supine, standing, sitting or other).

(c) Electrode placement:
  (i) Sampling site (intrinsic striated muscle of the urethra, periurethral striated muscle, bulbocavernosus muscle, external anal sphincter, pubococcygeus or other). State whether sites are single or multiple, unilateral or bilateral. Also state number of samples per site.
  (ii) Recording electrode: define the precise anatomical location of the electrode. For needle electrodes, include site of needle entry, angle of entry and needle depth. For vaginal or urethral surface electrodes state method of determining position of electrode.
  (iii) Reference electrode position.

Note: ensure that there is no electrical interference with any other machines, e.g. X-ray apparatus.

Technical Information

Specify

(a) Electrodes
  (i) Needle electrodes
    – design (concentric, bipolar, monopolar, single fibre, other)
    – dimensions (length, diameter, recording area).
    – electrode material (e.g. platinum).
  (ii) Surface electrodes
    – type (skin, plug, catheter, other)
    – size and shape
    – electrode material
    – mode of fixation to recording surface
    – conducting medium (e.g. saline, jelly)
(b) Amplifier (make and specifications)
(c) Signal processing (data: raw, averaged, integrated or other)
(d) Display equipment (make and specifications to include method of calibration, time base, full scale deflection in microvolts and polarity).
  (i) oscilloscope
  (ii) chart recorder
  (iii) loudspeaker
  (iv) other
(e) Storage (make and specifications)
  (i) paper
  (ii) magnetic tape recorder
  (iii) microprocessor
  (iv) other

(f) Hard copy production (make and specifications)
- (i)   chart recorder
- (ii) photographic/video reproduction of oscilloscope screen
- (iii) other

EMG Findings

(a) Individual motor unit action potentials – Normal motor unit potentials have a characteristic configuration, amplitude and duration. Abnormalities of the motor unit may include an increase in the amplitude, duration and complexity of waveform (polyphasicity) of the potentials. A polyphasic potential is defined as one having more than 5 deflections. The EMG findings of fibrillations, positive sharp waves and bizarre high frequency potentials are thought to be abnormal.

(b) Recruitment patterns – In normal subjects there is a gradual increase in "pelvic floor" and "sphincter" EMG activity during bladder filling. At the onset of micturition there is complete absence of activity. Any sphincter EMG activity during voiding is abnormal unless the patient is attempting to inhibit micturition. The finding of increased sphincter EMG activity, during voiding, accompanied by characteristic simultaneous detrusor pressure and flow changes is described by the term, detrusor-sphincter-dyssynergia. In this condition a detrusor contraction occurs concurrently with an in appropriate contraction of the urethral and or periurethral striated muscle.

5.2. Nerve Conduction Studies

Nerve conduction studies involve stimulation of a peripheral nerve, and recording the time taken for a response to occur in muscle, innervated by the nerve under study. The time taken from stimulation of the nerve to the response in the muscle is called the "latency". Motor latency is the time taken by the fastest motor fibres in the nerve to conduct impulses to the muscle and depends on conduction distance and the conduction velocity of the fastest fibres.

General Information

(also applicable to reflex latencies and evoked potentials – see below).

Specify

- (a) Type of investigation
    - (i)   nerve conduction study (e.g. pudendal nerve)
    - (ii) reflex latency determination (e.g. bulbocavernosus)
    - (iii) spinal evoked potential
    - (iv) cortical evoked potential
    - (v)   other

(b) Is the study a solitary procedure or part of urodynamic or neuro-physiological investigations?

(c) Patient position and environmental temperature, noise level and illumination.

(d) Electrode placement: Define electrode placement in precise anatomical terms. The exact interelectrode distance is required for nerve conduction velocity calculations.

    (i) Stimulation site (penis, clitoris, urethra, bladder neck, bladder or other).

    (ii) Recording sites (external anal sphincter, periurethral striated muscle, bulbocavernosus muscle, spinal cord, cerebral cortex or other).
When recording spinal evoked responses, the sites of the recording electrodes should be specified according to the bony landmarks (e.g. L4). In cortical evoked responses the sites of the recording electrodes should be specified as in the International 10–20 system.[6] The sampling techniques should be specified (single or multiple, unilateral or bilateral, ipsilateral or contralateral or other).

    (iii) Reference electrode position.

    (iv) Grounding electrode site: ideally this should be between the stimulation and recording sites to reduce stimulus artefact.

Technical Information

(also applicable to reflex latencies and evoked potential – see see below)

Specify

(a) Electrodes (make and specifications). Describe *separately* stimulus and recording electrodes as below.

    (i) design (e.g. needle, plate, ring, and configuration of anode and cathode where applicable).

    (ii) dimensions

    (iii) electrode material (e.g. platinum)

    (iv) contact medium

(b) Stimulator (make and specifications)

    (i) stimulus parameters (pulse width, frequency, pattern, current density, electrode impedance in Kohms. Also define in terms of threshold e.g. in case of supramaximal stimulation).

(c) Amplifier (make and specifications)

    (i) sensitivity (mV–μV)

    (ii) filters – low pass (Hz) or high pass (kHz)

    (iii) sampling time (ms)

(d) Averager (make and specifications)

    (i) number of stimuli sampled

(e) Display equipment (make and specifications to include method of calibration, time base, full scale deflection in microvolts and polarity).
   (i) oscilloscope
(f) Storage (make and specifications)
   (i) paper
   (ii) magnetic tape recorder
   (iii) microprocessor
   (iv) other
(g) Hard copy production (make and specification)
   (i) chart recorder
   (ii) photographic/video reproduction of oscilloscope screen
   (iii) XY recorder
   (iv) other

Description of Nerve Conduction Studies

Recordings are made from muscle and the latency of response of the muscle is measured. The latency is taken as the time to onset, of the earliest response.

(a) To ensure that response time can be precisely measured, the gain should be increased to give a clearly defined takeoff point. (Gain setting at least 100 μV/div and using a short time base e.g. 1–2 ms/div).

(b) Additional information may be obtained from nerve conduction studies, if, when using surface electrodes to record a compound muscle action potential, the amplitude is measured. The gain setting must be reduced so that the whole response is displayed and a longer time base is recommended (e.g. 1 mV/div and 5 ms/div). Since the amplitude is proportional to the number of motor unit potentials within the vicinity of the recording electrodes, a reduction in amplitude indicates loss of motor units and therefore denervation. (Note: A prolongation of latency is not necessarily indicative of denervation.)

5.3. Reflex Latencies

Reflex latencies require stimulation of sensory fields and recordings from the muscle which contracts reflexy in response to the stimulation. Such responses are a test of reflex arcs which are comprised of both afferent and efferent limbs and a synaptic region within the central nervous system. The reflex latency expresses the nerve conduction velocity in both limbs of the arc and the integrity of the central nervous system at the level of the synapse(s). Increased reflex latency may occur as a result of slowed afferent or efferent nerve conduction or due to central nervous system conduction delays.

General Information and Technical Information

The same technical and general details apply as discussed above under Nerve Conduction Studies (5.2).

Description of Reflex Latency Measurements

Recordings are made from muscle and the latency of response of the muscle is measured. The latency is taken as the time to onset, of the earliest response.

To ensure that response time can be precisely measured, the gain should be increased to give a clearly defined take-off point. (Gain setting at least 100 μV/div and using a short time base e.g. 1–2 ms/div.)

5.4 Evoked Responses

Evoked responses are potential changes in central nervous system neurones resulting from distant stimulation usually electrical. They are recorded using averaging techniques. Evoked responses may be used to test the integrity of peripheral, spinal and central nervous pathways. As with nerve conduction studies, the conduction time (latency) may be measured. In addition, information may be gained from the amplitude and configuration of these responses.

General Information and Technical Information

See above under Nerve Conduction Studies (5.2).

Description of Evoked Responses

Describe the presence or absence of stimulus evoked responses and their configuration.

Specify

(a) Single or multiphasic response.
(b) Onset of response: defined as the start of the first reproducible potential. Since the onset of the response may be difficult to ascertain precisely, the criteria used should be stated.
(c) Latency to onset: defined as the time (ms) from the onset of stimulus to the onset of response. The central conduction time relates to cortical evoked potentials and is defined as the difference between the latencies of the cortical and the spinal evoked potentials. This parameter may be used to test the integrity of the corticospinal neuraxis.
(d) Latencies to peaks of positive and negative deflections in multiphasic responses (Fig. A.1.2.6). P denotes positive deflections, N denotes negative deflections. In multiphasic responses, the peaks are numbered consecutively (e.g. P1, N1, P2, N2 ...) or according to the latencies to peaks in milliseconds (e.g. P44, N52, P6[[6]] ...).
(e) The amplitude of the responses is measured in μV.

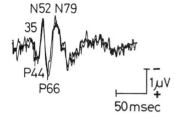

Fig. A.1.2.6 Multiphasic evoked response recorded from the cerebral cortex after stimulation of the dorsal aspect of the penis. The recording shows the conventional labelling of negative (N) and positive (P) deflections with the latency of each deflection from the point of stimulation in milliseconds.

5.5. Sensory Testing

Limited information, of a subjective nature, may be obtained during cystometry by recording such parameters as the first desire to micturate, urgency or pain. However, sensory function in the lower urinary tract, can be assessed by semi-objective tests by the measurement of urethral and/or vesical sensory thresholds to a standard applied stimulus such as a known electrical current.

General Information

Specify

(a) Patient's position (supine, sitting, standing, other)
(b) Bladder volume at time of testing
(c) Site of applied stimulus (intravesical, intraurethral)
(d) Number of times the stimulus was applied and the response recorded. Define the sensation recorded, e.g. the first sensation or the sensation of pulsing.
(e) Type of applied stimulus
    (i) electrical current: it is usual to use a constant current stimulator in urethral sensory measurement
       – state electrode characteristics and placement as in section on EMG.
       – state electrode contact area and distance between electrodes if applicable
       – state impedance characteristics of the system
       – state type of conductive medium used for electrode/epithelial contact. *Note: topical anaesthetic agents should not be used.*
       – stimulator make a specifications.
       – stimulation parameters (pulse width, frequency, pattern, duration, current density).
    (ii) other – e.g. mechanical, chemical.

Definition of Sensory Thresholds

The vesical/urethral sensory threshold is defined as the least current which consistently produces a sensation perceived by the subject during stimulation at the site under investigation. However, the absolute values will vary in relation to the site of the stimulus, the characteristics of the equipment and the stimulation parameters. Normal values should be established for each system.

6. A Classification of Urinary Tract Dysfunction

The lower urinary tract is composed of the *bladder* and *urethra*. They form a functional unit and their interaction cannot be ignored. Each has two functions, the bladder to store and void, the urethra to control and convey. When a reference is made to the hydrodynamic function or to the whole anatomical unit as a storage organ – the vesica urinaria – the correct term is the *bladder*. When the smooth muscle structure known as the m. detrusor urinae is being discussed then the correct term is *detrusor*. For simplicity the bladder/detrusor and the urethra will be considered separately so that a classification based on a combination of functional anomalies can be reached. Sensation cannot be precisely evaluated but must be assessed. This classification depends on the results of various objective urodynamic investigations. A complete urodynamic assessment is not necessary in all patients. However, studies of the filling and voiding phases are essential for each patient. As the bladder and urethra may behave differently during the storage and micturition phases of bladder function it is most useful to examine bladder and urethral activity separately in each phase.

Terms used should be objective, definable and ideally should be applicable to the whole range of abnormality. When authors disagree with the classification presented below, or use terms which have not been defined here, their meaning should be made clear.

Assuming the absence of inflammation, infection and neoplasm, *lower urinary tract dysfunction* may be caused by:

(a) Disturbance of the pertinent nervous or psychological control system.

(b) Disorders of muscle function.

(c) Structural abnormalities.

Urodynamic diagnoses based on this classification should correlate with the patient's symptoms and signs. For example the presence of an unstable contraction in an asymptomatic continent patient does not warrant a diagnosis of detrusor overactivity during storage.

6.1. The Storage Phase

6.1.1. Bladder Function During Storage

This may be described according to:
6.1.1.1 Detrusor activity
6.1.1.2 Bladder sensation

6.1.1.3 Bladder capacity
6.1.1.4 Compliance

6.1.1.1 *Detrusor activity* In this context detrusor activity is interpreted from the measurement of detrusor pressure (p_{det}).
Detrusor activity may be:

(a) Normal
(b) Overactive

(a) *Normal detrusor function* During the filling phase the bladder volume increases without a significant rise in pressure (accommodation). No involuntary contractions occur despite provocation.
A normal detrusor so defined may be described as "stable".

(b) *Overactive detrusor function* Overactive detrusor function is characterised by involuntary detrusor contractions during the filling phase, which may be spontaneous or provoked and which the patient cannot completely suppress. Involuntary detrusor contractions may be provoked by rapid filling, alterations of posture, coughing, walking, jumping and other triggering procedures. Various terms have been used to describe these features and they are defined as follows:

The *unstable detrusor* is one that is shown objectively to contract, spontaneously or on provocation, during the filling phase while the patient is attempting to inhibit micturition. Unstable detrusor contractions may be asymptomatic or may be interpreted as a normal desire to void. The presence of these contractions does not

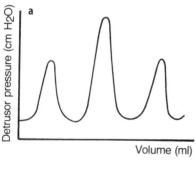

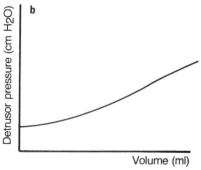

Fig. A.1.2.7 Diagrams of filling cystometry to illustrate:
a Typical phasic unstable detrusor contraction.
b The gradual increase of detrusor pressure with filling characteristic of reduced bladder compliance.

necessarily imply a neurological disorder. Unstable contractions are usually phasic in type (Fig. A.1.2.7a). A gradual increase in detrusor pressure without subsequent decrease is best regarded as a change of compliance (Fig. A.1.2.7b).

Detrusor hyperreflexia is defined as overactivity due to disturbance of the nervous control mechanisms. The term detrusor hyperreflexia should only be used when there is objective evidence of a relevant neurological disorder. The use of conceptual and undefined terms such as hypertonic, systolic, uninhibited, spastic and automatic should be avoided.

6.1.1.2. *Bladder Sensation* Bladder sensation during filling can be classified in qualitative terms (see 3.1) and by objective measurement (see 5.5). Sensation can be classified broadly as follows:

(a) Normal
(b) Increased (hypersensitive)
(c) Reduced (hyposensitive)
(d) Absent

6.1.1.3 *Bladder Capacity* (see 3.1.)

6.1.1.4 *Compliance* is defined as: $\Delta V/\Delta p$ (see 3.1.).
Compliance may change during the cystometric examination and is variably dependent upon a number of factors including:

(a) Rate of filling
(b) The part of the cystometrogram curve used for compliance calculation
(c) The volume interval over which compliance is calculated
(d) The geometry (shape) of the bladder
(e) The thickness of the bladder wall
(f) The mechanical properties of the bladder wall
(g) The contractile/relaxant properties of the detrusor

During normal bladder filling little or no pressure change occurs and this is termed "normal compliance". However at the present time there is insufficient data to define normal, high and low compliance.
When reporting compliance, specify:

(a) The rate of bladder filling
(b) The bladder volume at which compliance is calculated
(c) The volume increment over which compliance is calculated
(d) The part of the cystometrogram curve used for the calculation of compliance.

6.1.2. Urethral Function During Storage

The urethral closure mechanism during storage may be:

(a) Normal
(b) Incompetent

(a) The *normal urethral closure mechanism* maintains a positive urethral closure pressure during filling even in the presence of increased abdominal pressure. Immediately prior to micturition the normal closure pressure decreases to allow flow.

(b) *Incompetent urethral closure mechanism.* An incompetent urethral closure mechanism is defined as one which allows leakage of urine in the absence of a detrusor contraction. Leakage may occur whenever intravesical pressure exceeds intraurethral pressure (genuine stress incontinence) or when there is an involuntary fall in urethral pressure. Terms such as "the unstable urethra" await further data and precise definition.

6.1.3. Urinary Incontinence

Urinary incontinence is involuntary loss of urine which is objectively demonstrable and a social or hygienic problem. Loss of urine through channels other than the urethra is extraurethral incontinence.
　　Urinary incontinence denotes:

(a) A symptom
(b) A sign
(c) A condition

The symptom indicates the patient's statement of involuntary urine loss.
　　The sign is the objective demonstration of urine loss.
　　The condition is the urodynamic demonstration of urine loss.

Symptoms

Urge incontinence is the involuntary loss of urine associated with a strong desire to void (urgency).

Urgency may be associated with two types of dysfunction:

(a) Overactive detrusor function (*motor urgency*)
(b) Hypersensitivity (*sensory urgency*)

Stress incontinence: the symptom indicates the patient's statement of involuntary loss of urine during physical exertion.
　　"Unconscious" incontinence. Incontinence may occur in the absence of urge and without conscious recognition of the urinary loss.
　　Enuresis means any involuntary loss of urine. If it is used to denote incontinence during sleep, it should always be qualified with the adjective "nocturnal".
　　Post-micturition dribble and *Continuous leakage* denote other symptomatic forms of incontinence.

Signs

The sign stress-incontinence denotes the observation of loss of urine from the urethra synchronous with physical exertion (e.g. coughing). Incontinence may also be observed without physical exercise. Post-micturition dribble and continuous leakage denotes other signs of incontinence. Symptoms and signs alone may not disclose the cause of urinary incontinence. Accurate diagnosis often requires urodynamic investigation in addition to careful history and physical examination.

Conditions

Genuine stress incontinence is the involuntary loss of urine occurring when, in the absence of a detrusor contraction, the intravesical pressure exceeds the maximum urethral pressure.

Reflex incontinence is loss of urine due to detrusor hyperreflexia and/or involuntary urethral relaxation in the absence of the sensation usually associated with the desire to micturate. This condition is only seen in patients with neuropathic bladder/urethral disorders.

Overflow incontinence is any involuntary loss of urine associated with overdistension of the bladder.

6.2. The Voiding Phase

6.2.1. The Detrusor During Voiding

During micturition the detrusor may be:

- (a) acontractile
- (b) underactive
- (c) normal

(a) *The acontractile detrusor* is one that cannot be demonstrated to contract during urodynamic studies. *Detrusor areflexia* is defined as acontractility due to an abnormality of nervous control and denotes the complete absence of centrally coordinated contraction. In detrusor areflexia due to a lesion of the conus medullaris or sacral nerve outflow, the detrusor should be described as *decentralised* – not denervated, since the peripheral neurones remain. In such bladders pressure fluctuations of low amplitude, sometimes known as "autonomous" waves, may occasionally occur. The use of terms such as atonic, hypotonic, autonomic and flaccid should be avoided.

(b) *Detrusor underactivity.* This term should be reserved as an expression describing detrusor activity during micturition. Detrusor underactivity is defined as a detrusor contraction of inadequate magnitude and/or duration to effect bladder emptying with a normal time span. Patients may have underactivity during micturition and detrusor overactivity during filling.

(c) *Normal detrusor contractility*. Normal voiding is achieved by a voluntarily initiated detrusor contraction that is sustained and can usually be suppressed voluntarily. A normal detrusor contraction will effect complete bladder emptying in the absence of obstruction. For a given detrusor contraction, the magnitude of the recorded pressure rise will depend on the degree of outlet resistance.

6.2.2. Urethral Function During Micturition

During voiding urethral function may be:
- (a) normal
- (b) obstructive
  - – overactivity
  - – mechanical

(a) *The normal urethra* opens to allow the bladder to be emptied.

(b) *Obstruction due to urethral overactivity*: this occurs when the urethral closure mechanism contracts against a detrusor contraction or fails to open at attempted micturition. Synchronous detrusor and urethral contraction is *detrusor/urethral dyssynergia*. This diagnosis should be qualified by stating the location and type of the urethral muscles (striated or smooth) which are involved. Despite the confusion surrounding "sphincter" terminology the use of certain terms is so widespread that they are retained and defined here. The term *detrusor/external sphincter dyssynergia or detrusor-sphincter-dyssynergia* (DSD) describes a detrusor contraction concurrent with an involuntary contraction of the urethral and/or periurethral striated muscle. In the adult, detrusor sphincter dyssynergia is a feature of neurological voiding disorders. In the absence of neurological features the validity of this diagnosis should be questioned. The term *detrusor/bladder neck dyssynergia* is used to denote a detrusor contraction concurrent with an objectively demonstrated failure of bladder neck opening. No parallel term has been elaborated for possible detrusor/distal urethral (smooth muscle) dyssynergia.

Overactivity of the striated urethral sphincter may occur in the absence of detrusor contraction, and may prevent voiding. This is not detrusor/sphincter dyssynergia.

Overactivity of the urethral sphincter may occur during voiding in the absence of neurological disease and is termed *dysfunctional voiding*. The use of terms such as "non-neurogenic" or "occult neuropathic" should be avoided.

Mechanical obstruction: is most commonly anatomical e.g. urethral stricture.

Using the characteristics of detrusor and urethral function during storage and micturition an accurate definition of lower urinary tract behaviour in each patient becomes possible.

7. Units of Measurement

In the urodynamic literature pressure is measured in cmH_2O and *not* in millimetres of mercury. When Laplace's law is used to calculate tension in the bladder wall, it is often found that pressure is then measured in dyne cm^{-2}. This lack of uniformity in the systems used leads to confusion when other parameters, which are a function of pressure, are computed, for instance, "compliance", contraction force, velocity etc. From these few examples it is evident that standardisation is essential for meaningful communication. Many journals now require that the results be given in SI units. This section is designed to give guidance in the application of the SI system to urodynamics and defines the units involved. The principal units to be used are listed below (Table I).

Table I.

Quantity	Acceptable unit	Symbol
volume	millilitre	ml
time	second	s
flow rate	millilitres/second	$ml\ s^{-1}$
pressure	centimetres of water[a]	cmH_2O
length	metres or submultiples	m, cm, mm
velocity	metres/second or submultiples	$m\ s^{-1}$, $cm\ s^{-1}$
temperature	degrees Celsius	°C

[a]The SI Unit is the pascal (Pa), but it is only practical at present to calibrate our instruments in cmH_2O. One centimetre of water pressure is approximately equal to 100 pascals (1 cmH_2O = 98.07 Pa = 0.098 kPa).

Table II. List of symbols

Basic symbols		Urological qualifiers		Value	
Pressure	p	Bladder	ves	Maximum	max
Volume	V	Urethra	ura	Minimum	min
Flow rate	Q	Ureter	ure	Average	ave
Velocity	v	Detrusor	det	Isovolumetric	isv
Time	t	Abdomen	abd	Isotonic	ist
Temperature	T	External		Isobaric	isb
Length	l	stream	ext	Isometric	ism
Area	A				
Diameter	d				
Force	F				
Energy	E				
Power	P				
Compliance	P				
Work	W				
Energy per unit volume	e				

Examples:
$p_{det,max}$ = maximum detrusor pressure
e_{ext} = kinetic energy per unit volume in the external stream

Symbols

It is often helpful to use symbols in a communication. The system in Table II has been devised to standardise a code of symbols for use in urodynamics. The rationale of the system is to have a basic symbol representing the physical quantity with qualifying subscripts. The list of basic symbols largely conforms to international usage. The qualifying subscripts relate to the basic symbols to commonly used urodynamic parameters.

References

1. Abrams P, Blaivas JG, Stanton SL, Andersen JT, Fowler CJ, Gerstenberg T, Murray K (1986). Sixth report on the standardisation of terminology of lower urinary tract function. Procedures related to neurophysiological investigations: Electromyography, nerve conduction studies, reflex latencies, evoked potentials and sensory testing. World J Urol 4:2–5. Scand J Urol Nephrol 20:161–164
2. Bates P, Bradley WE, Glen E, Melchior H, Rowan D, Sterling A, Hald T (1976). First report on the standardisation of terminology of lower urinary tract function. Urinary incontinence. Procedures related to the evaluation of urine storage: Cystometry, urethral closure pressure profile, units of measurement. Br J Urol 48:39–42. Eur Urol 2:274–276. Scand J Urol Nephrol 11:193–196. Urol Int 32:81–87.
3. Bates P, Glen E, Griffiths D, Melchior H, Rowan D, Sterling A, Zinner NR, Hald T (1977). Second report on the standardisation of terminology of lower urinary tract function. Procedures related to the evaluation of micturition: Flow rate, pressure measurement, symbols. Acta Urol Jpn 27:1563–1566. Br J Urol 49:207–210. Eur Urol 3:168–170. Scand J Urol Nephrol 11:197–199.
4. Bates P, Bradley WE, Glen E, Griffiths D, Melchior H, Rowan D, Sterling A, Hald T (1980). Third report on the standardisation of terminology of lower urinary tract function. Procedures related to the evaluation of micturition: Pressure flow relationships, residual urine. Br J Urol 52: 348–350. Eur Urol 6:170–171. Acta Urol Jpn 27:1566–1568. Scand J Urol Nephrol 12:191–193.
5. Bates P, Bradley WE, Glen E, Melchior H, Rowan D, Sterling A, Sundin T, Thomas D, Torrens M, Turner-Warwick R, Zinner NR, Hald T (1981). Fourth report on the standardisation of terminology of lower urinary tract function. Terminology related to neuromuscular dysfunction of lower urinary tract. Br J Urol 52:333–335. Urology 17:618–620. Scand J Urol Nephrol 15:169–171. Acta Urol Jpn 27:1568–1571.
6. Jasper HH (1958). Report to the committee on the methods of clinical examination in electroencephalography. Electroencephalography in Clinical Neurophysiology 10:370–75.

Appendix 1, Part 3

Lower Urinary Tract Rehabilitation Techniques: Seventh Report on the Standardisation of Terminology of Lower Urinary Tract Function

Neurourol Urodyn 11:593–603 (1992) Published 1992 by Wiley-Liss, Inc.

J. T. Andersen (Chairman), J. G. Blaivas, L. Cardozo, and J. Thüroff

International Continence Society Committee on Standardisation of Terminology

1. Introduction

Lower urinary tract rehabilitation comprises non-surgical, non-pharmacological treatment for lower urinary tract dysfunction. The specific techniques defined in this report are listed in the contents above.

Most of the conditions for which rehabilitation techniques are employed have both a subjective and an objective component. In many instances, treatment is only capable of relieving symptoms, not curing the underlying disease. Therefore, symptoms should be quantified before and after treatment, and the means by which the physiology is altered should be clearly stated.

The applications of the individual types of treatment cited here are taken from the scientific literature and from current clinical practice. It is not within the scope of this committee to endorse specific recommendations for treatment, nor to restrict the use of these treatments to the examples given.

The standards set in this report are recommended to ensure the reproducibility of methods of treatment and to facilitate the comparison of results obtained by different investigators and therapists. It is suggested that acknowledgement of these standards, in written publications, should be indicated by a footnote to the section "Methods and Materials" or its equivalent, to read as follows:

"Methods, definitions and units conform to the standards recommended by the International Continence Society, except where specifically noted."

2. Pelvic Floor Training

2.1. Definition

Pelvic floor training is defined as repetitive selective voluntary contraction and relaxation of specific pelvic floor muscles. This necessitates muscle awareness in order to be sure that the correct muscles are being utilised, and to avoid unwanted contractions of adjacent muscle groups.

2.2. Techniques

2.2.1. Standard of Diagnosis and Implementation

The professional status of the individual who establishes the diagnosis must be stated as well as the diagnostic techniques employed. Also the professional status of the person who institutes, supervises and assesses treatment must be specified.

2.2.2. Muscle Awareness

The technique used for obtaining selective pelvic floor contractions and relaxations should be stated. Registration of electromyographic (EMG) activity in the muscles of the pelvic floor, urethral or anal sphincter, or the anterior abdominal wall, may be necessary to obtain this muscle awareness. Alternatively or additionally, registration of abdominal, vaginal, urethral or anal pressure may be used for the same purpose.

2.2.3. Muscle Training

It should be specified as to whether treatment is given on an inpatient or outpatient basis. Specific details of training must be stated:

1. Patient position
2. Duration of each contraction
3. Interval between contractions
4. Number of contractions per exercise
5. Number of exercises per day
6. Length of treatment programme (weeks, months)

2.2.4. Adjunctive Equipment

Adjunctive equipment may be employed to enhance muscle awareness or muscle training. The following should be specified:

1. Type of equipment
2. Mechanism of action
3. Duration of use
4. Therapeutic goals

Examples of equipment in current use are:

Perineometers and other pressure-recording devices
EMG equipment
Ultrasound equipment
Faradic stimulators
Interferential current equipment
Vaginal cones

2.2.5. Compliance

Patient compliance has three major components:

1. Appropriate comprehension of the instructions and the technique
2. Ability to perform the exercises
3. Completion of the training program

Objective documentation of both the patient's ability to perform the exercises and the result of the training programme is mandatory. The parameters employed for objective documentation during training should be the same as those used for teaching muscle awareness.

2.3. Applications

Pelvic floor training can be used as treatment on its own, or as an adjunctive therapy, or for prophylaxis. The indications, mode of action and the therapeutic goals must be specified. Examples of indications for therapeutic pelvic floor training are incontinence and descent of the pelvic viscera (prolapse). Examples of indications for prophylactic pelvic floor training are postpartum and following pelvic surgery.

3. Biofeedback

3.1. Definition

Biofeedback is a technique by which information about a normally unconscious physiological process is presented to the patient and the therapist as a visual, auditory or tactile signal. The signal is derived from a measurable physiological parameter, which is subsequently used in an educational process to accomplish a specific therapeutic result. The signal is displayed in a quantitative way and the patient is taught how to alter it and thus control the basic physiological process.

3.2. Techniques

The physiological parameter (e.g. pressure, flow, EMG) which is being monitored, the method of measurement and the mode by which it is displayed as a signal (e.g. light, sound, electric stimulus) should all be specified. Further, the specific instructions to the patient by which he/she is to alter the signal must be stated. The following details of biofeedback treatment must also be stated:

1. Patient position
2. Duration of each session
3. Interval between sessions
4. Number of sessions per day/week/month and intervals between
5. Length of treatment programme (weeks, months)

3.3. Applications

The indications, the intended mode of action and the therapeutic goals must be specified. The aim of biofeedback is to improve a specific lower urinary tract dysfunction by increasing patient awareness, and by alteration of a measurable physiological parameter. Biofeedback can be applied in functional voiding disorders where the underlying pathophysiology can be monitored and subsequently altered by the patient. The following are examples of indications and techniques for biofeedback treatment:

Motor urgency and urge incontinence: display of detrusor pressure and control of detrusor contractions

Dysfunctional voiding: display of sphincter EMG and relaxation of the external sphincter

Pelvic floor relaxation: display of pelvic floor EMG and pelvic floor training

4. Behavioral Modification

4.1. Definition

Behavioral modification comprises analysis and alteration of the relationship between the patient's symptoms and his/her environment for the treatment of maladaptive voiding patterns. This may be achieved by modification of the behaviour and/or environment of the patient.

4.2. Techniques

When behavioral modification is considered, a thorough analysis of possible interactions between the patient's symptoms, his general condition and his environment is essential. The following should be specified:

1. Micturition complaints; assessment and quantification:
   Symptom analysis
   Visual analogue score
   Fluid intake chart
   Frequency/volume chart (voiding diary)
   Pad-weighing test
   Urodynamic studies (when applicable)
2. General patient assessment:
   General performance status (e.g. Kurtzke disability scale[1])
   Mobility (e.g. chairbound)
   Concurrent medical disorders (e.g. constipation, congestive heart failure, diabetes mellitus, chronic bronchitis, hemiplegia)
   Current medication (e.g. diuretics)
   Psychological state (e.g. psychonalysis)
   Psychiatric disorders
   Mental state (e.g. dementia, confusion)
3. Environmental assessment:
   Toilet facilities (access)
   Living conditions
   Working conditions
   Social relations
   Availability of suitable incontinence aids
   Access to health care

For behavioral modification, various therapeutic concepts and techniques may be employed. The following should be specified:

1. Conditioning techniques:
   Timed voiding (e.g. hyposensitive bladder)
   Double/triple voiding (e.g. residual urine due to bladder diverticulum)
   Increase of intervoiding intervals/bladder drill (e.g. sensory urgency)
   Biofeedback (see above)
   Enuresis alarm
2. Fluid intake regulation (e.g. restriction)
3. Measures to improve patient mobility (e.g. physiotherapy, wheelchair)
4. Change of medication (e.g. diuretics, anticholinergics)
5. Treatment of concurrent medical/psychiatric disorders
6. Psychoanalysis/hypnotherapy (e.g. idiopathic detrusor instability)
7. Environmental changes (e.g. provision of incontinence pads, condom urinals, commode, furniture protection etc.)

Treatment is often empirical, and may require a combination of the above-mentioned concepts and techniques. The results of treatment should be objectively documented using the same techniques as used for the initial assessment of micturition complaints.

4.3. Applications

Behavioral modification may be used for the treatment of maladaptive voiding patterns in patients when:

The etiology and pathophysiology of their symptoms cannot be identified (e.g. sensory urgency)

The symptoms are caused by a psychological problem

The symptoms have failed to respond to conventional therapy

They are unfit for definitive treatment of their condition

Behavioral modification may be employed alone or as an adjunct to any other form of treatment for lower urinary tract dysfunction.

5. Electrical Stimulation

5.1. Definition

Electrical stimulation is the application of electrical current to stimulate the pelvic viscera or their nerve supply. The aim of electrical stimulation may be to directly induce a therapeutic response or to modulate lower urinary tract, bowel or sexual dysfunction.

5.2. Techniques

The following should be specified:

1. Access:
   Surface electrodes (e.g. anal plug, vaginal electrode)

Percutaneous electrodes (e.g. needle electrodes, wire electrodes)
Implants

2. Approach
Temporary stimulation
Permanent stimulation

3. Stimulation site
Effector organ
Peripheral nerves
Spinal nerves (intradural or extradural)
Spinal cord

4. Stimulation parameters
Frequency
Voltage
Current
Pulse width
Pulse shape (e.g. rectangular, biphasic, capacitatively coupled)
With monopolar stimulation, state whether the active electrode is anodic or cathodic
Duration of pulse trains
Shape of pulse trains (e.g. surging trains)

5. Mode of stimulation
Continuous
Phasic (regular automatic on/off)
Intermittent (variable duration and time intervals)
Single sessions: number and duration of, and intervals between, periods of stimulation
Multiple sessions: number and duration of, and intervals between sessions

6. Design of electronic equipment, electrodes and related electrical stimulation characteristics:
Electrodes (monopolar or bipolar)
Surface area of electrodes
Maximum charge density per pulse at active electrode surface
Impedance of the implanted system
Power source (implants):
  active, self-powered
  passive, inductive current

7. For transurethral intravesical stimulation
Filling medium
Filling volume
Number of intravesical electrodes

5.3. Units of Measurement and Symbols

Parameters related to electrical stimulation, units of measurement and the corresponding symbols are listed in Table I.

Table I. Parameters for electrical stimulation

Quantity	Unit	Symbol	Definition
Electric current	ampere	A	1 A of electric current is the transfer of 1 C of electric charge per second
Direct (DC), Galvanic			Steady unidirectional electric current Unidirectional electric current derived from a chemical battery
Alternating (AC)			Electric current that physically changes direction of flow in a sinusoidal manner
Faradic			Intermittent oscillatory current similar to alternating current (AC), e.g. as produced by an induction coil
Voltage (potential difference)	volt	V	1 V of potential difference between 2 points requires 1 J of energy to transfer 1 C of charge from one point to the other
Resistance	ohm	Ω	1 Ω of resistance between 2 points allows 1 V of potential difference to cause a flow of 1 A of direct current (DC) between them
Impedance (Z)	ohm	Ω	Analogue of resistance for alternating current (AC); vector sum of ohmic resistance and reactance (inductive and/or capacitative resistance)
Charge	coulomb	C	1 C of electric charge is transferred through a conductor in 1 s by 1 A of electric current
Capacity	farad	F	A condensor (capacitor) has 1 F of electric capacity (capacitance) if transfer of 1 C of electric charge causes 1 V of potential difference between its elements
Frequency	hertz	$Hs(s^{-1})$	Number of cycles (phases) of a periodically repeating oscillation per second
Pulse width	time	ms	Duration of 1 pulse (phase) of a phasic electric current or voltage
Electrode surface area	area	mm^2	Active area of electrode surface
Charge density per pulse	coulomb/ area/time	$\mu C\ mm^{-2}ms^{-1}$	Electric charge delivered to a given electrode surface area in a given time (one pulse width)

5.4. Applications

The aims of treatment should be clearly stated. These may include control of voiding, continence, defecation, erection, ejaculation or relief of pain. Specify whether electrical stimulation aims at:

A functional result completely dependent on the continuous use of electrical current

Modulation, reflex facilitation, reflex inhibition, re-education or conditioning with a sustained functional result even after withdrawal of stimulation

Electrical stimulation is applicable in neurogenic or non-neurogenic lower urinary tract, bowel or sexual dysfunction. Techniques and equipment vary widely with the type of dysfunction and the goal of electrical stimulation. If electrical stimulation is employed for control of a neuropathic dysfunction, and the chosen site of stimulation is the reflex arc (peripheral nerves, spinal nerves or spinal cord), this reflex are must be intact. Consequently electrical stimulation is not applicable for complete lower motor neuron lesions except when direct stimulation of the effector organ is chosen.

When ablative surgery is performed (e.g. dorsal rhizotomy, ganglionectomy, sphincterotomy or levatorotomy) in conjunction with an implant to achieve the desired functional effect, the following should be specified.

1. Techniques used to reduce pain or mass reflexes during stimulation
   Number and spinal level of interrupted afferents
   Site of interruption of afferents
   Dorsal rhizotomy (intradural or extradural)
   Ganglionectomy
2. Techniques to reduce stimulated sphincter dyssynergia:
   Pudendal block (unilateral or bilateral)
   Pudendal neurectomy (unilateral or bilateral)
   Levatorotomy (unilateral or bilateral)
   Electrically induced sphincter fatigue
   External sphincterotomy

If electrical stimulation is combined with ablative surgery, other functions (e.g. erection or continence) may be impaired.

5.4.1. Voiding

When the aim of electrical stimulation is to achieve voiding, state whether this is obtained by:

Stimulation of the afferent fibres to induce bladder sensation and thus facilitate voiding (transurethral intravesical stimulation)
Stimulation of efferent fibres or detrusor muscle to induce a bladder contraction (electromicturition)

5.4.2. Continence

Electrical stimulation may aim to inhibit overactive detrusor function or to improve urethral closure. State whether overactive detrusor function is abolished/reduced by reflex inhibition (pudendal to pelvic nerve) or by blockade of nerve conduction. When electrical stimulation is applied to improve urethral closure, state whether this is by:

A direct effect on the urethra during stimulation
Re-education and conditioning to restore pelvic floor tone.

5.4.3. Pelvic Pain

If electrical stimulation is applied to control pelvic pain, the nature and etiology of the pain should be stated. When pelvic pain is caused by pelvic floor spasticity, electrical stimulation may be effective by relaxing the pelvic floor muscles.

5.4.4. Erection and Ejaculation

If electrical stimulation is applied for the treatment of erectile dysfunction or ejaculatory failure, the etiology should be stated. Electrically induced erection requires an intact arterial supply and cavernous tissue, and a competent venous closure mechanism of the corpora cavernosa. Electroejaculation requires an intact reproductive system.

5.4.5. Defecation

Defecation may be obtained by electrical stimulation, either intentionally or as a side-effect of electromicturition.

At present, the mechanism of action of electrically induced control of pelvic pain, erection, ejaculation and defecation are not fully understood. The clinical applications of these techniques have not yet been fully established.

6. Voiding Manoeuvres

Voiding manoeuvres are employed to obtain/facilitate bladder emptying. For lower urinary tract rehabilitation, voiding manoeuvres may be used alone or in combination with other techniques such as biofeedback or behavioral modification. The aim is to achieve complete bladder emptying at low intravesical pressures. The techniques employed may be invasive (e.g. catheters) or non-invasive (e.g. triggering reflex detrusor contractions, increasing intra-abdominal pressure).

When reporting on voiding manoeuvres, the professional status of the individual(s) who establishes the diagnosis must be stated as well as the diagnostic techniques employed. Also the professional status of the person(s) who institutes, supervises and assesses treatment should be specified.

6.1. Catheterisation

6.1.1. Definition

Catheterisation is a technique for bladder emptying employing a catheter to drain the bladder or a urinary reservoir. Catheter use may be intermittent or indwelling (temporary or permanent).

6.1.2. Intermittent (in/out) Catheterisation

Intermittent (in/out) catheterisation is defined as drainage or aspiration of the bladder or a urinary reservoir with subsequent removal of the catheter. The following types of intermittent catheterisation are defined:

1. Intermittent self-catheterisation: performed by the patient himself/herself
2. Intermittent catheterisation by an attendant (e.g. doctor, nurse or relative)
3. Clean intermittent catheterisation: use of a clean technique. This implies ordinary washing techniques and use of disposable or cleansed reusable catheters.
4. Aseptic intermittent catheterisation: use of a sterile technique. This implies genital disinfection and the use of sterile catheters and instruments/gloves.

6.1.2.1 Techniques. The following should be specified:

1. Preparation used for genital disinfection
2. Preparation and volume of lubricant
3. Catheter specifications: type, size, material and surface coating
4. Number of catheterisations per day/week
5. Length of treatment (e.g. weeks, months, permanent)

6.1.2.2 Applications. Specify the indications and the therapeutic goals. Typical examples for the use of intermittent catheterisation are: neurogenic bladder with impaired bladder emptying, postoperative urinary retention and transstomal catheterisation of continent reservoirs.

6.1.3 Indwelling Catheter

An indwelling catheter remains in the bladder, urinary reservoir or urinary conduit for a period of time longer than one emptying. The following routes of access are employed:

Transurethral
Suprapubic

6.1.3.1 Techniques. The following should be specified:

1. Catheter specifications: type, size, material
2. Preparation and volume of lubricant
3. Catheter fixation: e.g. balloon (state filling volume), skin suture
4. Mode of drainage: continuous/intermittent. For intermittent drainage specify clamping periods
5. Intervals between catheter change
6. Duration of catheterisation (days, weeks, years)

6.1.3.2 Applications. The indications and the therapeutic goals should be specified. Examples of the use of temporary indwelling catheters are:

Suprapubic catheter: after major pelvic surgery
Transurethral catheter: in order to monitor urine output in a severely ill patient

Examples of the use of permanent indwelling catheters are:

Suprapubic: candidates for urinary diversion unfit for surgery
Transurethral: severe bladder symptoms from untreatable bladder cancer

6.2. Bladder Reflex Triggering

6.2.1. Definition

Bladder reflex triggering comprises various manoeuvres performed by the patient or the therapist in order to elicit reflex detrusor contractions by exteroceptive stimuli. The most commonly used maneuvers are: suprapubic tapping, thigh scratching and anal/rectal manipulation.

6.2.2. Techniques

For each manoeuvre the following should be specified:

1. Details of manoeuvre.
2. Frequency, intervals and duration (weeks, months, years) of practice

6.2.3. Applications

When using bladder reflex triggering manoeuvres, the etiology of the dysfunction and the goals of treatment should be stated. Bladder reflex triggering manoeuvres are indicated only in patient with an intact sacral reflex are (suprasacral spinal cord lesions).

6.3. Bladder Expression

6.3.1. Definition

Bladder expression comprises various manoeuvres aimed at increasing intravesical pressure in order to facilitate bladder emptying. The most commonly used manoeuvres are abdominal straining, Valsalva's manoeuvre and Credé's manoeuvre.

6.3.2. Techniques

For each manoeuvre, the following should be specified:

Details of the manoeuvre
Frequency, intervals and duration of practice (weeks, months, years)

6.3.3. Applications

When using bladder expression, the etiology of the underlying disorder and the goals of treatment should be stated. Bladder expression may be used in patients where the urethral closure mechanism can be easily overcome.

Reference

1. Kurtzke JF (1983). Rating neurological impairment in multiple sclerosis: an expanded disability status scale (EDSS). Neurology 33:1444–1452.

Appendix 1, Part 4

The Standardisation of Terminology of Female Pelvic Organ Prolapse and Pelvic Floor Dysfunction

Am J Obstet Gynec (1996) 175:10–17

Richard C. Bump, Anders Mattiasson, Kari Bø, Linda P. Brubaker, John O. L. DeLancey, Peter Klarskov, Bob L. Shull and Anthony R. B. Smith

Produced by the International Continence Society Committee on Standardisation of Terminology (Anders Mattiasson, chairman), Subcommittee on Pelvic Organ Prolapse and Pelvic floor Dysfunction (Richard Bump, chairman) in collaboration with the American Urogynecologic Society and the Society of Gynecologic Surgeons.

Condensation

A system of standard terminology for the description and evaluation of pelvic organ prolapse and pelvic floor dysfunction, adopted by several professional societies, is presented.

1. Introduction

The International Continence Society (ICS) has been at the forefront in the standardisation of terminology of lower urinary tract function since the establishment of the Committee on Standardisation of Terminology in 1973. This committee's efforts over the past two decades have resulted in the world-wide acceptance of terminology standards that allow clinicians and researchers interested in the lower urinary tract to communicate efficiently and precisely. While female pelvic organ prolapse and pelvic floor dysfunction are intimately related to lower urinary tract function, such accurate communication using standard terminology has not been possible for these conditions since there has been no universally accepted system for describing the anatomic position of the pelvic organs. Many reports use terms for the description of pelvic organ prolapse which are undefined; none of the many aspiring grading systems has been adequately validated with respect either to reproducibility or to the clinical significance of different grades. The absence of standard, validated definitions prevents comparisons of published series from different institutions and longitudinal evaluation of an individual patient.

In 1993, an international, multidisciplinary committee composed of members of the ICS, the American Urogynecologic Society (AUGS), and Society of Gynecologic Surgeons (SGS) drafted this standardisation document following the committee's initial meeting at the ICS meeting in Rome. In late 1994 and early 1995, the final draft was circulated to members of all three societies for a one-year review and trial. During that year several minor revisions were made and reproducibility studies in six centres in the United States and Europe were completed, documenting the inter- and intrarater reliability and clinical utility of the system in 240 women.[1-5] The standardisation document was formally adopted by the ICS in October 1995, by the AUGS in January 1996, and by the SGS in March 1996. The goal of this report is to introduce the system to clinicians and researchers.

Acknowledgement of these standards in written publications and scientific presentations should be indicated in the Methods Section with the following statement: "Methods, definitions and descriptions conform to the standards recommended by the International Continence Society except where specifically noted."

2. Description of Pelvic Organ Prolapse

The clinical description of pelvic floor anatomy is determined during the physical examination of the external genitalia and vaginal canal. The details of the examination technique are not dictated by this document but authors should precisely describe their technique. Segments of the lower reproductive tract will replace such terms as "cystocele, rectocele, enterocele, or urethrovesical junction" because these terms may imply an unrealistic certainty as to the structures on the other side of the vaginal bulge particularly in women who have had previous prolapse surgery.

2.1. Conditions of the Examination

It is critical that the examiner sees and describes the maximum protrusion noted by the individual during her daily activities. Criteria for the end point of the examination and the full development of the prolapse should be specified in any report. Suggested criteria for demonstration of maximum prolapse should include one or all of the following: (a) Any protrusion of the vaginal wall has become tight during straining by the patient. (b) Traction on the prolapse causes no further descent. (c) The subject confirms that the size of the prolapse and extent of the protrusion seen by the examiner is as extensive as the most severe protrusion which she has experienced. The means of this confirmation should be specified. For example, the subject may use a small hand-held mirror to visualise the protrusion. (d) A standing, straining examination confirms that the full extent of the prolapse was observed in other positions used.

Other variables of technique that should be specified during the quantitative description and ordinal staging of pelvic organ prolapse include the following: (a) the position of the subject; (b) the type of examination table or chair used; (c) the type of vaginal specula, retractors, or tractors used; (d) diagrams of any customised devices used; (e) the type (e.g., Valsalva manoeuvre, cough) and, if measured, intensity (e.g. vesical or rectal pressure) of straining used to develop the prolapse maximally; (f) fullness of bladder and, if the bladder was empty, whether this was by spontaneous voiding or by catheterisation; (g) content of rectum; (f) the method by which any quantitative measurements were made.

2.2. Quantitative Description of Pelvic Organ Position

This descriptive system is a tandem profile in that it contains a series of component measurements grouped together in combination, but listed separately in tandem, without being fused into a distinctive new expression or "grade". It allows for the precise description of an individual woman's pelvic support without assigning a "severity value". Second, it allows accurate site-specific observations of the stability or progression of prolapse over time by the same or different observers. Finally, it allows similar judgements as to the outcome of surgical repair of prolapse. For example, noting that a surgical procedure moved the leading edge of a prolapse from 0.5 cm beyond the hymeneal ring to 0.5 cm above the hymeneal ring denotes more meagre improvement than stating that the prolapse was reduced from Grade 3 to Grade 1 as would be the case using some current grading systems.

2.2.1. Definition of Anatomic Landmarks

Prolapse should be evaluated by a standard system relative to clearly defined anatomic points of reference. These are of two types, a fixed reference point and defined points which are located with respect to this reference.

(a) *Fixed Point of Reference.* Prolapse should be evaluated relative to a fixed anatomic landmark which can be consistently and precisely identified. The hymen will be the fixed point of reference used throughout this system of quantitative prolapse description. Visually, the hymen provides a precisely identifiable landmark for reference. Although it is recognised that the plane of the hymen is somewhat variable depending upon the degree of levator ani dysfunction, it remains the best landmark available. "Hymen" is preferable to the ill-defined and imprecise term "introitus". The anatomic position of the six defined points for measurement should be centimetres above or proximal to the hymen (negative number) or centimetres below or distal to the hymen (positive number) with the plane of the hymen being defined as zero (0). For example, a cervix that protruded 3 cm distal to the hymen would be + 3 cm.

(b) *Defined Points.* This site-specific system has been adapted from several classifications developed and modified by Baden and Walker.[6] Six points (two on the anterior vaginal wall, two in the superior vagina, and two on the posterior vaginal wall) are located with reference to the plane of the hymen.

Anterior Vaginal Wall. Because the only structure directly visible to the examiner is the surface of the vagina, anterior prolapse should be discussed in terms of a segment of the vaginal wall rather than the organs which lie behind it. Thus, the term "anterior vaginal wall prolapse" is preferable to "cystocele" or "anterior enterocele" unless the organs involved are identified by ancillary test two anterior sites are as follows:

Point Aa. A point located in the midline of the anterior vaginal wall three (3) cm proximal to the external urethral meatus. This corresponds to the approximate location of the "urethro-vesical crease", a visible landmark of variable prominence that is obliterated in many patients. By definition, the range of position of Point Aa relative to the hymen is –3 to + 3 cm.

Point Ba. A point that represents the most distal (i.e., most dependent) position of any part of the upper anterior vaginal wall from the vaginal cuff or anterior vaginal fornix to Point Aa. By definition, Point Ba is at –8 cm in the absence of prolapse and would have a positive value equal to the position of the cuff in women with total post-hysterectomy vaginal eversion.

Superior Vagina. These points represent the most proximal locations of the normally positioned lower reproductive tract. The two superior sites are as follows:

Point C. A point that represents either the most distal (i.e., most dependent) edge of the cervix or the leading edge of the vaginal cuff (hysterectomy scar) after total hysterectomy.

Point D. A point that represents the location of the posterior fornix (or pouch of Douglas) in a woman who still has a cervix. It represents the level of uterosacral ligament attachment to the proximal posterior cervix. It is included as a point of measurement to differentiate suspensory failure of the uterosacral-cardinal ligament complex from cervical elongation. When the location of Point C is significantly more positive than the location of Point D, this is indicative of cervical elongation which may be symmetrical or eccentric. Point D is omitted in the absence of the cervix.

Posterior Vaginal Wall. Analogous to anterior prolapse, posterior prolapse should be discussed in terms of segments of the vaginal wall rather than the organs which lie behind it. Thus, the term "posterior vaginal wall prolapse" is preferable to "rectocele" or "enterocele" unless the organs involved are identified by ancillary tests. If small bowel appears to be present in the rectovaginal space, the examiner should comment on this fact and should clearly describe the basis for this clinical impression (e.g., by observation of peristaltic activity in the distended posterior vagina, by palpation of loops of small bowel between an examining finger in the rectum and one in the vagina, etc.). In such cases, a "pulsion" addendum to the point Bp position may be noted (e.g., Bp = +5 [pulsion]; see Sections 3.1(a) and 3.1(b) for further discussion). The two posterior sites are as follows:

Point Bp. A point that represents the most distal (i.e., most dependent) position of any part of the upper posterior vaginal wall from the vaginal cuff or posterior vaginal fornix to Point Ap. By definition, Point Bp is at –3 cm in the absence of prolapse and would have a positive value equal to the position of the cuff in a women with total post-hysterectomy vaginal eversion.

Point Ap. A point located in the midline of the posterior vaginal wall three (3) cm proximal to the hymen. By definition, the range of position of Point Ap relative to the hymen is –3 to +3 cm.

(c) *Other Landmarks and Measurements.* The genital hiatus (GH) is measured from the middle of the external urethral meatus to the posterior midline hymen. If the location of the hymen is distorted by a loose band of skin without underlying muscle or connective tissue, the firm palpable tissue of the perineal body should be substituted as the posterior margin for this measurement. The perineal body (PB) is measured from the posterior margin of the genital hiatus to the mid-anal opening. Measurements of the genital hiatus and perineal body are expressed in centimetres. The total vaginal length (TVL) is the greatest depth of the vagina in cm when Point C or D is reduced to its full normal position. *Note:* Eccentric elongation of a prolapsed anterior or posterior vaginal wall should not be included in the measurement of total vaginal length. The points and measurements are represented in Fig. A.1.4.1.

2.2.2. Making and Recording Measurements

The position of Points Aa, Ba, Ap, Bp, C, and (if applicable) D with reference to the hymen should be measured and recorded. Positions are expressed as centi-

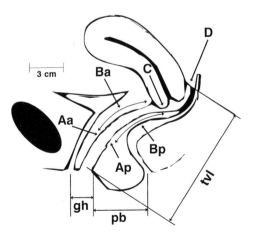

Fig. A.1.4.1 The six sites (*Aa, Ba, C, D, Bp* and *Bp*), the genital hiatus (*gh*), perineal body (*pb*) and total vaginal length (*tvl*) used of pelvic organ support quantitation.

metres above or proximal to the hymen (negative number) or centimetres below or distal to the hymen (positive number) with the plane of the hymen being defined as zero (0). While an examiner may be able to make measurements to the nearest half (0.5) cm, it is doubtful that further precision is possible. All reports should clearly specify how measurements were derived. Measurements may be recorded as a simple line of numbers (e.g., –3, –3, –7, –9, –3, –3, 9, 2, 2 for Points Aa, Ba, C, D, Bp, Ap, total vaginal length, genital hiatus, and perineal body respectively). Note that the last three numbers have no + or – sign attached to them because they denote lengths and not positions relative to the hymen. Alternatively, a three by three "tic-tac-toe" grid can be used to organise concisely the measurements as noted in Fig. A.1.4.2 and/or a line diagram of the configuration can be drawn as noted in Figs A.1.4.3 and A.1.4.4. Figure A.1.4.3 is a grid and line diagram contrasting measurements indicating normal support to those of post hysterectomy vaginal eversion. Figure A.1.4.4 is a grid and line diagram representing predominant anterior and posterior vaginal wall prolapse with partial vault descent.

2.3. Ordinal Stages of Pelvic Organ Prolapse

The tandem profile for quantifying prolapse provides a precise description of anatomy for individual patients. However, because of the many possible combinations, such profiles cannot be directly ranked; the many variations are too numerous to permit useful analysis and comparisons when populations are studied. Consequently they are analogous to other tandem profiles such as the TNM Index for various cancers. For the TNM description of individual patient's cancers to be useful in population studies evaluating prognosis or response to therapy, they are clustered into an ordinal set of stages. Ordinal stages represent adjacent categories that can be ranked in an ascending sequence of magnitude, but the categories are assigned arbitrarily and the intervals between them cannot be actually measured. While the committee is aware of the arbitrary nature of an ordinal staging system and the possible biases that it introduces, we conclude such a system is necessary if populations are to be described and compared, if

anterior wall **Aa**	anterior wall **Ba**	cervix or cuff **C**
genital hiatus **gh**	perineal body **pb**	total vaginal length **tvl**
posterior wall **Ap**	posterior wall **Bp**	posterior fornix **D**

Fig. A.1.4.2 A three-by-three grid for recording the quantitative description of pelvic organ support.

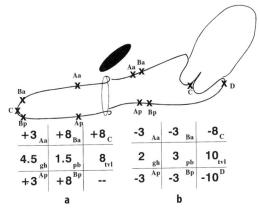

+3 Aa	+8 Ba	+8 C
4.5 gh	1.5 pb	8 tvl
+3 Ap	+8 Bp	--

a

-3 Aa	-3 Ba	-8 C
2 gh	3 pb	10 tvl
-3 Ap	-3 Bp	-10 D

b

Fig. A.1.4.3 a Example of a grid and line diagram of complete eversion of the vagina. The most distal point of the anterior wall (Point Ba), the vaginal cuff scar (Point C) and the most distal point of the posterior wall (Bp) are all at the same position (+8) and Points Aa and Ap are maximally distal (both at +3). The fact that the total vagina length equals the maximum protrusion makes this a Stage IV prolapse. **b** Example of normal support. Points Aa and Ba and Points Ap and Bp are all –3 since there is no anterior or posterior wall descent. The lowest point of the cervix is 8 cm above the hymen (–8) and the posterior fornix is 2 cm above this (–10). The vaginal length is 10 cm and the genital hiatus and perineal body measure 2 and 3 cm respectively. This represents Stage 0 support.

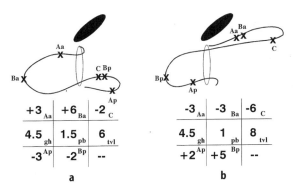

+3 Aa	+6 Ba	-2 C
4.5 gh	1.5 pb	6 tvl
-3 Ap	-2 Bp	--

a

-3 Aa	-3 Ba	-6 C
4.5 gh	1 pb	8 tvl
+2 Ap	+5 Bp	--

b

Fig. A.1.4.4 a Example of a grid and line diagram of a predominant anterior support defect. The leading point of the prolapse is the upper anterior vaginal wall, Point Ba (+6). Note that there is significant elongation of the bulging anterior wall. Point Aa is maximally distal (+3) and the vaginal cuff scar is 2 cm above the hymen (C = –2). The cuff scar has undergone 4 cm of descent since it would be at –6 (the total vaginal length) if it were perfectly supported. In this example, the total vaginal length is not the maximum depth of the vagina with the elongated anterior vaginal wall maximally reduced, but rather the depth of the vagina at the cuff with Point C reduced to its normal full extent as specified in Section 2.2.1(c). This represents Stage III-Ba prolapse. **b** Example of a predominant posterior support defect. The leading point of the prolapse is the upper posterior vaginal wall, Point Bp (+5). Point Ap is 2 cm distal to the hymen (+2) and the vaginal cuff scar is 6 cm above the hymen (–6). The cuff has undergone only 2 cm of descent since it would be at –8 (the total vaginal length) if it were perfectly supported. This represents Stage III-Bp prolapse.

symptoms putatively related to prolapse are to be evaluated, and if the results of various treatment options are to be assessed and compared.

Stages are assigned according to the most severe portion of the prolapse when the full extent of the protrusion has been demonstrated. In order for a stage to be assigned to an individual subject, it is essential that her quantitative description be completed first. The 2 cm buffer related to the total vaginal length in Stages 0 and IV is an effort to compensate for vaginal distensibility and the inherent imprecision of the measurement of total vaginal length. The 2 cm buffer around the hymen in Stage II is an effort to avoid confining a stage to a single plane and to acknowledge practical limits of precision in this assessment. Stages can be sub-grouped according to which portion of the lower reproductive tract is the *most distal* part of the prolapse using the following letter qualifiers: a = anterior vaginal wall, p = posterior vaginal wall, C = vaginal cuff, Cx = cervix, and Aa, Ap, Ba, Bp, and D for the points of measurement already defined. The five stages of pelvic organ support (0 through IV) are as follows:

Stage 0. No prolapse is demonstrated. Points Aa, Ap, Ba, and Bp are all at –3 cm and either Point C or D is between – TVL cm and – (TVL –2) cm (i.e., the quantitation value for point C or D is ≤ – (TVL –2) cm). Figure 3a represents Stage 0.

Stage I. The criteria for Stage 0 are not met but the most distal portion of the prolapse is more than 1 cm above the level of the hymen (i.e., its quantitation value is < –1 cm).

Stage II. The most distal portion of the prolapse is 1 cm or less proximal to or distal to the plane of the hymen (i.e., its quantitation value is ≥ –1 cm but ≤ + 1 cm).

Stage III. The most distal portion of the prolapse is more than 1 cm below the plane of the hymen, but protrudes no further than two centimetres less than the total vaginal length in cm (i.e., its quantitation value is > + 1 cm but < + (TVL –2) cm). Figure A.1.4.4a represents Stage III-Ba and Figure A.1.4.4b represents Stage III-Bp prolapse.

Stage IV. Essentially complete eversion of the total length of the lower genital tract is demonstrated. The distal portion of the prolapse protrudes to at least (TVL –2) cm (i.e., its quantitation value is ≥ + (TVL –2) cm). In most instances, the leading edge of stage IV prolapse will be the cervix or vaginal cuff scar. Figure 3B represents Stage IV-C prolapse.

3. Ancillary Techniques for Describing Pelvic Organ Prolapse

This series of procedures may help further characterise pelvic organ prolapse in an individual patient. They are considered ancillary either because they are not yet standardised or validated or because they are not universally available to all patients. Authors utilising these procedures should include the following information in their manuscripts: (a) Describe the objective information they intended to generate and how it enhanced their ability to evaluate or treat prolapse. (b) Describe precisely how the test was performed, any instruments that were used, and the specific testing conditions so that other authors can reproduce the study. (c) Document the reliability of the measurement obtained with the technique.

3.1. Supplementary Physical Examination Techniques

Many of these techniques are essential to the adequate pre-operative evaluation of a patient with pelvic organ prolapse. While they do not directly affect either the tandem profile or the ordinal stage, they are important for the selection and performance of an effective surgical repair. These techniques include, but are not necessarily limited to, the following: (a) performance of a digital rectal–vaginal examination while the patient is straining and the prolapse is maximally developed to differentiate between a high rectocele and an enterocele; (b) digital assessment of the contents of the rectal–vaginal septum during the examination noted in 3.1(a) to differentiate between a "traction" enterocele (the posterior cul-de-sac is pulled down with the prolapsing cervix or vaginal cuff but is not distended by intestines) and a "pulsion" enterocele (the intestinal contents of the enterocele distend the rectal–vaginal septum and produce a protruding mass); (c) Q-tip testing for the measurement of urethral axial mobility; (d) measurements of perineal descent; (e) measurements of the transverse diameter of the genital hiatus or of the protruding prolapse; (f) measurements of vaginal volume; (g) description and measurement of rectal prolapse; (h) examination techniques for differentiating between various types of defects (e.g., central versus paravaginal defects of the anterior vaginal wall).

3.2. Endoscopy

Cystoscopic visualisation of bowel peristalsis under the bladder base or trigone may identify an anterior enterocele in some patients. The endoscopic visualisation of the bladder base and rectum and observation of the voluntary constriction and dilation of the urethra, vagina and rectum has, to date, played a minor role in the evaluation of pelvic floor anatomy and function. When such techniques are described, authors should include the type, size and lens angle of the endoscope used, the doses of any analgesic, sedative or anaesthetic agents used, and a statement of the level of consciousness of the subjects in addition to a description of the other conditions of the examination.

3.3. Photography

Still photography of Stage II and greater prolapse may be utilised both to document serial changes in individual patients and to illustrate findings for manuscripts and presentations. Photographs should contain an internal frame of reference such as a centimetre ruler or tape.

3.4. Imaging Procedures

Different imaging techniques have been used to visualise pelvic floor anatomy, support defects and relationships among adjacent organs. These techniques may be more accurate than physical examination in determining which organs are involved in pelvic organ prolapse. However, they share the limitations of the other techniques in this section, i.e., a lack of standardisation, validation and/or availability. For this reason, no specific technique can be recommended but guidelines for reporting various techniques will be considered.

3.4.1. General Guidelines for Imaging Procedures

Landmarks should be defined to allow comparisons with other imaging studies and the physical examination. The lower edge of the symphysis pubis should be given high priority. Other examples of bony landmarks include the superior edge of the public symphysis, the ischial spine and tuberosity, the obturator foramen, the tip of the coccyx and the promontory of the sacrum. All reports on imaging techniques should specify the following: (a) position of the patient including the position of her legs; (Images in manuscripts should be oriented to reflect the patient's position when the study was performed and should not be oriented to suggest an erect position unless the patient was erect.) (b) specific verbal instructions given to the patient; (c) bladder volume and content and bowel content, including any pre-study preparations; and (d) the performance and display of simultaneous monitoring such as pressure measurements.

3.4.2. Ultrasonography

Continuous visualisation of dynamic events is possible. All reports using ultrasound should include the following information: (a) transducer type and manufacturer (e.g., sector, linear, MHz); (b) transducer size; (c) transducer orientation; and (d) route of scanning (e.g., abdominal, perineal, vaginal, rectal, urethral).

3.4.3. Contrast Radiography

Contrast radiography may be static or dynamic and may include voiding colpo-cysto-urethrography, defecography, peritoneography and pelvic fluoroscopy among others. All reports of contrast radiography should include the following information: (a) projection (e.g., lateral, frontal, horizontal, oblique); (b) type and amount of contrast media used and sequence of opacification of the bladder, vagina, rectum and colon, small bowel and peritoneal cavity; (c) any urethral or vaginal appliance used (e.g., tampon, catheter, bead-chain); (d) type of exposures (e.g., single exposure, video); and (e) magnification – an internal reference scale should be included.

3.4.4. Computed Tomography and Magnetic Resonance Imaging

These techniques do not currently allow for continuous imaging under dynamic conditions and most equipment dictates supine scanning. Specifics of the technique should be specified including: (a) the specific equipment used, including the manufacturer; (b) the plane of imaging (e.g., axial, sagittal, coronal, oblique); (c) the field of view (d) the thickness of sections and the number of slices; (e) the scan time; (f) the use and type of contrast; and (g) the type of image analysis.

3.5. Surgical Assessment

Intra-operative evaluation of pelvic support defects is intuitively attractive but as yet of unproven value. The effects of anaesthesia, diminished muscle tone and loss of consciousness are of unknown magnitude and direction. Limitations due to the position of the patient must also be evaluated.

4. Pelvic Floor Muscle Testing

Pelvic floor muscles are voluntarily controlled, but selective contraction and relaxation necessitates muscle awareness. Optimal squeezing technique involves contraction of the pelvic floor muscles without contraction of the abdominal wall muscles and without a Valsalva manoeuvre. Squeezing synergists are the intra-urethral and anal sphincteric muscles. In normal voiding, defecation and optimal abdominal-strain voiding, the pelvic floor is relaxed, while the abdominal wall and the diaphragm may contract. With coughs and sneezes and often when other stresses are applied, the pelvic floor and abdominal wall are contracted simultaneously.

Evaluation and measurement of pelvic floor muscle function includes (1) an assessment of the patient's ability to contract and relax the pelvic muscles selectively (i.e., squeezing without abdominal straining and vice versa) and (2) measurement of the force (strength) of contraction. There are pitfalls in the measurement of pelvic floor muscle function because the muscles are invisible to the investigator and because patients often simultaneously and erroneously activate other muscles. Contraction of the abdominal, gluteal and hip adductor muscles, Valsalva manoeuvre, straining, breath holding and forced inspirations are typically seen. These factors affect the reliability of available testing modalities and have to be taken into consideration in the interpretation of these tests.

The individual types of tests cited in this report are based both on the scientific literature and on current clinical practice. It is the intent of the committee neither to endorse specific tests or techniques nor to restrict evaluations to the examples given. The standards recommended are intended to facilitate comparison of results obtained by different investigators and to allow investigators to replicate studies precisely. For all types of measuring techniques the following should be specified: (a) patient position, including the position of the legs; (b) specific instructions given to the patient; (c) the status of bladder and bowel fullness; (d) techniques of quantification or qualification (estimated, calculated, directly measured); and (e) the reliability of the technique.

4.1. Inspection

A visual assessment of muscle integrity, including a description of scarring and symmetry, should be performed. Pelvic floor contraction causes inward movement of the perineum and straining causes the opposite movement. Perineal movements can be observed directly or assessed indirectly by movement of an externally visible device placed into the vagina or urethra. The abdominal wall and other specified regions might be watched simultaneously. The type, size and placement of any device used should be specified as should the state of undress of the patient.

4.2. Palpation

Palpation may include digital examination of the pelvic floor muscles through the vagina or rectum as well as assessment of the perineum, abdominal wall and/or other specified regions. The number of fingers and their position should be specified. Scales for the description of the strength of voluntary and reflex (e.g., with coughing) contractions and of the degree of voluntary relaxation should be clearly described and intra- and inter-observer reliability documented. Standardised palpation techniques could also be developed for the semi-quantitative estimation of the bulk or thickness of pelvic floor musculature around the circumference of the genital hiatus. These techniques could allow for the localisation of any atrophic or asymmetric segments.

4.3. Electromyography

Electromyography from the pelvic floor muscles can be recorded alone or in combination with other measurements. Needle electrodes permit visualisation of individual motor unit action potentials, while surface or wire electrodes detect action potentials from groups of adjacent motor units underlying or surrounding the electrodes. Interpretation of signals from these latter electrodes must take into consideration that signals from erroneously contracted adjacent muscles may interfere with signals from the muscles of interest. Reports of electromyographic recordings should specify the following: (a) type of electrode; (b) placement of electrodes; (c) placement of reference electrode; (d) specifications of signal processing equipment; (e) type and specifications of display equipment; (f) muscle in which needle electrode is placed; and (g) description of decision algorithms used by the analytic software.

4.4. Pressure Recording

Measurements of urethral, vaginal and anal pressures may be used to assess pelvic floor muscle control and strength. However, interpretations based on these pressure measurements must be made with a knowledge of their potential for artefact and their unproven or limited reproducibility. Anal sphincter contractions, rectal peristalsis, detrusor contractions and abdominal straining can affect pressure measurements. Pressures recorded from the proximal vagina accurately mimic fluctuations in abdominal pressure. Therefore it may be important to compare vaginal pressures to simultaneously measured vesical or rectal pressures. Reports using pressure measurements should specify the following: (a) the type and size of the measuring device at the recording site (e.g., balloon, open catheter, etc.); (b) the exact placement of the measuring device; (c) the type of pressure transducer; (d) the type of display system; and (e) the display of simultaneous control pressures.

As noted in Section 4.1, observation of the perineum is an easy and reliable way to assess for abnormal straining during an attempt at a pelvic muscle contraction. Significant straining or a Valsalva manoeuvre causes downward/caudal movement of the perineum; a correctly performed pelvic muscle contraction causes inward/cephalad movement of the perineum. Observation for perineal movement should be considered as an additional validation procedure whenever pressure measurements are recorded.

5. Description of Functional Symptoms

Functional deficits caused by pelvic organ prolapse and pelvic floor dysfunction are not well characterised or absolutely established. There is an ongoing need to develop, standardise, and validate various clinimetric scales such as condition-specific quality of life questionnaires for each of the four functional symptom groups thought to be related to pelvic organ prolapse.

Researchers in this area should try to use standardised and validated symptom scales whenever possible. They must always ask precisely the same questions regarding functional symptoms before and after therapeutic intervention. The description of functional symptoms should be directed toward four primary areas: (1) lower urinary tract, (2) bowel, (3) sexual, and (4) other local symptoms.

5.1. Urinary Symptoms

This report does not supplant any currently approved ICS terminology related to lower urinary tract function.[7] However, some important prolapse related symptoms are not included in the current standards (e.g., the need to manually reduce the prolapse or assume an unusual position to initiate or complete micturition). Urinary symptoms that should be considered for dichotomous, ordinal, or visual analogue scaling include, but are not limited to, the following: (a) stress incontinence, (b) frequency (diurnal and nocturnal), (c) urgency, (d) urge incontinence, (e) hesitancy, (f) weak or prolonged urinary stream, (g) feeling of incomplete emptying, (h) manual reduction of the prolapse to start or complete bladder emptying, and (f) positional changes to start or complete voiding.

5.2. Bowel Symptoms

Bowel symptoms that should be considered for dichotomous, ordinal or visual analog scaling include, but are not limited to, the following: (a) difficulty with defecation, (b) incontinence of flatus, (c) incontinence of liquid stool, (d) incontinence of solid stool, (e) faecal staining of underwear, (f) urgency of defecation, (g) discomfort with defecation, (h) digital manipulation of vagina, perineum or anus to complete defecation, (i) feeling of incomplete evacuation and (j) rectal protrusion during or after defecation.

5.3. Sexual Symptoms

Research is needed to attempt to differentiate the complex and multifactorial aspects of "satisfactory sexual function" as it relates to pelvic organ prolapse and pelvic floor dysfunction. It may be difficult to distinguish between the ability to have vaginal intercourse and normal sexual function. The development of satisfactory tools will require multidisciplinary collaboration. Sexual function symptoms that should be considered for dichotomous, ordinal, or visual analog scaling include, but are not limited to, the following: (a) Is the patient sexually active? (b) If she is not sexually active, why? (c) Does sexual activity include vaginal coitus? (c) What is the frequency of vaginal intercourse? (d) Does the patient experience pain with coitus? (e) Is the patient satisfied with her sexual activity? (f) Has there been any change in orgasmic response? (g) Is any incontinence experienced during sexual activity?

5.4. Other Local Symptoms

We currently lack knowledge regarding the precise nature of symptoms that may be caused by the presence of a protrusion or bulge. Possible anatomically based symptoms that should be considered for dichotomous, ordinal or visual analog scaling include, but are not limited to, the following: (a) vaginal pressure or heaviness; (b) vaginal or perineal pain; (c) sensation or awareness of tissue protrusion from the vagina; (d) low back pain; (e) abdominal pressure or pain; (f) observation or palpation of a mass.

Acknowledgements

The subcommittee would like to acknowledge the contributions of the following consultants who contributed to the development and revision of this document: W. Glenn Hurt, Bernhard Schüssler, L. Lewis Wall.

References

1. Athanasiou S, Hill S, Gleeson C, Anders K, Cardozo L (1995). Validation of the ICS proposed pelvic organ prolapse descriptive system. Neurourol Urodyn 14:414–415 (abstract of ICS 1995 meeting).
2. Schüssler B, Peschers U (1995). Standardisation of terminology of female genital prolapse according to the new ICS criteria: inter-examiner reproducibility. Neurourol Urodynamics 14:437–438 (abstract of ICS 1995 meeting).
3. Montella JM, Cater JR (1995). Comparison of measurements obtained in supine and sitting position in the evaluation of pelvic organ prolapse (abstract of AUGS 1995 meeting).
4. Kobak WH, Rosenberg K, Walters MD (1995). Interobserver variation in the assessment of pelvic organ prolapse using the draft International Continence Society and Baden grading systems.- (abstract of AUGS 1995 meeting).
5. Hall AF, Theofrastous JP, Cundiff GC, Harris RL, Hamilton LF, Swift SE, Bump RC (1996). Inter- and intra-observer reliability of the proposed International Continence Society, Society of Gynecologic Surgeons, and American Urogynecologic Society pelvic organ prolapse classification system. Am J Obstet Gynecol (submitted through the program of the Society of Gynecologic Surgeons 1996 meeting).
6. Baden W, Walker T (1992). Surgical repair of vaginal defects. Philadelphia: Lippincott, pp 1–7, 51–62
7. See this volume, Appendix 1, Part 2.

Appendix 1, Part 5

The Standardisation of Terminology and Assessment of Functional Characteristics of Intestinal Urinary Reservoirs

Neurourol Urodyn 15:499–511 (1996) © 1996 Wiley-Liss, Inc.

Joachim W. Thüroff, Anders Mattiasson, Jens Thorup Anderson, Hans Hedlund, Frank Hinman Jr., Markus Hohenfellner, Wiking Månsson, Anthony R. Mundy, Randall G. Rowland, and Kenneth Steven

Produced by the International Continence Society Committee on Standardisation of Terminology (Anders Mattiasson, chairman) Subcommittee on Intestinal Urinary Reservoirs (Joachim W. Thüroff, chairman)

1. Introduction

In 1993, the International Continence Society (ICS) established a committee for standardisation of terminology and assessment of functional characteristics of intestinal urinary reservoirs in order to allow reporting of results in a uniform fashion so that different series and different surgical techniques can be compared.

This report is consistent with earlier reports of the International Continence Society Committee on Standardisation of Terminology with special reference to the collated ICS report from 1988 (see Appendix 1, Part 2).

As the present knowledge about physiological characteristics of intestinal urinary reservoirs is rather limited in regard to normal and abnormal reservoir sensation, compliance, activity, continence, and other specifications, some of the definitions are necessarily imprecise and vague. However, it was felt that this report still would be capable of stipulating the standardised assessment of intestinal urinary reservoirs and reporting of the results in order to accumulate more information about physiological characteristics of intestinal urinary reservoirs and to establish precise definitions of normal and abnormal conditions. With increased knowledge and better understanding of intestinal urinary reservoirs, this report will have to be updated to become more specific.

It is suggested that in written publications, the acknowledgement of these standards is indicated by a footnote to the section Methods and Materials or its equivalent: "Methods, definitions and units conform to the standards recommended by the International Continence Society, except where specifically noted."

2. Terminology of Surgical Procedures

Up to now, when different surgical procedures for constructing an intestinal urinary reservoir are described, conflicting terminology is often used. This section defines the terminology of surgical procedures used throughout the report. These definitions may not be universally applicable to the published scientific literature to date, viewed in retrospect, but represent a standardised terminology for surgical procedures for the future.

Definitions

Bladder augmentation is a surgical procedure for increasing bladder capacity. This may be accomplished without other tissues (e.g., autoaugmentation) or with incorporation of other tissues such as intestine (enterocystoplasty, intestinocystoplasty), with or without changing the shape of such intestine (i.e., detubularisation and reconfiguration), and with or without resection of a portion of the original bladder.

Bladder replacement – see "Bladder Substitution."

Bladder substitution (Bladder Replacement) is a surgical procedure for in situ (orthotopic) total substitution/replacement of the bladder by other tissues such as isolated intestine. After subtotal excision of the original bladder (e.g., in interstitial cystitis) the intestinal urinary reservoir may be connected to the bladder neck (bladder substitution to bladder neck) and after complete excision of the original bladder (radical cystoprostatectomy), the reservoir may be connected to the urethra as a continent outlet (bladder substitution to urethra). If indicated, the urethral closure function may be surgically supported in addition (e.g., sling procedure, prosthetic sphincter, periurethral injections). Alternatively, an orthotopically placed urethral substitute/replacement, e.g., from intestine may be used as a continent outlet for a complete substitution of the lower urinary tract.

Continent anal urinary diversion is a surgical procedure for continent urinary diversion utilising bowel in continuity or isolated bowel as a reservoir and the anus as a continent outlet.

Continent cutaneous urinary diversion is a surgical procedure for continent urinary diversion providing an urinary reservoir, e.g., from intestine and a continence mechanism, e.g., from intestine for formation of a continent heterotopically placed (e.g., cutaneous) outlet (stoma).

Enterocystoplasty (bladder augmentation with intestine) – see "Bladder Augmentation".

Intestinocystoplasty (bladder augmentation with intestine) – see "Bladder Augmentation".

3. Assessment

3.1. Experimental Assessment

For reporting animal studies, the principles and standards for experimental scientific publications should be followed. Species, sex, weight, and age of the animals must be stated, as well as type of anesthesia. If chronic experiments are performed, the type of treatment between the initial experiment and the evaluation experiment should be stated. Raw data should be presented and, when applicable, the type of statistical analysis must be stated. For standardisation of urodynamic evaluation see 4 and 5.

3.2. Patient Assessment

The assessment of patients with intestinal urinary reservoirs should include history, frequency/volume chart, physical examination, and evaluation of the upper urinary tract.

3.2.1. History

The history must include etiology of the underlying disease (i.e., congenital anomaly, neurogenic bladder dysfunction, lower urinary tract trauma, radiation damage, bladder cancer or other tumours of the true pelvis) and indication for constructing an intestinal urinary reservoir (e.g., radical surgery for malignancy in the true pelvis, low bladder capacity/compliance, upper tract deterioration due to vesicoureteral obstruction or reflux, urinary incontinence). Information must be available on the duration of previous history of the underlying disease, previous urinary tract infections, and relevant surgery.

The history should also provide information on dexterity and ambulatory status of the patient (i.e., wheelchair bound, paraplegia, or tetraplegia). Information on sexual and bowel function must be reported in respect to the status prior to applying an intestinal urinary reservoir.

The urinary history must report symptoms related to both the storage and evacuation functions of the lower urinary tract with special reference to the technique of evacuation (i.e., spontaneous voiding with or without abdominal straining, Valsalva or Credé manoeuvres, intermittent catheterisation). Problems of evacuation due to mucus production or difficulty with catheterisation must be reported. Incidence of urinary infections must be reported in respect to the incidence prior to construction of an intestinal urinary reservoir.

3.2.2. Specification of Surgical Technique

The surgical technique must be specified stating the applied type of urinary reservoir and origin of gastrointestinal segments used (e.g., stomach, ileum, cecum, transverse colon, sigmoid colon, rectum), length and shape (e.g., tubular, detubularised) of bowel segments, the technique of urethral implantation (when applicable) and the type of the continent outlet (i.e., original urethra, functionally supported urethra, anal sphincter, catheterisable continent cutaneous outlet). If an intussusception nipple valve is applied, technique of fixation of the intussusception (i.e., sutures, staples) should be stated.

Additional and combined surgical procedures in the true pelvis must be reported, such as hysterectomy, colposuspension, excision of vaginal or rectal urinary fistulae, or resection of rectum. Information of adjuvant treatment, such as pharmacotherapy, physiotherapy, or electrical stimulation, must be available.

3.2.3. Frequency/Volume Chart

On the frequency/volume chart the time and volume of each micturition are reported along with quantities of fluid intake. It must be stated if evacuation was prompted by the clock or by sensation. In addition, episodes of urgency and incontinence have to be reported. The frequency/volume chart can be used for the primary assessment of symptoms of urgency, frequency, and incontinence and for follow-up studies.

3.2.4. Physical Examination

Besides general, urological, and, when appropriate, gynecological examination, the neurological status should be assessed with special attention to sensitivity of the sacral dermatomes, sacral reflex activity (anal reflex, bulbocavernosus reflex), and anal sphincter tone and control.

3.2.5. Evaluation of the Upper Urinary Tract

Evaluation of renal function and morphology must be related to the status prior to constructing an intestinal urinary reservoir. Studies of renal morphology can be based on renal ultrasound, intravenous pyelography, and radioisotope studies. Quantification of findings should be recorded by using accepted classifications of upper tract dilatation [Emmett and Witten, 1971], renal scarring [Smellie et al., 1975], and urethral reflux [Heikel and Parkkulainen, 1966]. Renal function should be assessed by measuring the serum concentration of creatinine and, if indicated, by creatinine clearance and radioisotope clearance studies.

3.2.6. Other Relevant Studies

Reported complications of urinary diversion into an intestinal reservoir include electrolyte and blood-gas imbalance, malabsorption syndromes, urolithiasis, urinary tract infection, and development of a secondary malignancy. Follow-up evaluation should include relevant tests when applicable and indicated, and reports should state the results of such studies as serum electrolyte concentrations, analysis of blood gases, serum levels of vitamins A, B12, D, E, K, and folic acid, serum levels of bile acids, urine osmolality and pH, urine excretion of calcium, phosphate, oxalate, and citrate, colonisation of urine, and findings on endoscopy and biopsy of the urinary reservoir.

4. Procedures Related to the Evaluation of Urine Storage in an Intestinal Urinary Reservoir

4.1. Enterocystometry

Enterocystometry is the method by which the pressure/volume relationship of the intestinal urinary reservoir is measured. All systems are zeroed at atmospheric pressure. For external transducers the reference point is the superior edge of the symphysis pubis for bladder augmentation, bladder substitution or continent anal urinary diversion, and the level of the stoma for continent cutaneous urinary diversion. Enterocystometry is used to assess reservoir sensation, compliance, capacity, and activity. Before filling is started, residual urine must be evacuated and measured. Enterocystometry is performed with the patient awake and unsedated, not taking drugs that may affect reservoir characteristics. In a urodynamic follow-up study for evaluation of adjutant treatment (e.g., pharmacological therapy) of an intestinal urinary reservoir, mode of action, dosage, and route of administration (enteral, parenteral, topical) of the medication have to be specified.

As an intestinal urinary reservoir starts to expand when permitted to store urine, time intervals between surgery for construction of the intestinal urinary reservoir, its first functional use for storage of urine and urodynamic testing must be stated. For reporting of functional characteristics of an intestinal urinary reservoir, the time interval between surgery and enterocystometric assessment must be stated to account for postoperative expansion of the reservoir.

As several intestinal segments used in urinary reservoirs react to gastric stimuli, time interval between food ingestion and the urodynamic evaluation should be stated. Reporting of pressure/volume relationships of an intestinal urinary reservoir should be obtained at standardised filling volumes or standardised pressures, which must be stated in absolute numbers.

Specify

a) Access (transurethral, transanal, transstomal, percutaneous);
b) Fluid medium;
c) Temperature of fluid (state in degrees Celsius);
d) Position of patient (supine, sitting or standing);
e) Filling may be by diuresis or catheter. Filling by catheter may be continuous or stepwise: the precise filling rate should be stated. When the stepwise filling is used, the volume increment should be stated. For general discussion, the following terms for the range of filling rate should be used:
    i)   up to 10 ml per minute is slow fill enterocystometry ("physiological" filling);
    ii) 10–100 ml per minute is medium fill enterocystometry;
    iii) over 100 ml per minute is rapid fill enterocystometry.

Technique

a) Fluid-filled catheter – specify number of catheters, single or multiple lumens, type of catheter (manufacturer), size of catheter, type (manufacturer), and specifications of external pressure transducer;
b) Catheter mounted microtransducer – list specifications;
c) Other catheters – list specifications;
d) Measuring equipment.

Definitions

Total reservoir pressure is the pressure within the reservoir.

Abdominal pressure is taken to be the pressure surrounding the reservoir. In current practice it is estimated from rectal or, less commonly, intraperitoneal or intragastric pressures.

Subtracted reservoir pressure is estimated by subtracting abdominal pressure from total reservoir pressure. The simultaneous recording of the abdominal pressure trace is essential for the interpretation of the subtracted reservoir pressure trace as artefacts of the subtracted reservoir pressure may be produced by intrinsic rectal contractions or relaxations.

Contraction pressure (amplitude) is the difference between maximum reservoir pressure during a contraction of an intestinal urinary reservoir and baseline reservoir pressure before onset of this contraction. Contraction pressures may be determined from the pressure curves of total reservoir pressure or subtracted reservoir pressure. For assessment of functional significance of such activity of an intestinal urinary reservoir, pressure and volume must be stated for the first, a typical, and the maximum contraction. The frequency of contractions should be stated at a specified volume.

Leak point pressure is the total reservoir pressure at which leakage occurs in the absence of sphincter relaxation. Leakage occurs whenever total reservoir pressure exceeds maximum outlet pressure so that a negative outlet closure pressure results.

Reservoir sensation is difficult to assess because of the subjective nature of interpreting fullness or "flatulence" from the bowel segments of the intestinal urinary reservoir. It is usually assessed by questioning the patient in relation to the sensation of fullness of the intestinal urinary reservoir during enterocystometry.

Commonly used descriptive terms are similar to conventional cystometry:

First desire to empty
Normal desire to empty (this is defined as the feeling that leads the patient to empty at the next convenient moment, but emptying can be delayed if necessary);
Strong desire to empty (this is defined as a persistent desire to empty without the fear of leakage);
Urgency (this is defined as a strong desire to empty accompanied by fear of leakage or fear of pain);
Pain (the site and character of which should be specified).

Maximum enterocystometric capacity is the volume at strong desire to empty. In the absence of sensation, maximum enterocystometric capacity is defined by the onset of leakage. If the closure mechanism of the outlet is incompetent, maximum enterocystometric capacity can be determined by occlusion of the outlet, e.g., by a Foley catheter. In the absence of both sensation and leakage, maximum enterocystometric capacity cannot be defined in the same terms and is the volume at which the clinician decides to terminate filling, e.g., because of a risk of over-distension.

Functional reservoir capacity or evacuated volume is assessed from a frequency/volume chart (urinary diary). If a patient empties the urinary reservoir by intermittent catheterisation, functional reservoir capacity will be dependent on presence or absence of sensation and/or leakage. Thus, when reporting functional reservoir capacity the following should be stated:

a) Mode of evacuation (e.g., spontaneous voiding, intermittent catheterisation);

b) Presence/absence of sensation of fullness;

c) Presence/absence of leakage;

d) Timing of evacuation (e.g., by sensation, by the clock, by leakage).

Maximum (anaesthetic) anatomical reservoir capacity is the volume measured after filling during a deep general or spinal/epidural anaesthetic, specifying fluid temperature, filling pressure and filling rate.

Compliance describes the change in volume over a related change in reservoir pressure. Compliance (C) is calculated by dividing the volume change (ΔV) by the change in subtracted reservoir pressure (ΔP_s) during that change in reservoir volume ($C = \Delta V/\Delta P_s$). Compliance is expressed as ml per cmH_2O.

4.2. Outlet Pressure Measurement

It should be noted that even under physiological conditions the evaluation of the competence of the closure mechanism of a continent outlet by measuring intraluminal pressures under various conditions is regarded as an idealized concept. Moreover, measurements of intraluminal pressures for functional evaluation of a continent outlet do not allow comparison of results between different closure mechanisms, which are in use with different types of intestinal urinary reservoirs. In addition, similar closure mechanisms may behave differently when used in different types of intestinal urinary reservoirs.

Therefore, urodynamic measurements of a continent outlet always have to be related to symptoms of the patient as assessed by history, frequency/volume chart, and, when applicable, measurement of urine loss.

The rationale of performing outlet pressure measurements is not to verify continence or degree of incontinence but to understand how different closure mechanisms work, which urodynamic parameters reflect their competence or dysfunction, and how their function is related to the characteristics of a reservoir.

In current urodynamic practice, intraluminal outlet pressure measurements are performed by a number of different techniques which do not always yield consistent values. Not only do the values differ with the method of measurement but there is often a lack of consistency for a single method – for example, the effect of catheter rotation when outlet pressure is measured by a catheter mounted microtransducer.

Measurements can be made at one point in the outlet (stationary) over a period of time, or at several points along the outlet consecutively during continuous or intermittent catheter withdrawal forming an outlet pressure profile (OPP). OPPs should be obtained at significant filling volumes of an intestinal urinary reservoir, which must be standardised and stated.

Two types of OPP can be measured:

a) Resting outlet pressure profile – with the urinary reservoir and the subject at rest;

b) Stress outlet pressure profile – with a defined applied stress (e.g., cough, strain, Valsalva manoeuvre).

The outlet pressure profile denotes the intraluminal pressure along the length of the closure mechanism. All systems are zeroed at atmospheric pressure. For external transducers the reference point is the level of the continence mechanism. For catheter mounted transducers the reference point is the transducer itself. Intrareservoir pressure should be measured to exclude a simultaneous reservoir contraction. The subtraction of total reservoir pressures from intraluminal outlet pressures produces the outlet closure pressure profile.

Specify

a) Infusion medium;

b) Rate of infusion;

c) Stationary, continuous or intermittent catheter withdrawal;

d) Rate of withdrawal;

e) Reservoir volume;

f) Position of patient (supine, sitting or standing);

g) Technique (catheters, transducers, measurement technique and recording apparatus are to be specified according to the 1988 ICS report; see Appendix 1, Part 2).

Definitions

Maximum outlet pressure is the maximum pressure of the measured profile.

Maximum outlet closure pressure is the difference between maximum outlet pressure and total reservoir pressure.

Functional outlet profile length is the length of the closure mechanism along which the outlet pressure exceeds total reservoir pressure.

Functional outlet profile length (on stress) is the length over which the outlet pressure exceeds total reservoir pressure on stress.

Pressure "transmission" ratio[1] is the increment in outlet pressure on stress as a percentage of the simultaneously recorded increment in the total reservoir

---

[1] The term "transmission" is in common usage and cannot be changed. However, transmission implies that forces transmitted to the closure mechanism are generated completely by extrinsic activities. Such an assumption is not yet justified by scientific evidence. A role for intrinsic muscle activity cannot be excluded for the urethra and the anus and their intrinsic sphincter mechanisms, while it is unlikely to be of significance in any of the surgically constructed closure mechanisms of a continent outlet.

The terms "passive transmission" and "active transmission" have been introduced to describe different processes in respect of the source of extrinsically generated forces and the mode of transmission. "Passive transmission" is taken to be the result of forces, which are generated by striated muscles distant from the closure mechanism (e.g., diaphragm, abdominal wall muscles) and are "passively" transmitted through surrounding tissues to the closure mechanism in the same way they are transmitted to all other intraabdominal tissues and organs. "Active transmission" is taken to be result of forces, which are generated by striated muscles in direct anatomical contact with the closure mechanism (e.g., pelvic floor muscles with urethra or anus, and abdominal wall muscles with a continent cutaneous outlet) and are directly "transmitted" to the closure mechanism.

pressure. For stress profiles obtained during coughing, pressure "transmission" ratios can be obtained at any point along the closure mechanism. If single values are given, the position in the closure mechanism should be stated. If several transmission ratios are defined at different points along the closure mechanism, a pressure "transmission" profile is obtained. During "cough profiles" the amplitude of the cough should be stated if possible.

4.3. Quantification of Urine Loss

On a frequency/volume chart, incontinence can be qualified (with/without urge or stress) and quantified by the number, type, and dampness (damp/wet/soaked) of pads used each day. However, subjective grading of incontinence may not completely disclose the degree of abnormality. It is important to relate the complaints of each patient to the individual urinary regimen and personal circumstances, as well as to the results of objective measurements.

In order to assess and compare results of different series and different surgical techniques, a simple standard test can be used to measure urine loss objectively in any subject. In order to obtain a representative result, especially in subjects with variable or intermittent urinary incontinence, the test should occupy as long a period as possible; yet it must be practical. The circumstances should approximate to those of everyday life, yet be similar for all subjects to allow meaningful comparison.

The total amount of urine lost during the test period is determined by weighing a collecting device such as a nappy, absorbent pad, or condom appliance. A nappy or pad should be worn inside waterproof underpants or should have a waterproof backing if worn over a continent stoma. Care should be taken to use a collecting device of adequate capacity.

Immediately before the test begins the collecting device is weighed to the nearest gram.

In the 1988 collated report on "Standardisation of Terminology of Lower Urinary Tract Function" (see Appendix 1, Part 2), the ICS has offered the choices to conduct a pad test either with the patient drinking 500 ml sodium-free liquid within a short period (max. 15 min) without the patient voiding before the test or after having the bladder filled to a defined volume. Because there is a great variation in the functional capacity of different types of intestinal urinary reservoirs and since some types of closure mechanism of the outlet physiologically have a leak point and others have no leak point, it is recommended that the reservoir is emptied by catheterisation immediately before the test and refilled with a reasonable volume of saline, which must be standardised and be stated in absolute numbers. A typical test schedule and additional procedures are described in the 1988 ICS report (Appendix 1, Part 2). Specifications for presentation of results, findings, and statistics from the 1988 ICS report are applicable (Appendix 1, Part 2).

5. Procedures Related to the Evaluation of Evacuation of an Intestinal Urinary Reservoir

5.1. Mode of Evacuation

The mode of evacuation of an intestinal urinary reservoir varies as some patients may have a surgically constructed closure mechanism requiring catheterisation (e.g., continent cutaneous urinary diversion) and some patients may have a reservoir with a physiological sphincter mechanism (e.g., bladder augmentation, bladder substitution to bladder neck or to urethra, continent anal urinary diversion), through which they may be able to evacuate urine spontaneously. However, as catheterisation may also be required after bladder augmentation or bladder substitution to bladder neck or to urethra, it must be stated by what means the reservoir is emptied (e.g., spontaneous evacuation with or without Valsalva or Credé manoeuvres and/or intermittent catheterisation).

If intermittent catheterisation is necessary, whether it is performed on a regular basis or only periodically, the intervals between catheterisations must be stated.

Measurements of urinary flow, reservoir pressures during micturition and residual urine apply only to patients with bladder augmentation or bladder substitution to bladder neck or to urethra who void spontaneously. However, as there is no volitional initiation of contraction of an intestinal urinary reservoir, spontaneous evacuation is different from voiding by a detrusor contraction.

In patients with an intestinal urinary reservoir, evacuation is initiated by relaxation of the urethral sphincteric mechanisms and/or passive expression of the reservoir by abdominal straining or Valsalva or Credé manoeuvres. Therefore, measurements of flow and micturition pressures must be interpreted with great caution in respect of the diagnosis of an outlet obstruction.

5.2. Measurements of Urinary Flow, Micturition Pressure, Residual Urine

For specifications of measurements of urinary flow, reservoir pressures during micturition and residual urine the 1988 ICS report is applicable (Appendix 1, Part 2). The specifications of patient position, access for pressure measurement, catheter type, and measuring equipment are as for enterocystometry (see 4.1).

6. Classification of Storage Dysfunction of an Intestinal Urinary Reservoir

Dysfunction of an intestinal urinary reservoir has to be defined in respect to indications and functional intentions of incorporating bowel into the urinary tract. The rationale of using an intestinal urinary reservoir is to improve or provide storage function by:

a)   Reducing bladder hypersensitivity;
b)   Providing/enlarging reservoir capacity;
c)   Providing/improving reservoir compliance;
d)   Lowering bladder pressures/providing low reservoir pressures;
e)   Improving/providing the closure function of the outlet.

It is not a primary goal of surgery to maintain or provide the capability of spontaneous voiding; intermittent catheterisation is required for evacuation of the reservoir in all cases of continent cutaneous diversion and in many other situations. The need to evacuate a urinary reservoir by intermittent catheterisation is not regarded as a failure in bladder augmentation and bladder substitution to bladder neck or to urethra, even though the majority of patients may evacuate urine spontaneously.

Consequently, the classification of dysfunctions of an intestinal urinary reservoir relates to the storage phase only. Problems of storing urine in an intestinal urinary reservoir may be related to dysfunction of the reservoir or dysfunction of the outlet. The classification is based on the pathophysiology of dysfunction as assessed by various urodynamic investigations. The urodynamic findings must be related to the patient's symptoms and signs. For example, the presence of reservoir contractions in an asymptomatic patient with normal upper tract drainage does not warrant a diagnosis of reservoir overactivity unless the contractions cause urine leakage or other problems defined below.

6.1. Reservoir Dysfunction

The symptoms of frequency, urgency, nocturia, and/or incontinence may relate to dysfunction of an intestinal urinary reservoir and should be assessed by enterocystometry, which is an adequate test for evaluation of the pathophysiology of a reservoir dysfunction (see 4.1). Abnormal findings may relate to sensation, compliance, capacity, and/or activity of an intestinal urinary reservoir.

6.1.1. Sensation

Sensations from an intestinal urinary reservoir as assessed by questioning the patient during enterocystometry can be classified in qualitative terms. Often these symptoms are associated with contractions of the reservoir as shown by enterocystometry or fluoroscopy. However, up to now there is insufficient information about an isolated hypersensitive state of the bowel of an intestinal urinary reservoir. If symptoms such as frequency, urgency, and nocturia are persisting after bladder augmentation or bladder substitution to bladder neck (e.g., in interstitial cystitis), they are likely to derive from remnants of the original lower urinary tract, which have not been replaced by intestine, if enterocystometry is otherwise normal.

6.1.2. Capacity/Compliance

Capacity of an intestinal urinary reservoir is determined by sensation and/or compliance. For definitions of reservoir capacity and compliance ($\Delta V/\Delta P$), see 4.1. Compliance describing the change in volume over a related change in reservoir pressure is likely to reflect a different physiology when determined in an intestinal urinary reservoir as compared to the urinary bladder. The calculation of compliance will reflect wall characteristics of an intestinal urinary reservoir such as distensibility only after a process of "unfolding" of an empty intestinal urinary reservoir has been completed and stretching of the walls begins to take place, which is different in the normal urinary bladder. Compliance may change during the enterocystometric examination and is variably dependent upon a number of factors including:

a) Rate of filling;
b) The part of the enterocystometrogram curve used for compliance evaluation;
c) The volume interval over which compliance is calculated;
d) The distensibility of the urinary reservoir as determined by mechanical and contractile properties of the walls of the reservoir.

During normal filling of an intestinal urinary reservoir little or no pressure changes occur and this is termed "normal compliance." However, at the present time there is insufficient data to define normal, high, and low compliance. When reporting compliance, specify:

a) The rate of filling;
b) The volume at which compliance is calculated;
c) The volume increment over which compliance is calculated;
d) The part of the enterocystometrogram curve used for the calculation of compliance.

The selection of bowel segments, the size of bowel (diameter, length), and the geometry (shape) of a reservoir after bowel detubularisation and reconfiguration determine capacity of an intestinal urinary reservoir [Hinman, 1988]. For a given length of bowel, reconfiguration into a spherical reservoir provides the largest capacity. The distensibility of bowel wall, as assessed in experimental models, varies between bowel segments (i.e., large bowel, small bowel, stomach) and with orientation (longitudinal, circumferential) of measurement within a bowel segment [Hohenfellner et al., 1993]. However, the relative contributions of wall distensibility (influenced by selection of bowel segments) and of geometric capacity (influenced by size of selected bowel and reservoir shape after detubularisation and reconfiguration) in determining the capacity of an intestinal urinary reservoir are not yet precisely understood. Low capacity of an intestinal urinary reservoir may relate to bowel size (diameter/length) and/or configuration of bowel segments in the reservoir (e.g., tubular, inadequate detubularisation, and reconfiguration).

6.1.3. Activity

In intact bowel segments, peristaltic contractions are elicited at a certain degree of wall distension. As a result of detubularisation and reconfiguration of bowel segments in an intestinal urinary reservoir, such contractions do not encompass the whole circumference of a reservoir. Net pressure changes in the reservoir are determined by the mechanical and muscular properties of both the contracting and the non-contracting segments of the reservoir. Contractions of segments of an intestinal urinary reservoir may be observed by fluoroscopy but may not increase subtracted reservoir pressure if the generated forces are counterbalanced by other segments of a urinary reservoir which relax and distend. Some contractile activity of an intestinal urinary reservoir is a normal finding on enterocystometry or fluoroscopy.

Overactivity of an intestinal urinary reservoir is defined as a degree of activity which causes lower urinary tract symptoms and/or signs of upper tract deterioration in the absence of other causes of upper tract damage such as urethral obstruction or reflux. Symptoms such as abdominal cramping, urgency, frequency, and/or leakage may be related to reservoir activity seen during enterocystometry and thus establish the diagnosis of an unacceptable degree of reservoir activity ("overactivity"). Signs of impaired upper tract drainage may be associated with elevated subtracted reservoir pressures on enterocystometry due to an early onset, high amplitudes, and/or frequency of contractions and thus establish the diagnosis of overactivity even if subjective symptoms are not experienced.

However, since a precise definition of normal and increased activity of a urinary reservoir from intestine is not yet established, the frequency of contractions should be reported at a specified volume and the pressure/volume relationships should be stated for the following defined contractions of the reservoir:

a) First contraction;
b) Contraction with maximum contraction pressure (amplitude);
c) Typical contraction.

The diagnosis of overactivity of an intestinal urinary reservoir should not be made until a reasonable interval – which must be stated – has elapsed after surgery, since an intestinal urinary reservoir expands after surgery, when permitted to store urine, and since some of the reservoir activity subsides with time with an increase of capacity.

6.2. Outlet Dysfunction

The symptoms of incontinence and/or difficulties with catheterisation may relate to dysfunction of the outlet of an intestinal urinary reservoir and should be assessed in terms of pathophysiology. Leakage may occur if total reservoir pressure exceeds outlet pressure so that the result is a negative outlet closure pressure as assessed by outlet pressure profiles (see 4.2). For such an event, volume and total reservoir pressure at onset of leakage (leak point pressure) must be stated.

Leakage may occur with a functioning closure mechanism because of an excessive reservoir pressure increase due to contractions of the intestinal urinary reservoir (overactivity) or overdistension of the reservoir (overflow).

The definition of incompetence of a closure mechanism is different for a closure mechanism which physiologically has a leak point from that for a closure mechanism without a leak point.

A closure mechanism which physiologically has a leak point (e.g., the urethral sphincter, some types of closure mechanism in continent cutaneous urinary diversion) is incompetent if it allows leakage or urine in the absence of contraction of the intestinal urinary reservoir (overactivity) or overdistension of the reservoir (overflow) as assessed by enterocystometry (see 4.1). A closure mechanism which normally has no leak point (e.g. an intussusception nipple) is incompetent if it permits leakage of urine independent of results of enterocystometry.

References

Emmett JL, Witten DM (1971). Urinary stasis: The obstructive uropathies, atony, vesicoureteral reflux, and neuromuscular dysfunction of the urinary tract. In: Emmett JL, Witten DM (eds): Clinical urography. An atlas and textbook of roentgenologic diagnosis. Vol. 1, 3rd edn. Philadephia, London, Toronto: Saunders, p 369.

Heikel PE, Parkkulainen KV (1966). Vesicoureteric reflux in children. A classification and results of conservative treatment. Ann Radiol 9:37.

Hinman F Jr (1988). Selection of intestinal segments for bladder substitution: physical and physiological characteristics. J Urol 139:519.

Hohenfellner M, Büger R, Schad H, Heimisch W, Riedmiller H, Lampel A, Thüroff JW, Hohenfellner R (1993). Reservoir characteristics of Mainz-pouch studied in animal model. Osmolality of filling solution and effect of Oxybutynin. Urology 42:741.

Smellie JM, Edwards D, Hunter N, Normand ICS, Prescod N (1975). Vesico-ureteric reflux and renal scarring. Kidney Int 8:65.

Appendix 1, Part 6
The Standardisation of Terminology of Lower Urinary Tract Function: Pressure–Flow Studies of Voiding, Urethral Resistance and Urethral Obstruction

Neurourol Urodyn (1997) in press

Derek Griffiths (subcommittee chairman), Klaus Höfner, Ron van Mastrigt, Harm Jan Rollema, Anders Spångberg, Donald Gleason and Anders Mattiasson (overall chairman)

International Continence Society Subcommittee on Standardisation of Terminology of Pressure–Flow Studies

1. Introduction

This report has been produced at the request of the International Continence Society. It was approved at the twenty-fifth annual meeting of the society in Sydney, Australia.

The 1988 version of the collated reports on standardisation of terminology, which appeared in *Neurourology and Urodynamics*, vol. 7, pp. 403–427, contains material relevant to pressure–flow studies in many different sections. This report is a revision and expansion of Sections 4.2 and 4.3 and parts of Sections 6.2 and 7 of the 1988 report. It contains a recommendation for a provisional standard method for defining obstruction on the basis of pressure–flow data.

2. Evaluation of Micturition

2.1. Pressure–Flow Studies

At present, the best method of analysing voiding function quantitatively is the pressure–flow study of micturition, with simultaneous recording of abdominal, intravesical and detrusor pressures and flow rate (Fig. A.1.6.1).

Direct inspection of the raw pressure and flow data before, during and at the end of micturition is essential, because it allows artefacts and untrustworthy data to be recognised and eliminated. More detailed analyses of pressure–flow relationships, described below, are advisable to aid diagnosis and to quantify data for research studies.

The flow pattern in a pressure–flow study should be representative of free flow studies in the same patient. It is important to eliminate artefacts and unrepresentative studies before applying more detailed analyses.

Pressure–flow studies contain information about the behaviour of the urethra and the behaviour of the detrusor. Section 2.2 deals with the urethra. Detrusor function is considered in Section 2.3.

2.1.1. Pressure and Flow Rate Parameters

Definitions See Fig. A.1.6.1 and Table II; see also Table II Appendix 1, Part 2.

Maximum flow rate is the maximum measured value of the flow rate. Symbol Q_{max}.

Maximum pressure is the maximum value of the pressure measured during a pressure–flow study. Note that this may be attained at a moment when the flow rate is zero. Symbols: $p_{abd, max}$, $p_{ves, max}$, $p_{det, max}$.

Pressure at maximum flow is the pressure recorded at maximum measured flow rate. If the same maximum value is attained more than once or if it is sustained for a period of time, then the point of maximum flow is taken to be where the detrusor pressure has its lowest value for this flow rate; abdominal, intravesical and detrusor pressures at maximum flow are all read at this same point. Flow delay (see Section 2.1.2) may have a significant influence and should be considered. Symbols: $p_{abd, Q_{max}}$, $p_{ves, Q_{max}}$, $p_{det, Q_{max}}$.

Opening pressure is the pressure recorded at the onset of measured flow. Flow delay should be considered. Symbols: $p_{abd, open}$, $p_{ves, open}$, $p_{det, open}$.

Closing pressure is the pressure recorded at the end of measured flow. Flow delay should be considered. Symbols: $p_{abd, clos}$, $p_{ves, clos}$, $p_{det, clos}$.

Minimum voiding pressure is the minimum pressure during measurable flow (see Fig. A.1.6.1). It may be, but is not necessarily, equal to the opening pressure or the closing pressure. Example: minimum voiding detrusor pressure, symbol: $p_{det, min, void}$.

2.1.2. Flow Delay

When a pressure–flow study is performed, the flow rate is measured at a location downstream of the bladder pressure measurement and so the flow rate measurement is delayed. The delay is partly physiological, but it also depends on the equipment. It may depend on the flow rate.

When considering pressure–flow relationships, it may be important to take this delay into account, especially if there are rapid changes in pressure and flow rate. In current practice an average value is estimated by each investigator, from observations of the delay between corresponding pressure and flow rate changes in a number of actual studies. Values from 0.5 to 1.0 s are typical.

Definition
Flow delay is the time delay between a change in bladder pressure and the corresponding change in measured flow rate.

2.1.3. Presentation of Results

Pressure–flow plots and the nomograms used for analysis should be presented with the flow rate plotted along the *x*-axis and the detrusor pressure along the *y*-axis (see Fig. A.1.6.2).

Specify
The value of the flow delay that is used.

2.2. Urethral Resistance and Bladder Outlet Obstruction

2.2.1. Urethral Function During Voiding

During voiding urethral function may be

(a) normal or
(b) obstructive as a result of
    (i)   overactivity or
    (ii) abnormal structure.

Obstruction due to urethral overactivity occurs when the urethral closure mechanism contracts involuntarily or fails to relax during attempted micturition in spite of an ongoing detrusor contraction. Obstruction due to abnormal structure has an anatomical basis, e.g., urethral stricture or prostatic enlargement.

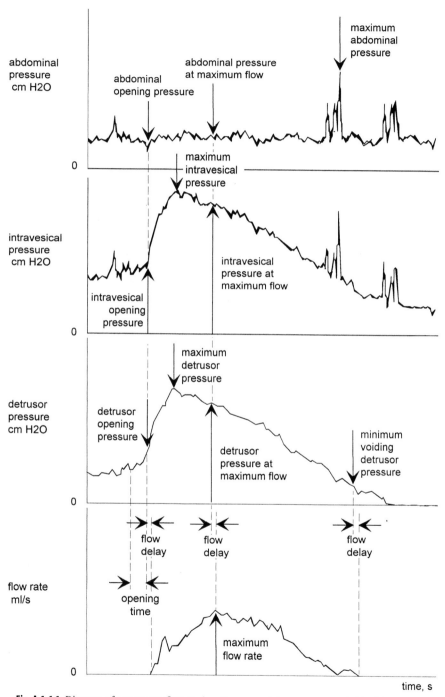

Fig. A.1.6.1 Diagram of a pressure–flow study with nomenclature recommended in this report.

2.2.2. Urethral Resistance

Urethral resistance is represented by a relation between pressure and flow rate, describing the pressure required to propel any given flow rate through the urethra. The relation is called the *urethral resistance relation* (URR).

An indication of the urethral resistance relation is obtained by plotting detrusor pressure against flow rate. The most accurate procedure, which requires a computer or an *x/y* recorder, is a quasi-continuous plot showing many pairs of corresponding pressure and flow rate values (Fig. A.1.6.2). A simpler procedure, which can be performed by hand, is to plot only two or three pressure–flow points connected by straight lines; for example, the points of minimum voiding pressure and of maximum flow may be selected. In whatever way the plot is made, flow delay should be considered.

A further simplification is to plot just one point showing the maximum flow rate and the detrusor pressure at maximum flow. Flow delay should be considered.

Methods of analysing pressure–flow plots are further discussed below.

2.2.3. Urethral Activity

Ideally, the urethra is fully relaxed during voiding. The urethral resistance is then at its lowest and the detrusor pressure has its lowest value for any given flow rate. Under these circumstances the urethral resistance relation is defined by the inherent mechanical and morphological properties of the urethra and is called the *passive urethral resistance relation* (Fig. A.1.6.2).

Urethral activity can only increase the detrusor pressure above the value defined by the passive urethral resistance relation. Therefore, any deviations of the pressure–flow plot from the passive urethral resistance relation toward higher pressures are regarded as due to activity of the urethral or periurethral muscles, striated or smooth.

2.2.4. Bladder Outlet Obstruction

Obstruction is a physical concept which is assessed from measurements of pressure and flow rate, made during voiding. Whether due to urethral over-activity or to abnormal structure, obstruction implies that the urethral resistance to flow is abnormally elevated. Because of natural variation from subject to subject, there cannot be a sharp boundary between normal and abnormal. Therefore the definition of abnormality requires further elaboration.

2.2.5. Methods of Analysing Pressure–Flow Plots

The results of pressure–flow studies may be used for various purposes, for example for objective diagnosis of urethral obstruction or for statistical testing of differences in urethral resistance between groups of patients. For these purposes methods have been developed to quantify pressure–flow plots in terms of one or

Table I. Methods of analysing pressure–flow plots

Method	Aim	Number of p/Q points	Assumed shape of URR	Number of parameters	Number of classes or continuous
Abrams–Griffiths nomogram[1]	diagnosis	1	n/a	n/a	3
Spångberg nomogram [2]	diagnosis	1	n/a	n/a	3
URA[3,4]	resistance	1	curved	1	continuous
linPURR[5]	resistance	1[a]	linear	1	7
Schäfer PURR[6]	resistance	many	curved	2	continuous
CHESS[7]	resistance	many	curved	2	16
OBI[8]	resistance	many	linear	1	continuous
Spångberg et al.	resistance	many	linear or curved	3	continuous + 3 categories
DAMPF[9]	resistance	2	linear	1	continuous
A/G number[10]	resistance	1	linear	1	continuous

[a]Schäfer uses 2 points to draw a linear relation but the point at maximum flow determines the resistance grade.

more numerical parameters. The parameters are based on aspects such as the position, slope or curvature of the plot. Some of these methods are primarily intended for use in adult males with possible prostatic hypertrophy.

Some methods of analysis are shown in Table I.

Quantification of Urethral Resistance In all current methods, urethral resistance is derived from the relationship between pressure and flow rate. A commonly used method of demonstrating this relationship is the pressure–flow plot. The lower pressure part of this plot is taken to represent the passive urethral resistance relation (see Fig. A.1.6.2). In general, the higher is the pressure for a given flow rate, and/or the steeper or more sharply curved upward is this part of the plot, the higher is the urethral resistance. The various methods differ in how the position, slope, and/or curvature of the plot are quantified and how and whether they are combined. Some methods grade urethral resistance on a continuous scale; others grade it in a small number of classes (Table I). If there are few classes, small changes in resistance may not be detected. Conversely, a small change on a continuous scale may not be clinically relevant.

Some methods result in a single parameter; others result in two or more parameters (Table I). A single parameter makes it easy to compare different measurements. A larger number of parameters makes comparison more difficult but potentially gives higher accuracy and validity. If there are too many parameters, however, accuracy may be compromised by poor reproducibility.

Choice of Method Some methods in Table I are intended primarily to quantify urethral resistance. Others are intended only for the diagnosis of obstruction. Methods that quantify urethral resistance on a scale can also be used to aid

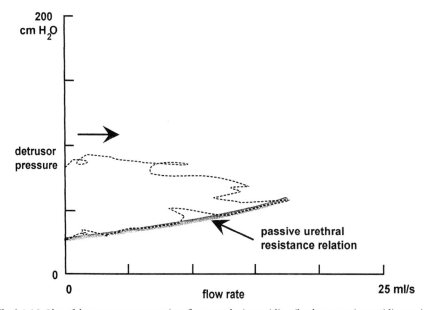

Fig. A.1.6.2 Plot of detrusor pressure against flow rate during voiding (broken curve), providing an indication of the urethral resistance relation (URR). The continuous smooth curve is an estimate of the passive urethral resistance relation.

diagnosis of obstruction by comparison with cutoff values. In every case an equivocal zone may be included.

Because of their underlying similarity, all the above methods classify clearly obstructed and clearly unobstructed pressure–flow studies consistently, but there is some lack of agreement in a minority of cases with intermediate urethral resistance.

Any of the methods of analysing pressure–flow studies may be useful for a particular purpose. In selecting a method, investigators should consider carefully what their aims are and which method is best suited to attain them.

Identification of Optimum Methods For a subsequent report the International Continence Society will compare the above methods with each other and may also develop new methods, with the aim of reaching a consensus on their use. The Society will continue to seek better ways of clinically validating these methods. The following procedure has been agreed on.

Making use of good-quality data stored in digital format, the following databases will be examined:

1. Pressure–flow studies in untreated men with lower urinary tract symptoms and signs suggestive of benign prostatic obstruction.
2. Pressure–flow studies repeated after a time interval with no intervention.
3. Pressure–flow studies before and after TURP.
4. Pressure–flow studies before and after alternative therapeutical intervention that causes a small change in urethral resistance.

Database 1 will be used to determine which existing or new methods adequately describe the actual pressure–flow plots of male patients with lower urinary tract symptoms. Database 2 will be used to determine the reproducibility of the various methods. Database 3 will be used to determine in which groups of patients TURP significantly reduces urethral resistance, and hence which patients are indeed obstructed. Database 4 will be used to test the sensitivity of the various methods to small changes of urethral resistance.

On the basis of these analyses, the International Continence Society will attempt to identify:

(i) A simple and reproducible method with high validity of diagnosing obstruction.

(ii) A sensitive and reproducible method with high validity of measuring urethral resistance and changes in resistance.

Provisional Recommendation Pending the results of these procedures, it is recommended that investigators reporting pressure–flow studies in adult males, particularly those with benign prostatic hyperplasia, use one simple standard method of analysis in addition to any other method that they have selected, so that results from different centres can be compared. For this provisional method it is recommended that urethral resistance is specified by the maximum flow rate and the detrusor pressure at maximum flow, i.e., by the pair of values (Q_{max}, $p_{det, Q_{max}}$). A provisional diagnostic classification may be derived from these values as follows:

- If ($p_{det, Q_{max}} - 2Q_{max}$) > 40 the pressure–flow study is obstructed.
- If ($p_{det, Q_{max}} - 2Q_{max}$) < 20 the pressure–flow study is unobstructed.
- Otherwise the study is equivocal.

In these formulae pressure and flow rate are expressed in cmH$_2$O and ml/s respectively. This method is illustrated graphically in Fig. A.1.6.3. It may be referred to as the *provisional ICS method for definition of obstruction*.

The equivocal zone of the provisional method (Fig. A.1.6.3) is similar but not identical to those of the Abrams–Griffiths and Spångberg nomograms and to the region defining linPURR grade II. For micturitions with low to moderate flow rates it is consistent with cutoff values used to define obstruction in the URA and CHESS methods.

2.3. The Detrusor During Micturition

During micturition the detrusor may be

(a) Acontractile
(b) Underactive
(c) Normal

(a) The acontractile detrusor is one that cannot be demonstrated to contract during urodynamic studies.
(b) Detrusor underactivity is defined as a detrusor contraction of inadequate magnitude and/or duration to effect complete bladder emptying in the

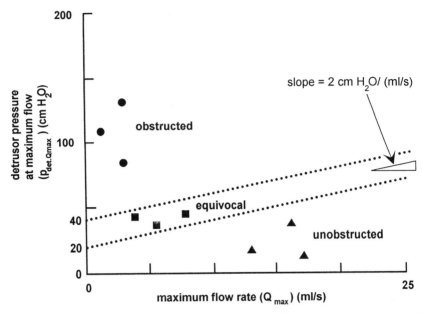

Fig. A.1.6.3 Provisional ICS method for definition of obstruction. The points represent schematically the values of maximum flow rate and detrusor pressure at maximum flow for 9 different voids, 3 in each class.

absence of urethral obstruction. (Concerning the elderly see (c). Both magnitude and duration should be considered in the evaluation of detrusor contractility.

(c) Normal detrusor contractility. In the absence of obstruction, a normal detrusor contraction will effect complete bladder emptying. Detrusor contractility in the elderly may need special consideration.

For a given detrusor contraction, the magnitude of the recorded pressure rise will depend on the outlet resistance. In general, the higher the detrusor pressure and/or the higher the flow rate, the stronger is the detrusor contraction. The magnitude of the detrusor contraction may be approximately quantified by means of a nomogram applied to the pressure–flow plot or by calculation.

3. Additional Symbols

Qualifiers that can be used to form symbols for variables relevant to voiding are shown in Table II. These are additions to those in Table II of the 1988 standardisation report.

Table II. Qualifiers that can be used to indicate pressure and flow variables relevant to voiding

Qualifiers	
At maximum flow	Q_{max}
During voiding	void
Opening	open
Closing	clos
Examples	
$p_{det,Q_{max}}$	Detrusor pressure at maximum flow
$p_{det\ min,\ void}$	Minimum voiding detrusor pressure
$p_{ves,\ open}$	Intravesical opening pressure
$p_{ves,\ clos}$	Intravesical closing pressure

When possible, qualifiers should be printed as subscripts (see above). Note that the preferred symbol for pressure is lower-case p, while the symbol for flow rate is capital (upper-case) Q.

References

1. Abrams PH, Griffiths DJ (1979). The assessment of prostatic obstruction from urodynamic measurements and from residual urine. Br J Urol 51:129–134.
2. Spångberg A, Teriö H, Ask P, Engberg A (1991). Pressure/flow studies preoperatively and post-operatively in patients with benign prostatic hypertrophy: estimation of the urethral pressure/flow relation and urethral elasticity. Neurourol Urodyn 10:139–167.
3. Griffiths D, Van Mastrigt R, Bosch R (1989). Quantification of urethral resistance and bladder function during voiding, with special reference to the effects of prostate size reduction on urethral obstruction due to benign prostatic hypertrophy. Neurourol Urodyn 8:17–27.
4. Rollema HJ, van Mastrigt R (1992). Improved indication and follow-up in transurethral resection of the prostate (TUR) using the computer program CLIM. J Urol 148:111–116.
5. Schäfer W (1990). Basic principles and clinical application of advance analysis of bladder voiding function. Urol Clin N Am 17:553–566.
6. Schäfer W (1983). The contribution of the bladder outlet to the relation between pressure and flow rate during micturition. In: Hinman F Jr (ed) Benign prostatic hypertrophy. New York: Springer-Verlag, pp. 470–496.
7. Höfner K, Kramer AEJL, Tan HK, Krah H, Jonas U (1995). CHESS classification of bladder outflow obstruction. A consequence in the discussion of current concepts. World J Urol 13:59–64.
8. Kranse M, Van Mastrigt R (1991). The derivation of an obstruction index from a three parameter model fitted to the lowest part of the pressure flow plot. J Urol 145:261A.
9. Schäfer W (1995). Analysis of bladder-outlet function with the linearized passive urethral resistance relation, linPURR, and a disease-specific approach for grading obstruction: from complex to simple. World J Urol 13:47–58.
10. Lim CS, Abrams P (1995). The Abrams–Griffiths nomogram. World J Urol 13:34–39.

Appendix: ICS Standard for Digital Exchange of Pressure–Flow Study Data

A1. Introduction

To facilitate exchange of digital urodynamic data a standard file format is required. In this document an ICS standard is summarised. Its primary purpose is to enable data from pressure–flow studies to be exchanged. Enough detail is given to allow exchange of other urodynamic data. Extensions may be made as described in Section A5.

A2. General Description of Signal Storage

For each pressure–flow study, urodynamic signals sampled equidistantly with an A/D converter, and other associated information, are stored in one binary MS-DOS compatible file on a 5.25 or 3.5 inch floppy disk. The stored signals start 10 seconds before a detectable change in the flow rate signal and continue until 10 seconds after the flow rate has finally returned to baseline. Whenever possible, all signals should be stored at the same sample rate. In this case all signals have the same length, i.e., contain the same number of bytes.

The file name and extension are A B C D E F G H. ICS, where A B C D E F G H stands for a unique measurement identification string. In the case of a multi-centre study requiring exchange of data, "unique" implies that this string is defined by the coordinating centre. In the ICS-BPH study for instance this would be a number consisting of (first) 3 digits for centre number, (next) 3 digits for patient number and (finally) 2 digits for identification of successive measurements made on this one patient in one or more sessions.

The file consists of a number of records of various types. In the ICSMFF proposal on which this document is partly based (see Section A8: Acknow-ledgements) 14 different types of record are defined, numbered –1 and 1 to 13. Existing record types may not be modified but extensions may be implemented by defining new types of record. For ICS purposes 6 additional types of record, types 14 to 19, are required and are defined in Section A5. In addition, the structures of records of types 8 and 9 are further elaborated in Section A5.

A3. Variable Values and Types

In this report actual values for bytes or words may be given in hexadecimal notation as follows: Hex:DD for 8-bit bytes, Hex:DDDD for 16-bit words, and so on, where D stands for a hexadecimal digit.

The following variable types are used in the definitions in the following sections:

byte	unsigned 8-bit value
word	unsigned 16-bit value
integer	signed 16-bit value
dword	unsigned 32-bit value
string [N]	N bytes including a terminating Hex:00
word [N]	N words

A4. General Structure of File and Records

Each file A B C D E F G H . ICS consists of a number of records. The number of records is not predefined. Records may be of different types, containing different kinds of data. For example a record may contain a description of a urodynamic signal or information about the patient.

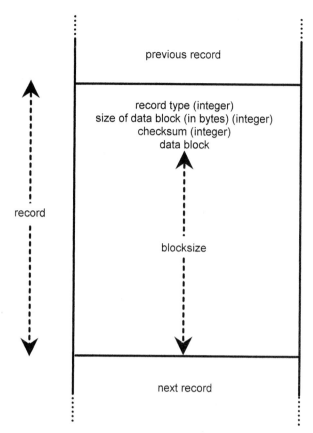

Fig. A.1.6.A1 Schematic structure of file and records.

Each record starts with a descriptor containing the record type, the size of the data block in bytes and a checksum. The descriptor is followed by the block containing the actual data (see Fig. A.1.6.A1).

The record type and the block size are integers. The checksum is an integer such that the 16-bit sum of the record type, the data block size and the checksum is zero.

A5. Definitions of Record Types

The record type defines what kind of data is contained by the data block in the record. The only constraint is that the record type is unique.

Backward compatibility is preserved by the requirement that previously defined record types may not be modified. Extensions are implemented by defining new types of record. New types of signal may be implemented by defining new signal IDs, together with signal names and units. Forward compatibility will be insured if the user does not try to handle unknown types of record or unknown signal IDs.

A register of the types of record in use, and a register of signal IDs, signal names and units, will be administered centrally by the ICS. This standard contains initial versions of the registers. Proposed extensions should be communicated to the ICS for registration.

Default Values

Empty fields are not permitted. Occasionally, the value for a certain field may not be available. In this case a default value should be stored (see below).

Signal ID

See Section A9: Addendum.

The following sections describe the types of record needed to implement this ICS standard. Other types are described in the document *ICS Measure File Format (ICSMFF)* version 1.00, dated 14.10.93 (see Section A8: Acknowledgements).

Record Type 8: The Measurement Marker Record

This type of record defines a marker within the measurement and an associated comment.

Record type	8	integer
Blocksize	$1 + N + 1 + 4 + M$	integer
Checksum	$-(8+\text{blocksize})$	integer
Data block	marker type	byte
	name	string $[N]$
	signal ID	byte
	position	dword
	comment	string $[M]$

The following information should be stored in these fields:

In the field:

marker type   0 = default value
                (other types are defined in the ICSMFF document)

name   empty string as default value
                (empty string contains only the terminating Hex:00, so
                that $N = 1$)

signal ID	as in Section A9: Addendum
position	the number of the sample (16-bit word) with which the marker and comment are associated
comment	the comment string, terminated with Hex:00

Record Type 9: The Measurement Comment Record

This record stores a comment. For the ICS standard it should be used to identify the patient and the type of the measurement.

Record type	9	integer
Blocksize	N	integer
Checksum	–(9 + blocksize)	integer
Data block	measurement comment	string [N]

The following information should be stored:

In the field:

measurement comment	a free format string, terminated with Hex:00, that uniquely identifies patient and measurement for the originating centre. This string would not only include a patient ID, e.g. from the local hospital information system, but also the relation of this measurement to a particular research study, e.g. "post-TURP investigation". For use in a specific multi-centre study, this string may be specified more strictly.

Record Type 14: The ICS Signal Property Record

This record type describes the properties of one stored signal, including its name, the unit of measurement, the zero and full scale values, and the sample rate (which if possible should be identical for all signals).

Record type	14	integer
Blocksize	$1 + N + M + 2 + 4$	integer
Checksum	–(14 + blocksize)	integer
Data block	signal id	byte
	signal name	string [N]
	unit	string [M]
	binzero	integer
	binsize	integer

fullscale	integer
sample rate	dword

The following information should be stored in these fields:

In the field:

signal ID	as specified in Section A9: Addendum
signal name	as specified in Section A9: Addendum
unit	as specified in Section A9: Addendum
binzero	the signal value represented in the data samples field of record type 18 by the word 0
binsize	the full scale binary sample value
fullscale	the signal value represented in the data samples field of record type 18 by the full scale binary value
sample rate	sample rate specification in samples/s (Hz). The sample rate is in 16.16 format: i.e., it is a long integer, where bits 16 through 31 specify the integer part of a fixed point number and bits 0 through 15 specify the decimal part.

The following values are recommended:

- Sample rate at least 10 samples/s.
- Pressure signals bipolar up to + 200 cmH$_2$O with a minimum resolution of 0.5 cmH$_2$O/bit.
- Flow rate signal unipolar up to 50 ml/s with a minimum resolution of 0.05 ml/s/bit.

Example showing how sample rate is to be specified:

Suppose the rate of sampling is 512.5 Hz. Then the value to be stored in the field sample rate is the 16.16 value Hex:02008000.

Example showing how binzero, binsize and fullscale are to be used:

Suppose the abdominal pressure is sampled bipolarly with a ten bit A/D converter. Then the binary value will range from 0 to 1023. Suppose the A/D converter is configured so that this range represents the pressure range from −50 to 200 cmH$_2$O, then the three values to be stored are:

binzero	−50
binsize	1023
fullscale	200

Record Type 15: The ICS Patient Data Record

This record type contains the basic demographic data of the patient. It contains the actual text and numerical fields plus an index table to facilitate location of a particular field. The index gives the relative position within the data block.

Record type	15		integer
Blocksize	$17 * 2 + N + M + O + P + Q + R + S +$		
	$T + U + V + W + X + Y + 3 + 2$		integer
Checksum	$-(15 + \text{blocksize})$		integer
Data block	surname index		word
	first name index		word
	maiden name index		word
	ID index		word
	street index		word
	housenumber index		word
	city index		word
	country index		word
	postcode index		word
	phone index		word
	height index		word
	weight index		word
	sex index		word
	comments index		word
	birth day index		word
	birth month index		word
	birth year index		word
	surname		string [N]
	first name		string [M]
	maiden name		string [O]
	ID		string [P]
	street		string [Q]
	housenumber		string [R]
	city		string [S]
	country		string [T]
	postcode		string [U]
	phone		string [V]
	height		string [W]
	weight		string [X]
	comments		string [Y]
	sex		byte*
	birth day		byte
	birth month		byte
	birth year		word[†]

* 0 = male, 1 = female.
[†] Birth year is expressed in full, e.g., 1895, 1995, 2005.

The first name field may contain a middle or other initial in addition to the first name.

As a default, an empty string (containing only Hex:00) may be stored in any of the string fields for which information is not available or may not be disclosed because of ethical considerations. In this case the length (N, M, etc.) of the string is 1.

The index fields contain the position (in bytes) of the corresponding text or numerical field, relative to the start of the data block. Thus the value to be stored in surname index is $17 * 2$; the value to be stored in first name index is $17 * 2 + N$; and so on. All the index fields must be completed.

Record Type 16: The ICS Source Record

This record type specifies the origin of the measurement. It consists of an index table together with the actual text fields.

Record type	16	integer
Blocksize	$10 * 2 + N + M + O + P + Q + R + S +$ $T + U + V$	integer
Checksum	$-(16 + \text{blocksize})$	integer
Data block	clinic name index	word
	investigator name index	word
	street index	word
	streetnumber index	word
	city index	word
	country index	word
	postcode index	word
	phone index	word
	fax index	word
	comments index	word
	clinic name	string [N]
	investigator name	string [M]
	street	string [O]
	streetnumber	string [P]
	city	string [Q]
	country	string [R]
	postcode	string [S]
	phone	string [T]
	fax	string [U]
	comments	string [V]

The phone and fax fields should include the area code as well as the local number.

An empty string may be stored in any of the string fields for which information is not available. In this case the length (N, M, etc.) of the string is 1.

The index fields contain the position (in bytes) of the corresponding text field, relative to the start of the data block. All the index fields must be completed.

Record Type 17: ICS Volume Record

This record contains the filling volume and the residual volume.

Record type	17	integer
Blocksize	4	integer
Checksum	–(17 + blocksize)	integer
Data block	filling volume	integer
	residual volume	integer

The following information should be stored:

In the field:

filling volume	the calculated volume in the bladder at the beginning of the pressure–flow study (in ml)
residual volume	the volume in the bladder at the end of the study, either calculated or measured directly (in ml); if the calculated volume is negative the value zero should be stored

Record Type 18: The ICS Signal Value Record

The ICS signal value record contains the actual data samples for one of the urodynamic signals. It includes a record number, allowing a signal that is too long to fit into one record to be divided so as to span several records. If the signal spans more than one record the number of the first record should be 1 and the following records should be numbered 2, 3, ... If there is only one record its record number should be 0.

Record type	18	integer
Blocksize	$2 + N * 2$	integer
Checksum	–(18 + blocksize)	integer
Data block	signal ID	byte
	record number	byte
	data samples	word [N]

The following information should be stored in these fields:

In the field:

signal ID	As specified in Section A9: Addendum.
record number	As described above.

data samples	The binary samples themselves, 1 word = 2 bytes = 1 sample, stored in the order low byte, high byte.

Record Type 19: The ICS Measurement Description Record

This record indicates that the file is an ICS standard file and describes the measurement's start date and time, the number of signals stored and the number of records in the file.

Record type	19		integer
Blocksize	$1 + N + 5 + 1 + 2$		integer
Checksum	$-(19 + \text{blocksize})$		integer
Data block	Measurement type		byte
	Name		string [N]
	Start	minute	byte
		hour	byte
		day	byte
		month	byte
		year	byte*
	Number of signals		byte
	Number of records		word

*Year is expressed modulo 100; e.g. 1995 = 95, 2005 = 05.
The following information should be stored in these fields:

In the field:

measurement type	the version number of this document, multiplied by 10 (e.g., for this version 70). (Note that the version number may not contain hundredths or smaller decimal fractions.)
name	the string "ICS standard pressure–flow study"
start	the starting time and date of the measurement (if any of these are unavailable, the default value Hex:00 should be stored in the corresponding position: minute, hour, day, month and/or year)
number of signals	the number of signals stored in this file (e.g., 3 if just intravesical pressure, abdominal pressure and flow rate are stored).
number of records	the total number of records stored in this file (including this measurement description record)

A6. Signals and Information to be Stored: Minimal Specification and Optional Extensions

Minimally the following 3 signals should be stored in 3 records of type 18:

intravesical pressure

abdominal pressure

flow rate

For each signal certain associated information should be stored in a record of type 14.

Optionally the following signals can also be stored in records of type 18, with associated information in records of type 14:

EMG envelope

voided volume

The voided volume signal may be useful if this is the signal measured by the urodynamic system, and the flow rate signal is derived from it.

In addition to the signals, further information about the patient and the measurements should be stored in records of types 16, 17 and 19. Full demographic data for the patient can be stored in a record of type 15. Optionally a free format comment can be stored in a record of type 9, and if detailed comments relating to events during the measurement are available they can be stored in records of type 8.

A7. Typical File Structure

Of the various record types, some are mandatory and some are optional. The structure of the file describing a particular measurement varies according to what records are stored.

The order of the records within the file is arbitrary in principle. However, it may be convenient to place records containing easily recognisable strings near the beginning, so that the file can quickly be identified if it is accidentally renamed or misplaced. In particular, record type 19 should preferably be the first one.

Thus a typical file structure might be:

Record type 19: ICS measurement description record (identifies file as an ICS standard file)

Record type 16: ICS source record (identifies originating clinic and investigator)

Record type 9: Measurement comment record (identifies patient and type of measurement)

Optionally, record type 15: ICS patient data record (contains full demographic data for patient)

Record type 14: ICS signal property record (describes properties of intravesical pressure signal)

Record type 14: ICS signal property record (describes properties of abdominal pressure signal)

Record type 14: ICS signal property record (describes properties of flow rate signal)

   Optionally, further records of type 14 for voided volume and EMG envelope

Record type 18: ICS signal value record (contains actual intravesical pressure data)

Record type 18: ICS signal value record (contains actual abdominal pressure data)

Record type 18: ICS signal value record (contains actual flow rate data)

   Optionally, further records of type 18 for voided volume and EMG envelope

   Optionally, record type 8: measurement marker record (identifies position and type of marker in data, the signal with which it is associated and a comment)

   Optionally, further records of type 8 with additional markers

Record type 17: ICS volume record (contains filling volume prior to pressure–flow study and residual urine volume after voiding)

A8. Acknowledgements

This draft proposal is based partly on the ICS Measure File Format (ICSMFF) version 1.00 of 14.10.93, which was written by Michael Gondy Jensen, formerly of the Wiest company and now of Andromeda Medical Systems, and also on an earlier proposal for a simple digital pressure–flow standard circulated by Ron van Mastrigt. The Dantec, Laborie, Life-Tech and Wiest companies have agreed in principle to support a standard similar to the ICSMFF. The Life-Tech company has agreed to support the approved ICS standard.

A9. Addendum: Signal IDs

In records of types 8, 14 and 18, a signal ID of the type byte is specified. Corresponding signal names and units of the type string are required in record type 14. The following signal ID values, signal names and units have been defined:

		Signal ID	Signal name	Unit
For	intravesical pressure	1	pves	cmH_2O
	abdominal pressure	2	pabd	cmH_2O
	flow rate	3	Q	ml/s
	EMG envelope	4	EMG_{env}	μV
	voided volume	5	V_{void}	ml

The following are reserved for possible future use:

	Signal ID	Signal name	Unit
For p_{det} acquired independently	6	p_{det}	cmH_2O
infused volume	7	V_{inf}	ml
direct EMG signal	8	EMG	μV
urethral pressure	9	p_{ura}	cmH_2O
urethral closure pressure	10	p_{clos}	cmH_2O

Additional signal IDs, signal names and units may be introduced; proposed additions should be communicated to the ICS for registration.

Appendix 2, Part 1
Frequency–Volume Chart

Please note the time you pass your water, and the volume passed. Any measuring jug will do for this purpose. Obviously when you are at work it may be inconvenient to measure the volume; in this case record only the time. However, at other times please try to record both.

If you wet yourself at any time record the time and underneath the letter "W".

Day-time means when you are up: Night-time when you are in bed.

An example is provided below to help you:-

EXAMPLE

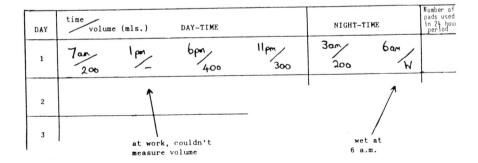

DAY	time / volume (mls.) DAY-TIME				NIGHT-TIME		Number of pads used in 24 hour period
1	7am / 200	1pm / –	6pm / 400	11pm / 300	3am / 200	6am / W	
2							
3			at work, couldn't measure volume		wet at 6 a.m.		

Name _____

Date of appointment _____

DAY	time ⁄ volume (mls.)	DAY-TIME	NIGHT-TIME	Number of pads used in 24 hour period
1				
2				
3				
4				
5				
6				
7				

AVERAGE DAILY FLUID INTAKE (in cups) = _____

* instructions on other side *

Patient Information Sheet

SOUTHMEAD HEALTH
Services —

A NATIONAL HEALTH SERVICE TRUST

URODYNAMIC
INVESTIGATIONS

Urodynamic Unit
Southmead Hospital
Bristol BS10 5NB

Telephone (0117) 9595181

Urodynamic tests will show how well your bladder is working

Why do you need these tests?

- Your Doctor or consultant needs more information about the cause of your bladder problems
- To be sure that you receive the correct treatment
- During your tests, a Doctor, Nurse or Technician will be with you. They will also answer your questions and tell you the results of your tests

Your appointment letter will say which tests you will be having. These may include:-

Flow Studies

- Takes approximately 2 to 3 hours
- This test will show how much your bladder can hold, and at what speed it empties
- After drinking some water you will be asked to wait until your bladder is full

- Then to pass water into a specially adapted toilet
- Afterwards your bladder will be scanned,using ultrasound, to see whether it has emptied completely
- This process will be repeated 2 or 3 times which is why this test takes a long time
- Following the flow studies you will be sent a further appointment to see the Consultant in the Outpatient Clinic

Transport (with flow studies appointments only)

- If hospital transport has been requested this will be arranged for you

Urodynamics (UDS)

- Takes approximately 1 hour
- This test will show how effectively your bladder is working
- A small soft plastic tube is passed into the bladder and used to fill it with fluid

- Pressure recordings are taken from the tube as your bladder fills and empties

Video urodynamics (VIDEO)

- Takes approximately 1-2 hours
- This test is similar to UDS above
- X-rays are taken during the test to show how the bladder is working

Ambulatory studies (LTM)

- Takes 3-4 hours
- A small, soft plastic tube is passed into your bladder and records what happens as your bladder fills
- Your bladder will be monitored whilst you are walking, exercising and relaxing
- You will be asked to fill and empty your bladder twice
- It is best to wear loose fitting clothes and please bring a book or knitting etc to do whilst 'relaxing'

Pad test

- Takes approximately 1-1$^1/_2$ hours
- This will measure any leakage of urine that you have
- After drinking some water, you will be given a weighed pad to wear
- Then you will be asked to do some exercises for one hour
- Afterwards the pad will be weighed again and any leakage calculated

After your tests

- The results will be sent to your Doctor and Consultant who will arrange your next appointment
- It is a good idea to increase the amount you drink for 24 hours after the tests
- You may notice a small amount of blood in your urine, and feel slightly uncomfortable
- This is nothing to worry about and should get better within 24 hours
- If it becomes a problem, please contact your family Doctor for advice

ud.1.March 96

Your rights as a Patient

- To know how, and why, you will be treated and what the alternatives are
- To be given enough information to make decisions about your care
- To have access to your health records
- To know that information about you will not be given to anyone who is not involved in your care
- To choose whether or not to take part in research or Medical Student training

If you have any comments on the service provided by the Unit, either good or bad, please speak to a member of staff or you can send them to;

The Clinical Director of the Urodynamic Unit or the Urology Services Manager

Sponsored by

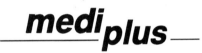

Produced by Potten, Baber & Murray Ltd., Tel: 0117 966 1126

Appendix 3, Part 1

Urodynamics Data Sheet: Full Version

U R O D Y N A M I C   U N I T
SOUTHMEAD HOSPITAL, BRISTOL

NOTE: —

(a) Number of entries Strictly dictated by number of boxes

(b) Where no information enter ☒

(c) − = not applicable

1. SURNAME: _____

FIRST NAME: _____

2. ADDRESS: _____

_____

Post Code _____ Tel. No. _____

3. DATE OF BIRTH:

4. SEX: (1 male; 2 female)

5. HOSPITAL NUMBER(S):

6. INITIAL REFERRAL: 1 Urol   2 Gynae   3 Surg   4 Geriatric
5 G.P.   6 Nurse   7 Other   8 Paediatrics

6a. 1 = in patient   2 = out-patient   3 = not known

7. CONSULTANT: (Name) _____

8. G.P.: (Name) _____

Address (not coded) _____

_____

9a. CIU NUMBER: 9b. INVESTIGATION NUMBER:

Presenting Complaint:

Previous Treatment:

HEIGHT	cms
WEIGHT	Kg
SMOKER YES / NO	............/Day

Examination:

Management:

Report sent to: Follow up arrangements: —

If enter 'other' in any question please describe on this sheet.

10. DATE: ⬜⬜ ⬜⬜ ⬜⬜

11. AGE: ⬜⬜

12. TRIAL IDENTIFICATION (see code) ⬜⬜

        X if not known
        — is not applicable

13. ENTER HISTORY   1 YES   ⬜
                           2 NO

    If NO go to 54

14. INVESTIGATOR: ⬜⬜⬜⬜

15. LENGTH HISTORY:
    (Enter figure if   0 = less than 1 yr
    1-9 years)   A = more than 9 years   ⬜
                         B = lifelong
                         X = not known

16. FREQUENCY OF MICTURITION: (from F/V chart)
    (Waking hours)   X = not known   ⬜⬜
                         — = not applicable (eg retention,
                                appliance, conduit)

17. NOCTURIA: XX = not known
    (from F/V chart)   — = not applicable (eg   ⬜ . ⬜
                            retention, appliance, conduit)

18. FLUID INTAKE:
    (litres per 24 hrs)   0 = less than 1L
    (Enter figure if intake   A = more than 9L   ⬜
      1-9 litres/24 hrs)   X = not known

19. ANALYSIS, VOIDED VOLUME/FREQUENCY/VOLUME CHART

                         X = not known
                         — = not applicable (eg retention,
                              appliance, conduit)
                         Maximum voided volume   ⬜⬜⬜ ml.

                         Average voided volume   ⬜⬜⬜ ml.

                         Maximum duration between daytime voids   ⬜ . ⬜ hrs.

20. PREMICTURITION SYMPTOMS

1 = normal
2 = decreased sensation
3 = absent sensation
4 = increased bladder sensation
5 = bladder pain
6 = urethral pain
7 = urgency, fear of leakage
8 = cannot void
X = unknown

If 1, 3, 8 or X in 20 go to 21

FREQUENCY (of premicturition symptoms)

1 = more than x 1/day
2 = x 1/day
3 = more than x 1/week
4 = x 1/week
5 = less than x 1/week
X = unknown

21. HESITANCY

1 = none
2 = only on full bladder
3 = occasional
4 = usually
5 = always strains to void urine
6 = cannot void urine
X = unknown

if 1, 5, 6 or X in 21 go to 22

FREQUENCY (of hesitancy)

1 = more than x 1/day
2 = x 1/day
3 = more than x 1/week
4 = x 1/week
5 = less than x 1/week
X = unknown

22. INCONTINENCE

1 = none
2 = present (or under treatment
        for incontinence, eg catheter)
X = unknown

if 1 or X in 22 go to 30

23. STRESS INCONTINENCE

1 = no
2 = yes
X = unknown

if 1 or X in 23 go to 24

FREQUENCY (of stress incontinence)

1 = more than x 1/day
2 = x 1/day
3 = more than x 1/week
4 = x 1/week
5 = less than x 1/week
X = unknown

24. URGE INCONTINENCE   1 = no
                                2 = yes   ▢
                                X = unknown

if 1 or X in 24 go to 25

      FREQUENCY (of urge incontinence)
                                1 = more than x 1/day
                                2 = x 1/day
                                3 = more than x 1/week   ▢
                                4 = x 1/week
                                5 = less than x 1/week
                                X = unknown

25. PATIENT: PRESENT HISTORY OF ENURESIS
                                1 = no
                                2 = present problem
                                3 = yes + past history (with enuresis   ▢
                                       free interval of years)
                                X = unknown

if 1 or X in 25 go to 26

      FREQUENCY (of enuresis)   1 = more than x 1/night
                                2 = x 1/night
                                3 = more than x 1/week   ▢
                                4 = 1/week
                                5 = less than 1/week
                                X = unknown

26. OTHER INCONTINENCE   1 = none
                                2 = post micturition dribbling
                                3 = continuous incontinence   ▢
                                4 = other
                                5 = Incontinence during sexual intercourse

if 1, 3 or X in 26 go to 27

      FREQUENCY   1 = more than x 1/day
                                2 = x 1/day
                                3 = more than x 1/week   ▢
                                4 = x 1/week
                                5 = less than x 1/week
                                X = unknown

27. DEGREE OF INCONTINENCE   1 = drops, wets underclothes
                                2 = 'floods', wets outer clothes
                                3 = 'floods', on floor   ▢
                                X = not known

28. MANAGEMENT OF INCONTINENCE
                                1 = no protective measures, no clothes change
                                2 = changes underwear/clothes
                                3 = pads for safety
                                4 = pads for necessity
                                5 = appliance   ▢
                                6 = catheter
                                7 = urinary diversion
                                8 = other
                                X = unknown

complete ONLY if 3 or 4 in 28

                                PADS PER DAY   ▢▢

                                PADS PER NIGHT   ▢▢

29. INCAPACITY DUE TO INCONTINENCE

1 = none
2 = minimal
3 = social restriction, e.g. length of time out
4 = physical restriction, e.g. tennis or dancing
5 = housebound
6 = hospitalised
7 = other
X = unknown

30. PHYSICAL INCAPACITY

1 = none
2 = minor, walks unaided
3 = walks with aids (e.g. sticks)
4 = partial use wheelchair
5 = wheelchair bound
6 = bedbound
7 = limited manual dexterity, otherwise mobile
X = unknown

31. HISTORY OF ENURESIS

(i) Patient (includes
present enuresis)

1 = no
2 = yes
X = not known

(ii) Family

1 = none
2 = yes, sibs
3 = yes, sibs & parents
4 = yes, parents
5 = unspecified family history
X = unknown

32. URINARY STREAM

1 = normal
2 = decreased
3 = decreased only on full bladder
4 = interrupted
5 = decreased and interrupted
6 = cannot void
7 = decreased with terminal dribble
X = unknown

33. POST MICTURITION SYMPTOMS

1 = normal
2 = persistent abdominal sensation
3 = persistent perineal sensation
4 = feeling of incomplete emptying
5 = cannot void
X = unknown

if 1, 5 or X in 33 go to 34

FREQUENCY

1 = more than 1 x/day
2 = x 1/day
3 = more than x 1/week
4 = x 1/week
5 = less than x 1/week
X = unknown

34. DYSURIA/U.T.I.

1 = none — no proven UTI
2 = occasional — no proven UTI
3 = frequent — no proven UTI
4 = occasional — proven UTI
5 = frequent — proven UTI
6 = none — proven UTI
X = unknown

34a. HAEMATURIA
                                       1 = yes
                                       2 = no
                                       X = not known

35. HISTORY OF RETENTION
    1 = none
    2 = spontaneous
    3 = acute retention after operation
    4 = acute retention after childbirth
    5 = chronic retention
    6 = retention secondary to acute neurological disease
    7 = other
    X = unknown

if 1 or X in 35 go to 37

36. PRESENT MANAGEMENT OF RETENTION
    1 = indwelling catheter
    2 = intermittent self-catheterisation
    3 = urinary diversion
    4 = drugs
    5 = other
    X = unknown

37. BOWEL FUNCTION
(if stoma code —)

(a) Control
    1 = normal
    2 = urgency
    3 = poor control (soiling)
    X = unknown

(b) Stool frequency
    1 = > 1/day
    2 = x 1/day
    3 = between alternate days and
          x 2/week
    4 = < x 2/week
    X = unknown

(c) Mechanics of defaecation
    1 = normal (no straining)
    2 = strains
    3 = suppositories
    4 = enemas
    5 = manual evacuation
    X = unknown

(d) Post-defaecation symptoms
    1 = none
    2 = feeling incomplete emptying
          (further evacuation gives relief)
    3 = Feeling incomplete emptying
          (further straining no relief)
    4 = Other
    X = unknown

(e) Bowel diagnosis
    1 = normal
    2 = irritable bowel syndrome
    3 = constipation
    4 = diarrhoea
    5 = constipation/diarrhoea
    6 = other
    X = unknown

38. PRESENT DRUG THERAPY

   (if on more than one
   drug, use left hand
   box for drug with
   most bladder/urethral
   effect)

1 = none
2 = anti-biotics
3 = bladder stimulants
4 = bladder depressants
5 = urethral relaxants
6 = urethral stimulants
7 = anti-depressants
8 = diuretics
9 = oral contraceptives
A = oestrogens
B = other
X = unknown

☐ ☐ ☐

39a. NEUROLOGICAL FEATURES

   (if more than one
   feature, use left
   hand box for condition
   with most bladder/
   urethral effect)

1 = none
2 = diabetes
3 = cervical disc/sp'osis
4 = lumbar disc/sp'osis
5 = paraplegia/tetraplegia
6 = M.S.
7 = C.V.A.
8 = dementia
9 = other cerebral disorders
A = spina bifida
B = epilepsy
C = Parkinsons
D = other neurological disease
X = unknown

☐ ☐ ☐

39b. SEXUAL FUNCTION

1 = normal
2 = abnormal
3 = unknown

☐

If 2 state abnormality on front sheet

40. MALE OPERATIONS/TRAUMA

   (i) For outflow tract problem

1 = none
2 = TUR
3 = RPP
4 = urethral dilatation
5 = artificial sphincter
6 = other urethral surgery
7 = bladder neck incision
X = unknown

☐ ☐

   (ii) Surgery with possible denervation

1 = none
2 = Helmsteins
3 = rectal resection
4 = denervation procedure
5 = other
X = unknown

☐ ☐

   (iii) Other procedures/factors

1 = none
2 = pelvic radiotherapy
3 = renal failure/transplantation
4 = cystoscopy
5 = trauma
6 = urinary diversion
7 = other
X = unknown

☐ ☐

Go to 46

FEMALE PATIENTS ONLY

41. FEMALE OPERATIONS/TRAUMA

(i) For stress incontinence

1 = none
2 = vaginal repair
3 = Marshall Marchetti
4 = colpo
5 = sling
6 = Stamey
7 = Teflon
8 = artificial sphincter
9 = other
X = unknown

□ □ □

(ii) For gynaecological symptoms including prolapse

1 = none
2 = vaginal repair
3 = abdominal hysterectomy
4 = vaginal hysterectomy
5 = laparotomy
6 = other
X = unknown

□ □

iii) Surgery with possible denervation effects

1 = none
2 = Wertheims hysterectomy
3 = A.P. resection
4 = Helmsteins
5 = denervation procedures
6 = other
X = unknown

□ □

(iv) Other factors

1 = none
2 = pelvic radiotherapy
3 = renal failure/transplant
4 = cystoscopy
5 = urethral dilatation
6 = other urethral surgery
7 = relevant trauma (spinal injuries & direct
                                        urinary tract trauma)
8 = diversions
9 = other
X = unknown

□ □

42. HORMONAL STATUS

1 = premenopausal
2 = probably premenopausal (hyst)
3 = menopausal
4 = probably menopausal (hyst)
5 = post-menopausal
6 = probably post-menopausal (hyst)
7 = pre menarche
X = unknown

□

if 5, 6 or X then go to 44
if 7 go to 46

43. SYMPTOMS RELATED TO MENSTRUATION

      1 = no relation to cycle
      2 = worse premenstrually
      3 = worse during menstruation
      4 = worse postmenstrually
      5 = worse mid-cycle
      6 = not relevant
      X = unknown

44. PARITY (Number of deliveries)

if 0 (zero) in 44 go to 46

45. COMPLICATIONS
     OF DELIVERY

     Code complications
     <u>NOT</u> each delivery.
     If all code 1 enter 111
     If 1 abnormal,
     eg 6 and others normal
     code 611 etc.

      1 = none
      2 = > 4 Kg baby
      3 = forceps
      4 = breech
      5 = lower segment caesar.
      6 = episiotomy
      7 = tears
      8 = other
      X = unknown

46. SYMPTOMATIC DIAGNOSIS

    (i) Bladder during filling

      1 = normal
      2 = unstable
      3 = hypersensitive
      4 = other
      X = unknown

    (ii) Urethra during filling

      1 = competent
      2 = incompetent e.g. stress incontinence
      3 = other
      X = unknown

    (iii) Bladder during voiding

      1 = normal
      2 = underactive
      3 = other
      X = unknown

    (iv) Urethra during voiding

      1 = normal
      2 = mechanical obstruction
      3 = neuropathic obstruction
      4 = urethral syndrome
      5 = other
      X = unknown

PHYSICAL EXAMINATION: if 1 in 4 (Male) answer 47, if 2 in 4 (Female) go to 48.

<u>MALE</u>

47(a). PROSTATE

1 = normal
2 = BPH +
3 = BPH + +
4 = BPH + + +
5 = malignant
6 = prostatitis
X = unknown

47(b). INCONTINENCE SEEN DURING PHYSICAL EXAMINATION

1 = none
2 = incontinence observed
X = unknown

go to 50

<u>FEMALE</u>

48. VAGINAL EXAMINATION

1 = normal vagina
2 = atrophic vaginitis
3 = infective vaginitis
X = unknown

49(a). PROLAPSE

(i) Uterine prolapse

1 = none
2 = uterine prolapse Gd.1
3 = uterine prolapse Gd.2
4 = uterine prolapse Gd.3
X = unknown

(ii) Cysto urethrocoele

1 = none
2 = slight cystocoele
3 = marked cystocoele
X = unknown

(iii) Gut prolapse

1 = none
2 = rectocoele
3 = enterocoele
X = unknown

(iv) Other factors

1 = none
2 = deficient perineum
3 = other
X = unknown

49(b). INCONTINENCE SEEN DURING PHYSICAL EXAMINATION

1 = none
2 = incontinence observed
X = unknown

50. NEUROLOGICAL SIGNS

    (i) Legs

        1 = normal
        2 = LMN
        3 = UMN
        4 = LMN/UMN
        5 = other
        X = unknown

    (ii) Anal reflex

        1 = normal
        2 = absent
        X = unknown

    (iii) Anal tone

        1 = normal
        2 = present but lax after p.r.
        3 = reduced throughout
        4 = absent
        X = unknown

    (iv) Perineal sensation

        1 = normal
        2 = patchy loss
        3 = absent
        X = unknown

51. OBESITY

        1 = slim
        2 = slight obesity
        3 = moderate obesity
        4 = gross obesity
        X = unknown

52. BLADDER

        1 = not palpable
        2 = palpable
        X = unknown

53. PELVIC FLOOR SQUEEZE

        1 = normal
        2 = decreased
        3 = absent
        X = unknown

53a. UPPER TRACT
     DILATATION
     Information from)
     I.V.P., ultrasound, etc)

        1 = normal
        2 = present
        X = unknown

CODE 54 — 66 as 1 = done
              2 = not done

54.   INVESTIGATION

      a = Full UDS

      b = FLOW RATES only

      c = PAD TESTS only

if 1 in 54a go to 55

if 1 in 54b complete 67 to 70 then go to end

if 1 in 54c complete 82 then go to end

if 1 in 54b and 1 in 54c complete 67 to 70 and 82 then go to end

55.   FLOW RATES (initial or multiple)

56.   STATIC UPP

57.   STRESS UPP

58.   SACRAL REFLEXES

59.   URETHRAL SENSITIVITY

60.   FILLING CMG

61.   FLUID BRIDGE TEST

62.   VOIDING CYSTOMETROGRAM

63.   EMG

64.   EMG (single fibre)

65.   QUANTITATIVE URINE LOSS (PAD TESTING)

66.   VIDEO

If 1 in 55 answer 67

FLOW RATES:— (if single flow, ie initial flow in full UDS, then code 67 only and go to 71)

	FLOW RATE		VOLUME VOIDED		RESIDUAL URINE
67.		ml/sec		mls	
68.		ml/sec		mls	
69.		ml/sec		mls	

70. FLOW RATES/ULTRASOUND RUs — DIAGNOSIS DERIVED FROM MULTIPLE FLOWS (67 to 69)

1 = normal
2 = obstructed
3 = equivocal
4 = dysfunctional voiding
5 = other
X = unknown

go to the end if 1 in 54(b) and 2 in 54(c) otherwise answer 82

if 1 in 4 and 1 in 56 (<u>MALE</u>) then go to 71, if 2 in 4 and 1 in 56 (<u>FEMALE</u>) go to 72

71. UPP STATIC (male)
X = unknown

Prostatic length	cms
Prostatic plateau height	cmH$_2$0
Prostatic area	cm.cm.H$_2$0
MUP	cmH$_2$0
MUCP	cmH$_2$0

Prostatic peak
1 = yes
2 = no

go to 74

72. UPP STATIC (female)
X = unknown

Absolute length	cms
Functional length	cms
MUP	cmH$_2$0
MUCP	cmH$_2$0
Total area	cm.cmH$_2$0
Increment on squeeze	cmH$_2$0

if 1 in 57 answer 73.

73. UPP STRESS
X = unknown

Transmission ratio at 100 mls	%
Transmission ratio at capacity	%

if 1 in 58 complete 74

74. SACRAL REFLEXES
    X = unknown

Anal stimulus, Anal response | | | | m.secs.

Urethral/BN stimulus, Anal response | | | | m.secs.

Penile stimulus, Anal response | | | | m.secs.

Anal stimulus, Urethral response | | | | m.secs.

if 1 in 59 complete 75

75. URETHRAL SENSITIVITY
    X = unknown

Mean threshold   ☐☐ m.Amps.

if 1 in 60 complete 76 and 77

76. FILLING CMG
    (Pdet.)
    X = unknown
    — = feature NOT seen

Filling speed ☐☐☐ ml/min

Empty resting pressure ☐☐☐ cm.H_2O

FDM ☐☐☐☐ ml

UDM ☐☐☐☐ ml

Vol. 1st unstable contraction ☐☐☐☐ ml

Leakage at (volume) ☐☐☐☐ ml

Leakage at (pressure) ☐☐☐ cm.H_2O

Cystometric capacity ☐☐☐☐ ml

Full resting pressure (if no detr. contr.) ☐☐☐ cm.H_2O

Pressure at capacity (if unstable) ☐☐☐ cm.H_2O

Old Instability Index (Pves) ☐ · ☐ cm.H_2O/ml

New Instability Index (Pdet) ☐ · ☐ cm.H_2O/ml

Compliance $\triangle V / \triangle P$ ☐☐☐

77. OBSERVED INCONTINENCE
    1 = none
    2 = stress
    3 = urge unstable
    4 = unstable urethra
    5 = stress/urge unstable
    6 = stress/unstable urethra
    7 = other
    X = unknown

if 1 in 61 complete 78

78. FLUID BRIDGE TEST
    1 = abnormal lying
    2 = abnormal erect
    3 = normal lying
    4 = normal erect
    X = unknown

if 1 in 62 complete 79

79. VOIDING CYSTOMETROGRAM
   X = unknown

Max. flow pressure (Pves)	☐☐☐	cm.H$_2$O
Max. flow pressure (Pdet)	☐☐☐	cm.H$_2$O
Max. flow rate (F)	☐☐	ml.sec.
P.det.iso	☐☐☐	cm.H$_2$O
Urethral Resistance (P.ves/F2)	☐ . ☐☐	
Volume passed	☐☐☐☐	ml
Residual urine	☐☐☐☐	ml

After contraction
1 = none
2 = present ☐

if 1 in 63 complete 80

80. EMG
   (i) Site
      1 = pelvic floor
      2 = urethra
      3 = anal
      4 = other
      X = unknown ☐

   (ii) Type
      1 = plug
      2 = needle
      3 = surface
      4 = catheter
      5 = other
      6 = unknown ☐

   (iii) Findings
      1 = normal
      2 = dyssynergia
      3 = reduced activity
      4 = other
      X = unknown ☐

if 1 in 64 complete 81

81. EMG (single fibre)
   X = unknown

      1 = normal
      2 = abnormal ☐

   Fibre density ☐ . ☐

if 1 in 65 complete 82

82. QUANTIFICATION URINE LOSS PER EXERCISE CYCLE
   X = unknown ☐☐☐ mls

if coded 1 in 54(c) go to end

ALL PATIENTS

if 1 in 56 complete 83

83. DIAGNOSIS UPP
    (i) Static profile

1 = normal
2 = low static UPP
3 = high static UPP
4 = increased prostatic area
5 = other
X = unknown

    (ii) Squeeze

1 = normal
2 = weak
3 = absent
X = unknown

84. STRESS UPP DIAGNOSIS
    (code severest abnormality)

1 = normal
2 = abnormal at 100 mls
3 = abnormal at capacity
4 = equivocal at 100 mls
5 = equivocal at capacity
X = unknown

If 1 in 60 complete 85 & 86

DIAGNOSIS FILLING PHASE

85. BLADDER
    (i) Sensation

1 = normal
2 = reduced
3 = increased (hypersensitive)
4 = absent
X = unknown

    (ii) Detrusor activity

1 = stable
2 = unstable (spontaneous)
3 = unstable (provoked)
4 = other
X = unknown

    (iii) Compliance

1 = normal
2 = low
3 = high
4 = other
X = unknown

if 1 in 66 complete (iv) and (v)

    (iv) Bladder shape

1 = normal
2 = trabeculation
3 = diverticula
4 = trabec/divertic
5 = other
X = unknown

    (v) Bladder base function

1 = normal
2 = bladder base descent
3 = other
X = unknown

86. URETHRA
    (i) Urethral sensation on
    catheterisation

1 = normal
2 = increased
3 = absent
X = unknown

if no video (2 in 66) complete (ii), if video (1 in 66) complete (iii)

(ii) Urethral behaviour

1 = normal urethra
2 = incompetent urethra (Genuine Stress Incontinence)
3 = unstable urethra with leakage
4 = unstable urethra without leakage
5 = other
X = unknown

(iii) Video: BN/urethral
function (filling)

1 = normal
2 = BN beaking at rest
3 = BN beaking on strain
4 = BN and urethra open at rest with leak
5 = BN and urethra open on stress with leak
6 = BN beaking at rest + stress incontinence
7 = unstable urethra with leakage
8 = unstable urethra without leakage
X = unknown

if 1 in 62 complete 87 & 88

DIAGNOSIS VOIDING PHASE

87. DETRUSOR

1 = normal detrusor contraction (normal flow)
2 = sustained low detrusor pressure (with low flow)
3 = fluctuating detrusor pressure (with intermittent flow)
4 = sustained high detrusor pressure (with low flow)
5 = acontractile detrusor (voids by straining)
6 = detrusor contraction — with strain
7 = acontractile detrusor (no voiding)
8 = detrusor contraction (no voiding)
9 = normal void — no detrusor contraction
A = normal void — no detrusor contraction — Piso present
B = other
X = unknown

88. URETHRA

if no video (2 in 66) complete (i), if video (1 in 66) performed complete (ii)

(i) Standard UDS

1 = normal
2 = dyssynergic
3 = obstructed
4 = other
X = unknown

(ii) Video UDS

1 = normal
2 = BN obstruction
3 = detrusor/BN/dyssynergia
4 = detrusor/urethral/dyssynergia
5 = static distal sphincter obstruction
6 = mechanical prostatic obstruction
7 = mechanical urethral obstruction
8 = other
X = unknown

if 1 in 66 complete 89

89.   OTHER VIDEO FEATURES

1 = none
2 = VU reflux
3 = prostatic duct reflux
4 = no milk back
5 = other
X = unknown

90.   URODYNAMIC
      Technical Aspects

1 = no problems
2 = unable to catheterise
3 = catheter voided
4 = undue anxiety (including fainting)
5 = other
X = unknown

91.   CLINICAL URODYNAMIC DIAGNOSIS

1 = interstitial cystitis
2 = urethral syndrome
3 = prostatodynia
4 = other
5 = diagnosis as above
X = unknown

Urodynamics Data Sheet: Shortened Version

U R O D Y N A M I C   U N I T
SOUTHMEAD HOSPITAL, BRISTOL

M 1337

NOTE:—

(a) Number of entries Strictly dictated by number of boxes

(b) Where no information enter ☒

(c) N = not applicable

1. SURNAME: _____

    FIRST NAME: _____

2. ADDRESS: _____

    _____

    Post Code _____ Tel. No. _____

3. DATE OF BIRTH:

4. SEX: (1 male; 2 female)

5. HOSPITAL NUMBER(S):

6. INITIAL REFERRAL:
    1 Urol   2 Gynae   3 Surg   4 Geriatric
    5 G.P.   6 Nurse   7 Other   8 Paediatrics

6a. 1 = in patient   2 = out-patient   3 = not known

7. CONSULTANT: (Name) _____

8. G.P.: (Name) _____

    Address (not coded) _____

    _____

9a. CIU NUMBER: 9b. INVESTIGATION NUMBER:

Presenting Complaint:

Previous Treatment:

HEIGHT _____ cms

WEIGHT _____ Kg

SMOKER | YES / NO | ..../Day

Examination:

Management:

Report sent to: Follow up arrangements:—

If enter 'other' in any question please describe on this sheet.

10.	Date	25.	Enuresis	(b) Stool Freq.
11.	Age		Freq.	(c) Defaecation
12.	Trial I.D.	26.	Other I.	(d) Post defaec. symp.
13.	Enter Hist.		Freq.	(e) Diagnosis
14.	Inv.	27.	Degree	38. Drugs
15.	Length Hist.	28.	Management	39a. Neuro. feat.
16.	Freq. (day)		Pads/day	39b. Sexual Function.
17.	Noct.		Pads/night	MALE ONLY
18.	Fluid Intake	29.	Incapacity	40. Operations/Trauma
19.	F/V chart	30.	Physical Incap.	(i) outflow
	Max. vol.	31.	Hist. Enuresis	(ii) denervation
	Av. vol.		(i) Patient	(iii) Other
	Duration		(ii) Family	FEMALE ONLY
20.	Pre. mict.	32.	Stream	41. Operations/Trauma
	Freq.	33.	Post. Mict.	(i) for stress Inc.
21.	Hest.		Freq.	(ii) gynae. symp/prolapse
	Freq.	34.	Dysuria	(iii) denervation
22.	Incontinence	34a.	Haematuria	(iv) Other
23.	Stress I.	35.	Hist. Retention	42. Hormone
	Freq.	36.	Management Retn.	43. Symp. Mense
24.	Urge I	37.	Bowel Function	44. Parity
	Freq.		(a) Control	45. Delivery

ALL PATIENTS

46. Symptomatic diag.

   (i) Bladder fill ☐

   (ii) Urethra fill ☐

   (iii) Bladder void ☐

   (iv) Urethra void ☐

PHYSICAL EXAMINATION

MALE ONLY

47a. Prostate ☐

47b. Incont. seen ☐

FEMALE ONLY

48. Vag. exam. ☐

49a. Prolapse

   (i) Uterine prolapse ☐

   (ii) Cysto. urethra ☐

   (iii) Gut prolapse ☐

   (iv) Other ☐

49b. Incont. seen ☐

ALL PATIENTS

50. Neuro. signs

   (i) Legs ☐

   (ii) Anal reflex ☐

   (iii) Anal Tone ☐

   (iv) Perineal sens. ☐

51. Obesity ☐

52. Bladder ☐

53. P.F. squeeze ☐

53a. Upper tract dilatation ☐

54. Investigations

   (a) Full UDS ☐

   (b) Flowrates ☐

   (c) Pad Test ☐

55. Flow rates ☐

56. Static UPP ☐

57. Stress UPP ☐

58. Sacral reflex ☐

59. Urethral sens. ☐

60. Fill CMG ☐

61. F.B.T. ☐

62. Void CMG ☐

63. EMG ☐

64. EMG (single fibre) ☐

65. Pad Test ☐

66. Video ☐

FLOW RATES

	Flow	Volvoid	R.U.
67.	☐☐☐	☐☐☐	☐☐☐
68.	☐☐☐	☐☐☐	☐☐☐
69.	☐☐☐	☐☐☐	☐☐☐

70. Ultrasound/F.R. diag. ☐

71. Static UPP (MALE)

   Length ☐ . ☐

   plat. ☐☐

   area ☐☐

   MUP ☐☐

   MUCP ☐☐☐

   Peak

72. Static UPP (FEMALE)

   Abs. length ☐ . ☐

   Function length ☐ . ☐

   MUP ☐☐☐

   MUCP ☐☐☐

   area ☐☐☐

   sq. ☐☐

73. Stress UPP

   Tr. 100 ml ☐☐☐

   Tr. cap ☐☐☐

Appendix 4
Drugs Active on the Lower Urinary Tract

α-Blockers

Alfuzosin
Doxazosin
Ergoloid mesylates
Ergotamine tartrate
Indoramin
Methysergide maleate
Phenoxybenzamine
Prazosin
Tamsalosin
Terazosin

α/β-Blockers

Labetalol

α-Agonists

Amphetamine
Benzphetamine
Clonidine
Dextroamphetamine sulphate
Dietheylproprion
Ephedrine
Epinephrine

Guanabenz acetate
Mazindol
Methamphetamine
Methyldopa
Methylphenidate
Pemoline
Phendimetrazine
Phenmetrazine
Phenylephrine
Phenylpropanolamine
Pseudoephedrine

Drugs with Anticholinergic Activity

Amitriptyline
Amoxapine
Anistropine
Atropine
Azatadine
Belladonna alkoids
Benztropine
Biperiden
Brompheniramine
Carbinoxamine
Chlorpheniramine
Chlorpromazine
Chlorprothixene
Clemastine
Clidinium
Cyproheptadine
Desipramine
Dicylomine
Diphenhydramine
Diphenylpyraline
Doxepin
Doxylamine
Emepromium
Flavoxate
Fluphenazine
Glycopyrrolate
Haloperidol
Hexocyclium
Homatropine
Hyoscyamine

Imipramine
Isopropamide
Loxapine
Mepenzolate
Mesoridazine
Methscopolamine
Molindone
Nortriptyline
Orphenadrine
Oxybutynin
Pimozide
Prochlorperazine
Procyclidine
Promazine
Promethazine
Propantheline
Protriptyline
Scopolamine
Terfenadine
Thiothixene
Thoridazine
Trazodone
Trifluoperazine
Tridihexethyl chloride
Trimeprazine
Trimipramine
Trihexyphenidyl hydrocholoride
Tripelennamine
Triprolidine
Trospium

Parasympathomimetics and Cholinergics

Bethanechol
Carbachol
Distigmine bromide

Neostigmine
Pyridostigmine

Index

Ranges of numbers in bold refer to entire chapters